CHARLES E. BROWN-SEQUARD

COURS OF LECTURES

ON THE

PHYSIOLOGY AND PATHOLOGY

OF THE

CENTRAL NERVOUS SYSTEM

Elibron Classics
www.elibron.com

Elibron Classics series.

ISBN 1-4021-9818-3 (paperback)
ISBN 1-4212-9889-9 (hardcover)

This Elibron Classics Replica Edition is an unabridged facsimile of the edition published in 1860, Philadelphia.

COURSE OF LECTURES

ON THE

PHYSIOLOGY AND PATHOLOGY

OF THE

CENTRAL NERVOUS SYSTEM.

DELIVERED AT THE

Royal College of Surgeons of England in May, 1858.

BY

C. E. BROWN-SÉQUARD, M. D., F. R. S.,

FELLOW OF THE ROYAL COLLEGE OF PHYSICIANS, OF LONDON; HON. FELLOW OF THE FACULTY OF PHYSICIANS AND SURGEONS, GLASGOW; LAUREATE OF THE INSTITUTE OF FRANCE (ACADEMY OF SCIENCES); PHYSICIAN TO THE NATIONAL HOSPITAL FOR THE PARALYZED AND THE EPILEPTIC; EX-PROFESSOR OF THE INSTITUTES OF MEDICINE AT THE MEDICAL COLLEGE OF VIRGINIA, U. S.; FELLOW OF THE ROYAL MEDICO-CHIRURGICAL SOCIETY OF LONDON; EX-SECRETARY AND VICE-PRESIDENT OF THE SOCIÉTÉ DE BIOLOGIE, OF PARIS, ETC.

PHILADELPHIA:

COLLINS, PRINTER, 705 JAYNE STREET.

1860.

TO

HENRY J. FELTUS, Esq.,

OF PHILADELPHIA, U. S.,

AND

JULES CHAUVIN, Esq.,

OF PORT-LOUIS, MAURITIUS.

My Dear Friends:—

Had it not been for the assistance I owe to your extreme kindness, it is probable that the publication of the present edition of these Lectures, in book form, would have been much delayed; I therefore take, with great pleasure, this opportunity of publicly expressing to you my very best thanks.

Your devoted friend,

C. E. BROWN-SÉQUARD.

London, September, 1860.

PREFACE.

THESE Lectures contain the results of the work of almost all my life, since I began to study medicine. From the year 1838 to the year 1858, when I had the honor of delivering them at the Royal College of Surgeons, in London, and ever since, I have devoted all the time I could to the study of the great questions, the solution of which I have tried to give in these Lectures. If I have not succeeded in my endeavors, I can at least have this consolation, that it is not because I have proceeded hastily. But, however prolonged my researches have been, I am afraid I must have come to erroneous conclusions on several points, because the questions discussed in these Lectures are as difficult as they are important, and also because many of these questions are quite new, and I had not, therefore, the views of other authors to guide me in their examination. I will be thankful to any one who will show me on what points I have erred. It is in the power of most medical practitioners to prove or to disprove the views I hold. Out of the millions of patients yearly treated by the medical men who may peruse this book, there are, indeed, many thousands whose cases may throw light, and often a decisive light, on the questions discussed in the following pages. As most of these questions are of the greatest importance, both in a practical and in a scientific point of view, I hope that those who will peruse this work will not let the cases pass unrecorded that may be the means of settling what is yet undecided in these questions, or of giving more strength to the proofs of the views held by myself or by my opponents.

C. E. BROWN-SÉQUARD.

London, 81 Wimpole Street,
Cavendish Square,
W.

TABLE OF CONTENTS.

LECTURE I.

LECTURE II.

LECTURE III.

PLACE OF DECUSSATION OF THE CONDUCTORS OF SENSITIVE IMPRESSIONS, IN THE CEREBRO-SPINAL AXIS.

LECTURE IV.

ON VARIOUS QUESTIONS RELATING TO THE TRANSMISSION OF SENSITIVE IMPRESSIONS AND OF THE ORDERS OF THE WILL TO MUSCLES, THROUGH THE SPINAL CORD AND THE MEDULLA OBLONGATA.

LECTURE V.

CONCLUSIONS FROM THE FACTS MENTIONED IN THE PRECEDING LECTURES, AND PATHOLOGICAL CASES SHOWING THAT THE TRANSMISSION OF SENSITIVE IMPRESSIONS SEEMS NOT TO TAKE PLACE THROUGH THE POSTERIOR COLUMNS OF THE SPINAL CORD.

LECTURE VI.

SOLUTION, BY PATHOLOGICAL CASES, OF VARIOUS QUESTIONS RELATING TO THE TRANSMISSION OF SENSITIVE IMPRESSIONS THROUGH THE SPINAL CORD.

LECTURE VII.

PATHOLOGICAL CASES SHOWING THAT THE CONDUCTORS OF SENSITIVE IMPRESSIONS FROM THE TRUNK AND LIMBS DECUSSATE IN THE SPINAL CORD AND NOT IN THE ENCEPHALON, AND THAT THE CONDUCTORS OF THE ORDERS OF THE WILL TO MUSCLES DECUSSATE IN THE LOWER PART OF THE MEDULLA OBLONGATA AND NOT IN THE PONS VAROLII.

LECTURE VIII.

CONCLUSIONS FROM THE PATHOLOGICAL CASES RELATED IN THE PRECEDING LECTURES AND FROM SEVERAL OTHER CASES, AS REGARDS THE DIAGNOSIS OF ALTERATIONS OF THE VARIOUS PARTS OF THE SPINAL CORD.

LECTURE IX.

ON THE PHYSIOLOGICAL AND MORBID ACTIONS DUE TO THE GREAT SYMPATHETIC NERVE.

LECTURE X.

ON THE INFLUENCE OF THE NERVOUS SYSTEM UPON NUTRITION AND SECRETION; WITH REMARKS ON THE IMPORTANCE OF THE KNOWLEDGE OF THIS INFLUENCE FOR THE TREATMENT AND THE EXPLANATION OF THE PRODUCTION OF MANY DISEASES.

LECTURE XI.

ON THE ETIOLOGY, NATURE, AND TREATMENT OF EPILEPSY, WITH A FEW REMARKS ON SEVERAL OTHER AFFECTIONS OF THE NERVOUS CENTRES.

LECTURE XII.

ON THE MEDULLA OBLONGATA, THE PONS VAROLII, AND SOME PARTS OF THE SPINAL CORD, IN THEIR RELATIONS WITH RESPIRATORY MOVEMENTS; WITH VERTIGINOUS OR ROTATORY CONVULSIONS; WITH THE TRANSMISSION OF SENSITIVE IMPRESSIONS AND OF THE ORDERS OF THE WILL TO MUSCLES, AND WITH THE VASO-MOTOR NERVES AND ANIMAL HEAT.—GENERAL CONCLUSIONS OF THE COURSE.

APPENDIX.

THE

CENTRAL NERVOUS SYSTEM.

LECTURE I.[1]

TRUTH OF SIR CHARLES BELL'S THEORY AS REGARDS THE EXISTENCE OF TWO DISTINCT SETS OF NERVOUS CONDUCTORS; THE SENSITIVE AND THE MOTOR.

Importance of comparing experiments upon animals with pathological cases observed in man.—Discovery of Sir Charles Bell; removal of the last objections to his views in regard to the roots of the spinal nerves.—The pretended recurring sensibility of Magendie. Causes of the pain produced by the irritation of the anterior roots of nerves, of the pain of cramps, of certain "contractures," of the spasm of the sphincter ani, and of the contractions of the uterus during parturition, &c.—Are the sensitive nerve-fibres of muscles contained in the anterior roots of the spinal nerves?—Theories concerning the transmission of the sensitive impressions in the spinal cord and the medulla oblongata.

MR. PRESIDENT AND GENTLEMEN: The subject of the lectures which I propose delivering here is a very vast one, as it includes, directly or indirectly, most of the principal questions concerning the Physiology and Pathology of the Nervous System. But vast as it is, this subject may be considered as composed of only three essential parts, which relate to the sensitive, the motor, and the vaso-motor nerve-fibres. In other words, I propose to examine successively the principal facts and views concerning the normal actions, and the consequences of the excess or of the absence of action, of these three kinds of nerve-fibres.

[1] Although six lectures only were delivered at the Royal College of Surgeons, I will publish here twelve lectures, covering just the same ground as those of the College, but differing from them in this respect, that I give here details concerning experiments and pathological cases, which, for the sake of brevity, I was obliged to omit when lecturing.

To try to solve the very important but complicated questions which are so numerous in both the physiological and the pathological history of the parts of these nerve-fibres which are in the nervous centres, it is necessary to make use of all the means that science may furnish, and particularly of the two best, which are: experimentation upon living animals, and observation of pathological cases. When employed together, these means of scientific research have allowed errors to be made; but, of course, the chance of committing errors is by far greater when either of them is employed alone. The danger of making use of one of these means exclusively is very strikingly illustrated by the many errors, concerning the cerebellum, committed by experimental physiologists, who mistook the effects of certain circumstances of their experiments for the results of injuries or of the absence of the cerebellum. Had they taken the trouble of comparing the phenomena they saw with those observed by medical men in cases of disease of the cerebellum, they would not have introduced in science a number of hypotheses which impede its progress. It is by so doing that experimentalists have thrown discredit on the means of scientific inquiry of which they have made so much use and abuse, and have given ground to many critics to blame their means of research, while the fault was in the men who employed those means, and not in the means themselves.

If erroneous views have been arrived at by the exclusive use of one of the means of scientific research we have named, we find that, on the contrary, many great advances in the medical sciences are due to the combined use of vivisections and clinical observation. Perhaps I may be allowed to say that the lectures I am about delivering will afford some proof of the advantage of a comparison of pathological cases observed in man, with the result of experiments upon living animals.

The great discovery of Sir Charles Bell gives a good instance of the importance of making use comparatively of clinical observation and vivisections. In fact, had Sir Charles had recourse to experiments upon living animals, he probably would have succeeded, at once, in proving the correctness of his theory concerning the roots of the spinal nerves.

Before him, already, many physiologists had, more or less distinctly, foreseen that the nervous conductors for voluntary movements and those for sensation form two distinct sets of nerves. Galen, Boerhaave, Lamarck, Alex. Walker, and others, had had this idea. To Alex. Walker the credit is due of having first published this opinion, that there is a difference in the functions of the anterior and posterior roots of the spinal nerves, one set being employed for volition and the other for sensation; but he did not try to prove, either by experiments or by pathological facts, the correctness of his views; and, led by erroneous ideas concerning the function of the cerebellum, he imagined that the anterior roots of the spinal nerves are for sensation and the posterior for motion. (See the *Archives of Universal Science* for April and July, 1809.)

It was only two years after the publication of this hypothesis of Walker, that Sir Charles Bell's first views received some publicity, in the celebrated little pamphlet, entitled, "*An Idea of a New Anatomy of the Brain*, submitted for the Observation of the Author's friends."[1] In this work, as far as we know, he did not try to prove that the anterior roots of the spinal nerves are employed as conductors of volition, and that the posterior roots are the conductors of the sensitive impressions. He seems not to have yet had (at that time) the idea of this difference. He admitted that the posterior roots of nerves come from the cerebellum, which he considered as an organ employed for the organic or vital functions of the body, while the anterior roots are in communication with the cerebrum, which he thought to be the organ for both volition and sensitive perceptions. But, however erroneous may be some of these views, we look upon this first work of Sir Charles Bell on the nervous system, as an admirable production of the genius of this great physiologist. The idea of the distinction between the nervous elements employed in the different functions of the nervous system is there clearly and forcibly presented, and we may safely state that the greatest part of the recent progress of our knowledge of the nervous system, both in a practical and in a scientific point of view, has its source in this idea. There is another important thing in this little pamphlet; it is the result of Sir Charles Bell's experiments on the roots of the spinal nerves. He found, on a dying animal, that the irritation of the anterior roots caused muscular contractions, while there was no effect produced by the irritation of the posterior roots. Of course this experiment could not show what are the functions of these roots, but it was sufficient to prove

[1] As only a few copies of this pamphlet were printed, it is now almost impossible to procure it. I speak of it after the numerous extracts published by Mr. Alexander Shaw and by Sir Charles Bell himself.

that there is a notable difference between the anterior and the posterior roots.

Long after this first publication, Sir Charles brought forward several facts, experimental and pathological, showing that the nervous conductors for motion are distinct from those for sensation. He showed that the facial nerve is motor, and that the ganglionic root of the trigeminal is for sensation. But although these facts had given good grounds to the hypothesis that the posterior or ganglionic roots of the spinal nerves are used for sensation, while the anterior roots are for motion, positive evidences of the exactitude of this distinction were still wanted. To Mr. Magendie belongs the merit of having furnished the proofs that were needed. He showed that the section of all the posterior roots of the nerves of one limb destroys the sensibility in the limb, while a section of the anterior roots of the nerves of a limb abolishes voluntary movements, leaving sensibility unaltered. He also found that strychnia, in this last case, does not excite convulsions in the paralyzed limb, while there are convulsions, in the limb deprived of sensibility, after the section of the posterior roots. So far as these experiments alone are studied, it seems quite certain that the anterior roots are motor and not sensitive, and that the posterior roots are sensitive and not motor; but Magendie tried other experiments, and, not being aware of a singular fact, which he discovered only in 1839, he arrived at conclusions which were quite different from those just exposed. The irritation of the anterior roots he found evidently to induce pain, though in a less degree than that of the posterior. On another side he found sometimes that local movements took place when he irritated the posterior roots. Here, then, are two facts which seem in direct opposition to the theory of Sir Charles Bell.

In 1839, Magendie made a step forward, and discovered a very important fact, which has removed the objection against Sir Charles Bell's theory as regards the anterior roots of the spinal nerves. He found that these roots really cause pain when they are irritated, but that if they are divided (see Fig. 1), the distal end (*d*) alone may give pain. He ascertained also that if the posterior roots of any of the spinal nerves are divided, the irritation of the anterior roots of the same nerve no longer causes pain. He concludes, from these facts and some others, that there is what he calls, erroneously, a *recurring* sensibility, which, on the irritation of the anterior roots, manifests itself in this way: The nervous irritation which causes the pain goes, at first, from the parts of the anterior roots (see the arrows in Fig. 1, A), in which it has begun, towards the trunk of the nerve, in which it goes to the periphery of the body, and then comes back towards the spinal cord, which it reaches in being conveyed by the ganglion (*g*) and the posterior roots (P); so that the current which proceeds from the cord along the anterior roots returns towards it and into it along the posterior ones. We must say that the name of *recurrent* sensibility is a very bad one, because sensibility is a vital property which cannot *move* from a place towards any other, and therefore cannot be *recurring*. It is the cause, whatever it may be, of the painful sensation, which is *recurring*, and not sensibility.

What is the channel of the nervous irritation generated when the anterior roots are excited? In the first place, we think it is necessary to repeat, that the current is not towards the spinal cord, inasmuch as Magendie has well proved that after the section of the anterior roots of a spinal nerve, we may irritate the central part (Fig. 1, C) without causing the least manifestation of any kind of sensation. It results, therefore, and as positively as possible, that the anterior roots have not the property of sensibility in the same manner as the really sensitive parts. On the contrary, pain is caused by the irritation of the parts of the anterior roots in appearance separated from the nervous centres. (See Fig. 1, A, *d*.) But if the trunk of the nerve is divided, the irritation of the anterior roots on either end remains completely painless; it results, therefore, that the current which causes the pain passes in this trunk. But how far does the current extend towards the periphery of the body, before returning upon itself in order to reach the spinal cord and the sensorium? This has not been positively determined. It seems, however, already, from the experiments of Magendie, of Professor Cl. Bernard, of Volkmann, of Schiff, and from my own, that the return takes place at the peripheric extremity of the nerve-fibres. Kronenberg and Pappenheim have erroneously admitted that the current merely passes from the anterior roots to the posterior, at the place where they meet to form the trunk of the spinal nerves.

The channel of the current which gives the pain when an anterior root is irritated, is, consequently, at first towards the trunk of the nerve; then in this trunk towards the periphery, where the *recurrence* seems to take place, and thence the current returns along the sensitive fibres of the nerve towards the ganglion of the posterior roots, and, at last, passes through the ganglion and these roots, and into the spinal cord. (See the upper roots in Fig. 1.)

What is the cause of the pain produced by the irritation of the anterior roots of nerves? According to Carus, the nervous loops, which he thought existed in the muscles, give an easy explanation of the facts discovered by Magendie. Unfortunately for this explanation (which Mr. Flourens has again proposed quite recently), the existence of nervous loops in muscles is now disproved. Indeed, even in the skin there is good ground to doubt the presence of many loops. Some experiments, which we have made, render it probable that the pain caused by the irritation of the anterior roots is exactly of the same nature as that of cramps, and that both the pain of cramps and the pain which we will call *recurrent*, to avoid circumlocutions, depend upon a peculiar kind of irritation of the sensitive nerves of muscles. The theory we will propose is also applicable to many pathological and physiological phenomena, which have puzzled for a long while both practitioners and physiologists, and which seem, indeed, to be very plain and natural now that we have the key to their explanation.

Professor Matteucci, nearly twenty years ago, found that when a nerve going to a muscle (Fig. 2, *m* 2) is put upon another muscle, a contraction takes place in the first one when the second contracts. In this case the nerve receives an *excitation* at the time the muscle, upon which it lies, contracts. The cause of the excitation of the nerve, according to Professor Matteucci, is a galvanic discharge which accompanies the muscular contraction. Dubois-Reymond explains otherwise the excitation of the nerve. He thinks it is due to a diminution of the galvanic current of the muscle when it contracts, and that the changes occurring, in consequence, in the nerve irritate it. But whatever be the right explanation, it seems certain that it is *some change in the galvanic state* of the muscle which causes the excitation of the nerve. We will, therefore, call it a galvanic excitation. Now, I have tried to prove, in 1849, that the sensitive nerve-fibres which are in muscles, receive that peculiar galvanic excitation which acts upon the motor nerves in the case of the preceding experiment, so that there is a galvanic cause of sensation in muscular contractions. (See Figs. 3 and 4, and their explanations.) I have also tried to show, elsewhere, that our faculty of guiding our movements depends upon the sensations that we have of the state of our muscles, from the galvanic excitation which accompanies our muscular contractions. I cannot dwell at length here upon this explanation, which is only slightly connected with my subject; but

I will try, at least, to show that several experiments and pathological cases agree perfectly with this theory.

If we fix a thread to the tendon of a muscle of a frog (see Fig. 2, *t*), and attach to this thread a weight, capable of entirely preventing the contraction of the muscle, which is fixed by its other extremity, we find that every time the muscle (Fig. 2, *m*) *tends* to contract, there is an excitation of the nerve (*n*) lying upon it, and a contraction of the muscle (*m* 2) to which this nerve is distributed. Hence it is not necessary for a muscle to contract in order to produce in nerves in contact with it a galvanic excitation. I repeat that it is sufficient that they *tend* to contract. Now, I have found that the greater is the resistance to the contraction of a muscle, the greater is the galvanic excitation that it gives to nerves in contact with its tissue. On the contrary, if there is no resistance at all, as already shown by Professor Matteucci, after the section of the tendon, then the galvanic excitation of nerves in contact with the contracting muscle no longer exists.

If we compare these results with the following pathological facts, we find that the phenomena are much alike in the two series of facts that we compare, and, therefore, that they seem to depend on the same causes. I suppose a case of painful contracture of the anterior muscles of the thigh; the pain is increased very much every time the contracted muscles are elongated, *i. e.*, when the resistance to the contraction is augmented; on the contrary, it diminishes when the resistance to the contraction is rendered less than it was, and, at last, *it disappears entirely, or almost entirely, when the resistance is completely, or almost completely, destroyed*, after tenotomy. Surgeons, till our researches, had not been able to explain this apparently strange cessation of pain; now it seems quite simple to understand that such should be the case.

In cases of *fissura in ano*, it is very well known that the pain due to the spasm of the sphincter is increased when there is a resistance to the contraction, and that the greater the elongation of the muscular fibres, the greater also the resistance to their contraction and the degree of pain. At last, when the muscular fibres can contract freely, and almost without resistance, the pain disappears, as is the case after the operation of Boyer (the section of the sphincter). Of course the pain depending upon the fissure persists, but that due to the muscular spasm disappears. In this case, also, surgeons could not explain the cessation of pain. We find here, as in the preceding case, that the excitation of the nerves due to the muscular contraction augments, decreases, and disappears in the same circumstances, concerning the degree or the absence of resistance, which produce analogous phenomena in the experiments above mentioned.

In cases of neuralgia, when the sensibility of nerves in muscles is increased, there is pain produced or increased every time the muscles contract.

The contractions of the uterus, which are the more painful the more there is resistance opposed to them, cause also pain in the same way as the spasm of the anus or the contraction of the muscles of the thigh. The relation between the degree of contraction of the uterus and that of pain is so evident, that the word "pains" is employed for that of "contraction."

Every muscular contraction seems to generate a galvanic excitation of the sensitive nerves in the neighborhood of the muscular fibres; and, the degree of excitation being in proportion to the degree of energy of the contraction, we have, in this way, an excellent means of judging of the state of the muscles. When the contraction acquires the degree which it has in cramps, then it causes pain, which is also in proportion to the energy of the spasm. If we succeed when we have a cramp in making it cease by elongating the contracted muscle, we find that the pain often increases at first, and disappears only when the contraction has ceased. I regret not to be able to bring forward all the reasons which have led me to admit the views I have just proposed, but I must keep within my programme.

If, now, we examine what takes place in the apparently paradoxical experiment of Magendie, we find that nothing is more easily explained. When the anterior roots of a spinal nerve are excited, a cramp is produced in the muscles in which the nerve-fibres of the roots are distributed, and the pain which belongs to a *cramp* is generated. I think this pain is due, as I have said for cramps, to a galvanic excitation of the sensitive nerve-fibres existing in the muscles which contract; but whether this theory be true or not is, in a measure, indifferent as regards the general cause of pain in the experiment of Magendie. In fact, there is then the same cause which exists in a cramp; and this cannot fail to be so inasmuch as a real cramp is generated by the irritation of the anterior roots. So, then, we can conclude: 1st, that the *recurrent* sensation is only in appearance recurrent; 2d, that the anterior roots of the spinal nerves cause pain when they are irritated, because they produce a cramp: 3d, that, consequently, *there is no sensibility of any kind in the anterior roots, and that it is because they are motor, and not because they are sensitive, that they cause pain when they are irritated.*

Therefore, the objection which has been urged against the views of Sir Charles Bell, and which was founded upon the fact that the anterior roots cause pain when irritated, is unfounded. We will now say a few words of the objection originating from the fact that there are, sometimes, some local movements when the posterior roots are excited. These local movements are proved to be only reflex movements. In the first place, there is no contraction whatever when the distal part of a posterior root is irritated; and, certainly, if there were motor nerve-fibres in this root, contractions should be produced. (See Fig. 1, *d*, *g*.) In the second place, the irritation of the central part of a divided posterior root is sometimes followed by local contractions, a fact which implies that to reach muscles, the irritation passes through the spinal cord. In the third place, after having cut the anterior roots of the pair of nerves of which we irritate a posterior root, we do not see any local contraction following this irritation. From these experiments it clearly results that, when a posterior root of a spinal nerve is irritated, if we see contractions of the muscles to which this nerve goes, they arise from the passage of the excitation to the spinal cord, and, from thence, to the muscles through the anterior roots. In other words, we must admit that it is only by a reflex action that the posterior roots act upon muscles.

It would seem from what we have just said, and from the explanation above given of the *recurring sensibility*, that no further objection to the views of Sir Charles Bell can be made; but this is not the case. J. W. Arnold[1] has tried to show that the anterior roots of nerves contain the nerve-fibres which convey to the sensorium the impressions which give the knowledge of the state of the muscles. The chief fact on which he grounds his opinion is, that after the section of the posterior roots of the posterior extremities of a frog, it can make use of its hind legs almost as well as if nothing had been done to the posterior roots. This experiment is certainly of some value,

[1] Ueber die verrichtung des Rueckenmarksnerven, &c., Heidelberg, 1845. Analyzed in the "British and Foreign Medical Review," April, 1845, p. 558, and p. 575.

and we must acknowledge that it is difficult to explain it otherwise than Arnold has done. Moreover, we have found that, after the section of *all* the posterior roots of the spinal nerves in frogs, the voluntary movements seem to be very nearly as perfect as if no operation had been performed, and that if the skin of the head is pinched on one side, the posterior limb on the same side tries to repel the cause of the pain as well as if no injury had been made. I have also ascertained that in frogs rendered blind, these experiments give the same results.

It seems very probable, from these facts, that there is at least a part of the sensations giving to the mind the idea of the state of a muscle, which passes along the anterior roots to go to the sensorium. But, although I agree so far with Arnold, I do not admit with him that it is only through the anterior roots that impressions are conveyed from the muscles to the brain. When a galvanic current is applied to the muscles of a limb of a frog, on which the posterior roots of the nerves of this limb have been divided, no trace of pain is produced, and all the other causes of pain are also unable to cause it, when applied either to the skin or to the muscles. When I examine, in another lecture, the correlation of pathological cases with experimental facts, I will speak again of the views of Arnold. I dismiss actually the subject, contenting myself in saying that, even if muscles have *peculiar* nerve-fibres, which go up to the brain along the anterior roots, to give there some special sensations in correspondence with the degree of contraction, it seems nevertheless quite certain that the nerves of touch and those which convey painful impressions, do not pass by the anterior roots, and that, therefore, the theory of Sir Charles Bell, as regards these nerves, remains entire. In another lecture I will show, also, that all, or at least almost all, the motor nerve-fibres which go to the bloodvessels, pass in the anterior roots.

But, if Sir Charles Bell's views concerning the roots of nerves are now based upon irrefragable experiments, it is not so as regards either of the views that he successively proposed concerning the columns of the spinal cord. We will prove by anatomical, experimental, and pathological facts, that his ideas concerning the channels for sensation and volition are not exact. But, at the same time that we show the mistakes he has committed in this respect, we will bring forward a great many proofs of a theory of this eminent physiologist, which is by far of greater importance than the views he held respecting the place of passage of the sensitive impressions, and the orders of the will in the spinal cord. The great theory of Sir Charles Bell was, not that volition and sensation have their conductors in this or that place, but that these conductors are distinct one from the other, all along from the brain to the periphery. It is this principle of a complete distinction between the elements of the nerves and of the spinal cord, which are employed in motion and in sensation, which is the great thing that science particularly owes to him. Others had had this idea, but no one so powerfully as he had; and, also, no one tried to prove it, as he did. But, the principle being imagined, it remained to find out, first, positive proofs of its existence; and, secondly, whether the conductors—though distinct one from the other—are congregated together in the same sheath (as in the trunks of the spinal nerves), or are separated in distinct bundles, as they seem to be in the roots of the spinal nerves. Now we must say that, had the various conductors been everywhere placed in contact one with the other, the theory could not have been proved. As regards the spinal cord, when we began our researches, the most positive facts amongst those that were known, seemed to be quite in opposition to the great view of Sir Charles Bell, as they seemed to show that the same part of the spinal cord is employed both in voluntary movements, and in sensations. I have tried to show that the same conductors cannot be the agents for both voluntary movements and sensations, inasmuch as those for sensations make their decussation in the spinal cord, whilst those for motion decussate in the medulla oblongata. In this respect, then, instead of being in opposition to the great principle, to the demonstration of which Sir Charles had employed his whole life, I have brought a striking fact in proof of the truth of this principle. But I repeat that, as regards the channels of conveyance of the sensitive impressions and the orders of the will in the spinal cord, Sir Charles has been completely mistaken. This will be fully demonstrated hereafter.

The idea first proposed by Bell was, that the posterior columns of the spinal cord are the continuations of the posterior roots, and that they convey the sensitive impressions to the brain. He thought also that the anterior columns convey the orders of the will to muscles. This theory received no other support from its author than the following attempt at experimenting, which we record in the words of Sir Charles: "I found that injury to the anterior portion of the spinal marrow convulsed the animal more certainly than injury to the posterior portion; but I found it difficult to make the experiment, without injuring both portions."[1]

The theory of Sir Charles Bell was opposed by Bellingeri, Schoeps, Rolando, Calmeil, Fodera, and several others, before it found a very ardent supporter in Mr. Longet. All the experimenters which we have just named, except Mr. Longet, agreed upon one fact, which is, that a section of the posterior columns of the spinal marrow is not followed by a loss of sensibility. Such was the state of science, when Longet undertook to prove that the theory of Sir Charles Bell concerning the columns of the spinal cord, was as exact as that concerning the roots of the spinal nerves. In the next lecture we will show how Longet has been mistaken.

[1] The Nervous System of the Human Body. By Sir Charles Bell. Third edition. London, 1844. Appendix, p. 443.

LECTURE II.

EXPERIMENTS SHOWING THAT THE TRANSMISSION OF THE SENSITIVE IMPRESSIONS, IN THE SPINAL CORD, TAKES PLACE CHIEFLY IN ITS CENTRAL PART—I. E., IN THE GRAY MATTER.

Experiments and views of Longet. Objections by Dr. R. B. Todd, Mr. Lockhart, Clarke, and the Lecturer. Causes of error in experimenting upon the spinal marrow.—Experiments proving that a part may be a conductor of the sensitive impressions, though not endowed with sensibility.—Experiments showing, 1st, that a transversal section of the posterior columns of the spinal cord, instead of causing anæsthesia, is followed by hyperæsthesia; 2d, that a transversal section of the whole spinal cord, except the posterior columns, is followed by a complete anæsthesia. Anatomical and experimental facts showing the relative share of the gray matter, and of the various columns of white matter, in the transmission of the sensitive impressions.

Mr. President and Gentlemen: Although extremely numerous, the theories concerning the transmission of the sensitive impressions in the spinal cord may be considered as mere varieties of two principal ones, according to which the transmission takes place chiefly, or exclusively in the posterior columns, or in the gray matter. Longet is the principal advocate of the first of these two theories. He thinks:—

1st. That all the nerve-fibres of the spinal nerves which are employed in the transmission of the sensitive impressions, enter the posterior columns of the spinal cord, and go up to the brain in these columns, and, therefore, that the Sensorium receives sensitive impressions only from these parts of the spinal cord, and their prolongations in the encephalon.

2dly. That in the medulla oblongata, the restiform bodies being the direct continuations of the posterior columns of the spinal cord, are also the only channels for the transmission of the sensitive impressions.

3dly. That the sensitive impressions going to the sensorium have to pass chiefly across the cerebellum, as the restiform bodies chiefly pass across this organ.

Longet did not adduce any proof of the correctness of this theory. He merely tried to show that the posterior columns of the spinal cord are the only parts of this organ which are sensitive—*i. e.*, which cause pain when irritated. We will show hereafter, that, even admitting this as true, it was wrong to draw the conclusion that the posterior columns are the only conductors of sensitive impressions. Before we pass to this demonstration, we must say, as we think that it may prove useful to do so, that, had the theory of Longet been criticized, even in taking notice only of the facts mentioned by this physiologist, it would have been easy to show the utter impossibility of admitting this theory; but science has no critics, and this *impossible doctrine* was received in France as perfectly demonstrated, and was admitted in England, by almost every one, as being the theory of Sir Charles Bell, while Sir Charles had already repudiated it, five or six years before the first publications of Longet. It has been a curious spectacle to see men of great learning admitting that Longet had proved the truth of Sir Charles Bell's views, while, had Longet given real proofs, he would have demonstrated that Sir Charles was mistaken. In April, 1835, Bell read a paper before the Royal Society,[1] in which he says: "Formerly I believed that the nerves of sensation—that is to say, the posterior roots of the spinal nerves, came from the posterior columns of the spinal marrow, and, consequently, from the cerebellum. Whilst entertaining this belief, I found my progress barred; for it appeared to me incomprehensible that motion could result from an organ like the cerebrum, and sensation from the cerebellum, for there was no agreement between them. They conformed neither in size, shape, nor subdivisions." In the same paper, Sir Charles tries to show that the lateral columns of the spinal marrow must be the parts transmitting sensitive impressions, because they go to the cerebrum, and because he thought that the posterior roots are united with them. There was, therefore, a complete disagreement between Longet and Sir Charles Bell, as regards the function of two out of the three columns of the spinal cord—the posterior and the lateral columns.

We owe to Dr. R. B. Todd the first serious objections made in England against the views of Longet.[2] These objections are par-

[1] Philosophical Transactions, Part I., 1835; and "The Nervous System of the Human Body," by Sir Ch. Bell, third edition, 1844, pp. 238, 239.

[2] See his and Mr. Bowman's admirable work, "The Physiological Anatomy and

ticularly grounded upon anatomical and pathological facts. Of these last facts we will speak elsewhere, and of the first we will say that they relate—first, to the size of the posterior columns, which are not, as they should be, according to the theory, larger and longer, the higher they are examined in the spinal cord; secondly, to the insertions of the posterior roots, which do not seem to be attached to the posterior columns.

In 1851 and 1853, Mr. Lockhart Clarke published his important papers "On the Structure of the Spinal Cord,"[1] in which he clearly showed, as Stilling and others had already done, that the posterior roots of nerves are in continuation with the gray matter, and not with the posterior columns; and he tried to show—as had been already done by Sir Charles Bell and Dr. Todd—that the posterior columns, being united with the cerebellum, could not be considered as the only conductors of the sensitive impressions.

As long as twelve years ago, I began to oppose the views of Longet.[2] I shall not here criticize at length this doctrine, as the very arguments which I shall give in support of the theory that I propose will be found easily, and without my showing it, to be decisive objections to the views of Longet. I will merely try to show the contradictions which exist between various parts of the system of this physiologist, and also try to explain how he has been mistaken.

1*st Contradiction.*—Mr. Longet thinks that the gray matter of the spinal cord cannot be a conductor of sensitive impressions, because it is not endowed with sensibility; and his single argument to prove that the posterior columns are the sole conductors of the sensitive impressions is, that they are the only sensitive parts of the spinal cord. On another side, he admits that the cerebellum, which he rightly believes not to be sensitive, is the principal channel for the transmission of the sensitive impressions. Of course, if the gray matter of the spinal cord cannot be a conductor, because it is not sensitive, the cerebellum also cannot be a conductor; and if it is, the gray matter also can be.

2*d Contradiction.*—Longet admits that the extirpation of the cere-

Physiology of Man," Part II., 1845, pp. 316–319; and the article "Nervous System," in the Cyclopædia of Anatomy and Physiology.

[1] Philosophical Transactions, 1851, Part II., p. 607, and 1853, Part I., p. 347.

[2] See my Inaugural Dissertation for the Degree of M. D.—Recherches et Expér. sur la Physiologie de la Moelle Epinière. Paris, 3 Janvier, 1846.

bellum does not diminish the sensibility of any part of the body, and he admits also that the cerebellum is the principal channel of the transmission of sensitive impressions to the brain.

3d Contradiction.—There are several pathological cases mentioned by Longet which show that an alteration of a lateral half of the pons Varolii produces a complete loss of sensibility of the opposite half of the body; Longet, however, admits that there are but a small number of the sensitive nerve-fibres of the body which enter the pons Varolii. On another side, Longet relates pathological cases showing that the cerebellum may be altered very deeply without any diminution of sensibility, whilst he admits that most of the conductors of sensitive impressions pass through this nervous centre.

4th Contradiction.—Longet has proposed this view: that the pons Varolii is the centre for the perception of the sensitive impressions; and he admits that most of these impressions do not reach this organ, and pass through the cerebellum going up to the brain.

These contradictions are certainly sufficient to show the untenableness of the systematic views of Longet, and it might seem useless to speak any more of these views; but as they have, for a long while, been admitted as correct by almost every one in France and in England, we must say a few words on the causes of the errors committed by that able physiologist.

There are two means of ascertaining by experiments the functions of a nerve, or of a part of the nervous centres. One of these means consists in exciting the part, and in finding out what action takes place in consequence of the excitation; the other consists in a section or the extirpation of the part, and in examining what are the actions then missing. The first one, therefore, may give the action of a part, whilst the other shows what is its action when we see what is missing. Of these two means, Longet has made use of the first one only, and he declares that it is impossible to employ the second on the spinal cord. We shall see, on the contrary, that the first one could not be employed alone with success; whilst the second may very easily be employed, and furnish positive and direct facts.

Causes of Errors in experimenting upon the Spinal Cord.—Longet declares that it is impossible to lay bare the spinal cord of a mammal without producing, at once, such a debility in the posterior limbs that they lose, more or less completely, both voluntary movements and sensibility. Of course, if mammals were always in this condition after the opening of the spinal canal, it would be quite impossible to perform any valuable experiment on the spinal cord, to find out what are the parts employed in the two functions which are then lost. Fortunately, animals may not have any apparent diminution of either voluntary movements or sensibility after the exposure of the spinal cord to the air. They may walk about and run as fast as if nothing had been done to them, and, except the little change in the movements of the spine due to the section of some of its muscles, no difference may be observed between them and animals which have not been operated upon. As regards sensibility, it soon becomes increased, as I have stated in a paper read last year to the Royal Society. (See "Proceedings of the Royal Society," 1857, No. 26.) Longet has been mistaken, for the reason, that he opened the spinal canal in a considerable portion of its length, and in so doing produced a state of exhaustion by a great loss of blood and by the excessive pain. When the operation is made quickly, even if a very considerable part of the cord is laid bare, if the hæmorrhage has not been great and if pain has been avoided by the exhibition of chloroform, there is no notable diminution of sensibility, and there is no other diminution in the voluntary movements, except that depending upon the section of the muscles of the back.[1]

Another cause of error committed by some experimenters was in thinking that the absence of sensibility in the gray matter of the spinal cord is a proof that this matter is not a conductor of the sensitive impressions. A distinction between the property of conduction or transmission, and the property of being sensitive or impressionable, would have prevented such a mistake. The nerve-fibres of the cerebral lobes are *conductors*, but they are not *excitable*, not *impressionable;* and so is the gray matter of the spinal cord; when it exists alone, establishing the communication between two parts of the spinal cord, after a transversal section of the whole of the white

[1] Animals usually survive after the laying bare of the spinal cord, while they usually die after the laying bare of the brain. Indeed, if the susceptibility to inflammation is not greater in the spinal cord and its membranes in man than in animals, I think that Clive, Tyrrell, Laugier, and others, who have applied the trephine to the spine after fractures, should have imitators. In dogs, I have ascertained that the fracture of the posterior part of the vertebræ causes death, unless the broken pieces be removed and the effused liquid evacuated. Even in adult animals, the pieces of bone taken away are usually reproduced in a few months, and the injured spinal cord may also recover its functions.

matter, it *conducts*, it *transmits* to the brain the sensitive impressions made on *impressionable* organs *behind* the section, but when irritated it does not transmit anything because it is not itself impressionable. I have found that even the most sensitive nerve in the body, the trigeminal, loses its sensibility, its impressibility, in a part of its length. It is well known that a very considerable root of the trigeminal nerve goes down in the medulla oblongata towards the nib of the calamus scriptorius, being there between the anterior pyramid and the restiform body. Magendie has shown that a transversal section of one-half of the medulla oblongata dividing this root causes the loss of sensibility of the face, so that this root is positively a channel for the transmission of the sensitive impressions to the sensorium. Now, I have found that if a pin (even a large one) be introduced slowly and perpendicularly (see Fig. 5, *p*) through the restiform body and the root of the trigeminal nerve in the medulla oblongata, there is no sign of pain, so that the impressibility of this root in that part of its length is lost, or at least notably diminished. This fact proves that the power of conducting sensitive impressions may exist in parts deprived of sensibility. Even when we compare the various parts of the length of the roots and of the trunk of the spinal nerves, from the skin to the spinal cord, we find great differences in the degree of sensibility, while the conducting power seems to be the same everywhere. (See my paper on this subject in my work, *Experimental Researches applied to Physiology and Pathology*, 1853, p. 98.)

Of the means of experimenting, of which we have already spoken, the one which consists in employing excitations is certainly unable to give any decisive result, as regards the question of the channel by which the sensitive impressions are conveyed to the brain, in the spinal cord. All that may legitimately be deduced from the effects of the excitation of the various parts of the spinal cord is, that a certain part is sensitive, or seems to be, while others seem not to be. Another cause of error exists when we try to find out if a part is sensitive or not. If galvanism is employed, as was the case in the experiments of Longet, it is indeed impossible to have a current applied to the posterior columns, which will not pass by the posterior roots, and as the sensibility of the roots, particularly at the place where they are in connection with the spinal marrow, is excessive, the signs of pain given by the animals do not prove that the posterior columns are sensitive. Experiments in which an irritation is made with the point of a needle or a pin may be considered as insufficient, because the degree of pain, then, is not very great. However, so far as we may draw conclusions from this kind of experiment, it seems very doubtful whether the posterior columns possess any sensibility, and the causes of the mistake which has been made in this respect are, that the posterior roots have been irritated, and that the excitability for reflex action is very great in the posterior columns, and the movements due to the reflex faculty have been considered as signs of pain.[1]

I pass now to the exposition of the facts upon which I ground the theory I have proposed concerning the channels of transmission of sensitive impressions.

The first fact I have to speak of is, that a transversal section of the posterior columns, instead of being followed by the loss, or even a diminution, of sensibility, seems to produce an increase in the amount of this property; in other words, I have found that the section of these pretended only channels of the sensitive impressions, instead of preventing them from passing, allows them, on the contrary, to pass more freely, so that instead of *anæsthesia* there is *hyperæsthesia.* In certain animals, and especially in rabbits and sheep, it is very easy to ascertain that there is a very great increase in sensibility in the various parts behind the section. Before the operation, in rabbits, the most energetic pinching of the skin produces agitation, but no shrieking; after the operation, on the contrary, the least pinching produces shrieking, and a much greater agitation. Sometimes the hyperæsthesia is so considerable that the least pressure upon the skin makes the animal shriek. Whether the operation is performed in the lumbar, the dorsal, or the cervical region, the phenomena are always the same; that is, there is a manifest hyperæsthesia in the various parts of the body which receive their nerves from the part of the spinal cord which is behind the section. It has been so in all the animals I have operated upon,

[1] Although the reflex excitability of the posterior columns of the spinal cord is very great, the reflex movements observed when we irritate these columns alone, in a decapitated animal, are not so powerful as when we irritate at the same time the posterior roots and the posterior columns. But whatever may be admitted concerning this difference, it is quite certain, as first pointed out by the learned translator of Müller (Physiol., p. 796), Dr. Baly, that the irritation of the posterior columns of the spinal cord produces more movement than the excitation of the anterior columns. In cases of tumours pressing upon the spinal cord there is also more spasmodic action when the pressure is on the posterior than when it is on the anterior columns.

and I have already made this experiment upon animals belonging to more than twenty species.

As long as the animals live after the section of the posterior columns, hyperæsthesia continues to exist, except in the cases where reunion takes place between the two surfaces of the section; but hyperæsthesia is greater during the first week after the operation than it is after a month or many months.

Laying aside the curious fact of the existence of hyperæsthesia, a fact which is observed also in man, when the posterior columns of the spinal marrow are altered or injured, in a small part of their length, it results from the experiments consisting in a transverse section of these columns that the transmission of sensitive impressions to the encephalon does not take place only along the posterior columns. If a complete transverse section is made upon any part of the restiform bodies, sensibility becomes very much increased in every part of the limbs and trunk.

Hyperæsthesia is also, but in a less degree, one of the results of a transversal incision in the cerebellum, in the processus cerebelli ad testes, and in the tubercula quadrigemina.

If we carefully dissect the two restiform bodies so as to separate them from the neighboring parts, and if we divide them transversely at their two extremities, and then remove them, we find that the animal, instead of losing its sensibility in the different parts of the limbs and trunk, becomes hyperæsthetic.

It results from these experiments, that the restiform bodies, which are the direct continuations of the posterior columns of the spinal cord, are not the only channels for the transmission of sensitive impressions to the sensorium.

It seems certain, therefore, *that the posterior columns of the spinal cord and of the medulla oblongata are not the only channels for the transmission of the sensitive impressions from the limbs and trunk to the sensorium.*

But we can go farther, and prove that the posterior columns do not seem to transmit the least part of the sensitive impressions to the encephalon.

I have ascertained that after almost a complete transverse section of the spinal cord, leaving undivided only the posterior columns, the transmission of sensitive impressions from almost all the parts of the body behind the section does not take place. This experiment, performed by Stilling almost exclusively upon frogs, led him to affirm that sensibility is then entirely lost in all the parts behind the section. Much more recently, M. Schiff, repeating this experiment, found, on the contrary, that sensibility is not lost in any of the various parts behind the section. Messrs. Vulpian and Philipeaux, who made this experiment some time after Schiff, positively declare that sensibility is completely and definitely lost. I have ascertained that the differences in the results of this experiment depend upon various circumstances. At first, if the least quantity of the central gray matter of the spinal cord is left undivided, sensibility persists (although much diminished) almost everywhere behind the section. Besides, there are parts in the neighborhood of the section, and behind it, which always remain sensitive. I will explain afterwards what is the cause of this partial persistence of sensibility. Whatever is this cause, if we perform the following experiment, we may obtain the most decisive results: The spinal cord having been laid bare in a large mammal, in the dorsal region, I divide transversely the whole of it, except only the two posterior columns (see Fig. 8, *d*), and, after ten or fifteen minutes, or a little more, I find that all the usual means of exciting pain are applied in vain to the posterior limbs, so that these parts seem to be entirely deprived of sensibility. It results from this experiment, and from many others, in which the section was made nearer to the medulla oblongata, that the sensitive impressions do not pass along the posterior columns in their way to the encephalon.

If the transmission of sensitive impressions does not take place along the posterior columns, it remains to be found what is the channel of this transmission. Is it the gray matter or some part of the lateral or anterior columns, or all or several of these constituents of the spinal cord? As regards the lateral columns, if we divide them transversely in the dorsal region, we find that sensibility, instead of being lost, seems to be increased in the two posterior limbs. But if, in performing this experiment, the knife goes farther than the limits of the lateral columns, and divides a part of the central gray matter on the two sides, sensibility is then diminished in the two posterior limbs. From these experiments, and from another one, which consists in a transverse section of the whole spinal cord except one of the lateral columns, it results that these columns, like the posterior, are not the channels of transmission of any part of the sensitive impressions to the encephalon.

It is not so with regard to the gray matter, as the following experiments show:—

1st. A transversal section of the whole posterior half of the spinal cord is made, in the dorsal region, so that the posterior columns and the posterior half of the lateral columns and of the gray matter are divided, and then sensibility is found diminished in the two posterior limbs. Of course we cannot attribute this diminution to the section of the posterior or of the lateral columns, as we know that these divisions cause an increase of sensibility, and not a diminution.

2d. A transversal section of the whole anterior half of the spinal cord, in the dorsal region, is made, so that the anterior columns and the anterior half of the lateral columns and of the gray matter are divided, and then sensibility is found diminished in the two posterior limbs. We cannot attribute this diminution to the section of a part of the lateral columns, as we know that such an injury to the cord would increase, and not diminish, sensibility; nor can we admit that the section of the anterior columns is the only cause of diminution of sensibility, as, when these columns are alone divided, there is no marked alteration of sensibility.

3d. If the anterior, the lateral, and the posterior columns of the spinal cord are divided transversely, at the dorsal region, one set at one place, another at a distance of one or two inches, and the third also at the same distance from the second, so that the only channel of communication between the posterior limbs and the sensorium is the gray matter, of which, however, several parts have, unavoidably, been divided (such as the anterior and the posterior gray cornua, and also more or less of the central gray matter), we find that the posterior limbs are still sensitive, though evidently less than in the normal condition.

4th. If the section is made so as to divide only a small part of one of the lateral columns, and almost the whole of the gray matter, sensibility is very much diminished in the parts of the body behind the section.

These facts prove that the gray matter is the principal conductor of the sensitive impressions in the spinal cord.

But, amongst the white columns, there are some, besides the posterior ones, which have been considered, by two or three physiologists, as organs of transmission of the sensitive impressions; I mean the anterior columns. Calmeil and Nonat thought that these parts share in this function. Although I admit their view, I believe they were mistaken in their experiments, which consisted in a transversal section of the whole spinal cord, except the anterior columns, as they state that immediately, or shortly after the operation, they found sensibility persisting. This is not the case when the whole of the gray matter has been cut transversely, and it is extremely probable that they had left a good part of it undivided. But if the operation be made so as to leave no gray matter at all, sensibility, which at first seems to be lost, after a time reappears, and many hours after, it evidently exists everywhere, though in a slight degree only.[1] It is evident, therefore, that the anterior columns have a share, but only a small one, in the transmission of the sensitive impressions to the sensorium.

From all the facts above related, it results that the transmission of sensitive impressions takes place chiefly by the gray matter, and, for a small part only, by the anterior columns, while the lateral and the posterior columns do not participate in the same way as the preceding parts of the cord, in this function. We shall see, in a moment, that they have a peculiar kind of share in this transmission.

Which part of the gray matter is employed in the transmission of sensitive impressions? This substance is composed of parts surrounding the central canal of the cord, of lateral masses, and of two anterior and two posterior horns, which separate the lateral columns from the anterior and the posterior ones. I call central gray matter the lateral masses, the bases of the anterior and posterior horns, and all the substance around the central canal, and I think that the transmission of the sensitive impressions takes place chiefly by this central gray matter. As regards the anterior horns of gray matter, I am not prepared to affirm that they have no share at all in this function; but I may state the posterior horns do not participate in it, in the same way as the central portion of gray matter.

Which elements of the central gray matter are employed in the transmission of sensitive impressions? This difficult question has not yet received a positive solution; but it cannot be doubted, at least, that the transmission takes place by both cells and nerve-fibres united together, and not by cells alone acting at a distance upon their neighbors. Most of the nerve-fibres of the roots of the spinal nerves, after having reached the gray matter, attach themselves to the nerve-cells, and, as has been well demonstrated by R. Wagner, and by Bidder, and several of his pupils, these cells communicate with others in such a way that two kinds of transmission are possible, one across the cord, and another towards or from

[1] See my paper in the "Proceedings of the Royal Society," No. 26, 1857.

the encephalon. But, besides the nerve-cells and their nervous fibrils of communication, there are, in the gray matter, several collections of longitudinal nerve-fibres, forming very minute white columns, surrounded by the gray substance. These white columns, first well described by Mr. Lockhart Clarke, and, after him, by Prof. Schrœder van der Kolk, cannot be considered as the only channels, in the gray matter, for the sensitive impressions or for the orders of the Will to muscles. The number of fibres they contain is too small for them to have these functions alone, but it is probable that they participate in it. Are they employed for a peculiar kind of sensitive impressions while the other impressions would be transmitted by nerve-cells and their communications? This is a question that experiments upon animals cannot solve. We will speak of it again when we give the history of the pathological cases relating to the subjects discussed here.

We must now examine if the posterior and lateral columns have not a peculiar share in the transmission of sensitive impressions. As regards the posterior columns, the following experiments will show that there are conductors of sensitive impressions passing through them. Long ago I found that after a transversal section of the columns, the inferior surface of the section, that which seems no more to be connected with the encephalon, appears to be highly sensitive. I have since ascertained that the posterior roots in the neighborhood of that surface are the parts which then give the sensation of pain. But whether sensibility exists only in the roots or in the fibres of the posterior columns, it is a fact that pain is produced when this inferior surface is irritated. In 1852, I was led still more to admit that there are nerve-fibres coming from the posterior roots, and passing in two opposite directions in the posterior columns (see the arrows in Fig. 6), some going upwards and some going downwards, or, in other words, some going direct towards the encephalon and some going away from it. The following experiment was the first which led me to the conclusion that there are fibres of the posterior roots *descending* in the posterior columns: I introduced a very sharp bistoury between the posterior and the anterior parts of the spinal cord, and by cutting from above downwards, or in the opposite direction, I separate a part of the length of the posterior columns of the cord from the anterior parts of this organ. This being done, I divide transversely and in its middle the part of the posterior columns separated from the anterior parts of the spinal cord, so as to obtain (see Fig. 6) two segments, one superior, the other inferior. The superior I will call cephalic segment, and the other caudal segment. Now, when there are some little parts of the posterior gray horns and some fibres of the posterior roots attached to these segments, we obtain this apparently strange and surely unforeseen result, that not only the caudal segment is sensitive, but that it seems to be more sensitive than the cephalic segment. But whatever may be the real amount of sensibility in these two segments, there is one capital conclusion to be drawn from this experiment, and this is, that *a number of the conductors of sensitive impressions in the posterior roots pass in the posterior columns, in which some go upwards towards the encephalon* (*centripetal or ascending fibres*), *while others go in the opposite direction—i. e., downwards or backwards* (*centrifugal or descending fibres*).

Now the question arises—*What become of these ascending and descending conductors?* By a great many experiments of various kinds, I have ascertained that they pass along the posterior columns only a little way, and leave them to enter the central gray matter. I will relate a few of the most striking experiments, which prove that such is truly the disposition of these conductors. If, after having ascertained that the roots attached to the upper or cephalic segment (see Fig. 6) are sensitive, I divide transversely the posterior columns at a very short distance above the extremity of the segment, I find that it loses its sensibility, which fact shows that the transmission takes place by these columns. Now if the section is made higher, sensibility persists, though diminished, showing that some of the conductors must, at this distance, have left the posterior columns and entered another part of the cord; at last, if the section is made far above the extremity of the segment, sensibility persists entire in the roots attached to that extremity, which shows that the conductors, at a certain distance from the point of their entrance into the posterior columns, leave these columns to pass into another part of the cord. This part is the central gray matter, as is proved by the fact that if we divide it transversely at four or five inches above the cephalic segment, this segment loses its sensibility.

With the inferior, or caudal segment, analogous experiments show that the conductors coming from the posterior roots descend in the posterior columns, and, after a very short distance, pass into the central gray matter. There the transmission takes place towards the encephalon; so that there are *recurrent* conductors in the spinal cord.

An excellent experiment, showing the share of the gray matter in the transmission of sensitive impressions may be made after we have prepared two segments of the posterior columns, as we have said already. We ascertain that the caudal, or lower segment, is very sensitive, and then we divide gradually the laid-bare gray matter (see Fig. 6, *g*), and we find that gradually, also, sensibility disappears in this segment.

Experiments, which it is useless to describe, seem to show also that there are some fibres from the posterior roots which *ascend*, and others which *descend*, in the lateral columns, and in the posterior horns, both of which soon reach the central gray matter, by which part the transmission to the encephalon is at last performed.

Their existence in the posterior columns, and also probably in the posterior horns and a part of the lateral columns, receives additional evidence from the following experiment: If the posterior half of the spinal cord is divided in two places, in one case very near, and in another very far, one from the other (see Fig. 7), we find that there is a loss of sensibility in the posterior roots which are between the two sections, when they are very near one to the other; while, on the contrary, sensibility remains, and seems to be increased, in the posterior roots which are between the two sections, when they are at a great distance one from the other. In admitting that before reaching the central gray matter the fibres of the posterior roots go up and down the cord along the posterior columns, and along the parts (gray or white) which are in the neighborhood of these columns, and which have been divided with them, we have the explanation of the loss of sensibility in the first case; and in admitting that these conductors, after a short distance, enter the central gray matter, we explain the persistence of sensibility in the second case.

With this knowledge of the mode of distribution of the sensitive conductors in the spinal cord, we may explain the differences in the results arrived at by different experimenters after the operation consisting in a transversal section of the totality of the spinal cord, except the posterior columns. If, for instance, this operation has been made at the level of the second or third lumbar vertebræ, very little *above* the place where the roots of the nerves going to the abdominal limbs begin to originate, we find that the extremities of these limbs seem to be completely deprived of sensibility, but that when the upper parts of the limbs are irritated, there are evident signs of sensibility. The reason of this difference is obvious, if we admit that the fibres from the roots of the nerves going to the extremities of the limbs leave the posterior columns of the spinal cord below the section, and pass into the gray matter, and, also, in the anterior columns, which parts are divided; while some of the fibres from the roots of the nerves going to the upper parts of the limbs, pass into the posterior columns at the level where the other parts of the cord are divided, and still transmit the sensitive impressions. To prove that they pass only a short way in and along the posterior columns, I have performed the following additional experiment. In one case I divide transversely the posterior columns at a very short distance above the place where the antero-lateral parts of the cord have been cut, and I find, then, that sensibility is entirely lost in all the parts of the posterior limbs (see Fig. 8, *d*, *s*), in the other case I divide transversely the posterior columns at a great distance from the other section, and I find that sensibility of the upper parts of the posterior limb persists.

There are many facts which I could mention, in addition to the preceding, which show that the posterior columns of the spinal cord afford passage to several of the conductors of sensitive impressions, but that, after a short distance, they leave these columns to enter the gray matter. I refrain speaking of these facts, because I think that the above experiments are sufficient. It is useless to try to show that these experiments prove that the idea that there are sensitive fibres going to the encephalon in the posterior columns must be abandoned.

As a general conclusion, we will say that the conductors of sensitive impressions, at their arrival in the spinal cord, either enter directly the central gray matter, or go up or down a little way in the posterior columns, and also, most likely, in the posterior gray cornua, and in the posterior part of the lateral columns, and entering afterwards the central gray matter, by, or in which, the impressions conveyed by these two sets ascend towards the encephalon.

I will add, that many experiments, some of which are related in this lecture, prove that the restiform bodies, which are the continuations of the posterior columns, seem not to give passage to any of the conductors of the sensitive impressions of either the various parts of the trunk and limbs, or of the head, and that, therefore, the cerebellum, with which the restiform bodies are connected, does not receive from them any of such conductors.

In another lecture, I will speak of the singular hyperæsthesia which exists in so high a degree after the section of the posterior columns of the spinal cord, and also after a deep section of the following parts on the posterior side of the encephalon: the restiform bodies, the cerebellum, the anterior crura cerebelli, and the tubercula quadrigemina.

LECTURE III.

PLACE OF DECUSSATION OF THE CONDUCTORS OF SENSITIVE IMPRESSIONS, IN THE CEREBRO-SPINAL AXIS.

The celebrated experiments of Galen, which had been universally considered as showing that there is no decussation of the conductors of sensitive impressions, in the spinal cord, do not prove anything in this respect.—Experiments showing that the conductors of sensitive impressions from the various parts of the trunk and limbs make their decussation in the spinal cord, and not in the encephalon, as was admitted.

MR. PRESIDENT AND GENTLEMEN: The question I am about treating has had a singular fate; considered as solved for a great many centuries, it has hardly been the object of the attention of scientific men in our days. Until 1849, when I first published the discovery I had just made, that there is a decussation of the conductors of sensitive impressions in the spinal cord, it had been universally admitted that Galen had proved that there is no such crossing in the spinal cord, and that, therefore, these conductors must make their decussation in the encephalon. Physiologists and pathologists agreed in attributing to Galen the merit of having given a demonstration, in this respect, although he seems never to have tried to solve the question. In detailing his experiments on the spinal cord,[1] he does not say a single word concerning sensibility, and it is upon the falsely understood results of these experiments, that, for a great many centuries, medical men have based their opinions that there is no decussation of the conductors of sensitive impressions in the spinal cord.

Haller[2] also speaks of voluntary movements, and not of sensibility in mentioning the effects of a section of a lateral half of the

[1] See his following works: "De Locis affectis," Lib. III. cap. xiv., et "De Anatomicis administrationibus," Lib. VIII. sect. vi.

[2] "Elementa Physiologiæ," vol. iv. pp. 326 and 334. In one of these places he says just the reverse of what he affirms in the other, as regards voluntary movements.

spinal cord. Lorry, Fodéra, Flourens, Calmeil, and many other physiologists, have studied the effects of an injury to one half of the medulla oblongata, but none of them has directly examined if there is a decussation of the sensitive fibres in the spinal cord; and in their experiments on the medulla oblongata they looked almost only at the effects on movements (paralysis and convulsions), and they hardly mention the state of sensibility.

Sir Charles Bell is the first biologist who has tried to determine the real place of decussation of the conductors of sensitive impressions in the cerebro-spinal axis. He imagines that it is in a small part of the length of the floor of the fourth ventricle above, and near the crossing of the pyramids;[1] but he does not give any reason in proof of his idea, except the results of a deceptive anatomical dissection, quite in opposition with the results of the important researches of John Reid, of Solly, of Valentin, and other anatomists.

Longet also has tried to show the place of decussation of the conductors of sensitive impressions.[2] He admits that the sensitive fibres, after having passed through the cerebellum, go towards the tubercula quadrigemina, along the *processus cerebelli ad testes*, and that they make their decussation below the tubercles. The erroneousness of this view is pretty evident from the fact that the sensitive fibres do not pass through the cerebellum, so that the fibres, which really seem to make a decussation where the anterior peduncles of the cerebellum coalesce, below the tubercula quadrigemina, cannot be the continuation of the sensitive fibres of the body.

We will try to prove that the conductors of sensitive impressions make their decussation in the neighborhood of the place of insertion of the sensitive nerves, or roots of nerves, in the cerebro-spinal axis. As regards the sensitive fibres of the trunk and limbs, we will try to show that their decussation takes place in the spinal cord. The following experiments seem to be decisive in this respect:—

1st. The spinal cord of a mammal is laid bare at the level of the two or three last dorsal vertebræ, and a lateral half of this organ (including the posterior, the lateral, and the anterior columns, and

[1] See the "Nervous System of the Human Body," 3d edition. London, 1844, pp. 231–40.

[2] "Anatomie et Physiol. du Syst. Nerveux," 1843, vol. i. pp. 385 and 421.

all the gray matter on one side) is divided transversely. (See Fig. 9, *s*.) The animal is left at rest for a little while, and then it is ascertained that sensibility seems to be much increased in the posterior limb on the side of the section, while it seems to be lost, or extremely diminished, in the posterior limb on the opposite side. There seems to be, therefore, *hyperæsthesia* behind and *on the side* of a transversal section of a complete lateral half of the spinal cord; while, on the contrary, there seems to be *anæsthesia* behind the section, and *on the opposite side.*

This experiment is one of the two made by Galen; but he seems not to have looked at all at the condition of sensibility, and he simply states that there is a paralysis on the side of the section, and no paralysis on the opposite side.

Sir Astley Cooper, under the suggestion of Dr. Yelloly,[1] has made a similar experiment, except that the section was higher; the state of sensibility is not mentioned, and, as regards movements, there was paralysis on the side operated upon.

Schœps, Van Deen, and Stilling have observed that sensibility is not lost in the limb or limbs behind, and on the side of the section of a lateral half of the spinal cord; but they have not remarked the most important fact, that on the opposite side there is anæsthesia. They also do not mention this curious result of this experiment, the existence of hyperæsthesia on the side of the injury.

Fodéra was very near discovering that there is a decussation of the sensitive fibres in the spinal cord. He says he has found in some cases, that a section of one of the posterior columns caused a diminution of sensibility in the opposite side of the body; but he states that in other cases he has seen the reverse. He also has sometimes remarked that the section of one of the posterior columns causes hyperæsthesia in the same side, and that a section of these two columns produces hyperæsthesia in the two sides, but he declares, also, that he has seen the reverse.[2]

Two explanations for some of the results of a section of a lateral half of the spinal cord may be proposed, as regards sensibility. Either it may be imagined, as it has been by several German physiologists, that the gray matter has the power of transmitting sensitive impressions in such a manner that one lateral half of this substance is sufficient for the two sides of the body, or that the

[1] Medico-Chirurgical Transactions, vol. i. p. 200, et seq.

[2] See his paper in Magendie's Journal de Physiologie, vol. iii. p. 191–217.

conductors of sensitive impressions decussate in the spinal cord, so that those which come from the left side of the body pass into the right side of the spinal cord, and *vice versâ*. The hypothesis of the Germans may explain the fact that sensibility persists on the side of the section, but it is proved to be absolutely inadmissible by the fact that there is anæsthesia on the opposite side. We will see that the other experiments we have to mention are also in opposition to the view of the Germans (Stilling, Schiff, and others). On the contrary, all the facts concur to prove the existence of a decussation.

2d. If, after having made a first section of a lateral half of the spinal cord in the dorsal region, on the right side, for instance (see Fig. 9, *s*), and after having ascertained that the *right* posterior limb is hyperæsthetic, or at least extremely sensitive, we divide the *left* lateral half of the spinal cord in the cervical region (Fig. 9, *s'*), we find then that the *right* posterior limb loses entirely, or almost entirely, its sensibility. This experiment shows clearly that the sensitive impressions coming from the *right* posterior limb, after the first section, passed across the spinal cord from the right into the left side, along which they were transmitted to the encephalon.

3d. To obtain a very striking result from the experiment which consists in only one section of a lateral half of the spinal cord, it is better to make it after the posterior columns have been divided. We know that after this division there is hyperæsthesia in the parts of the body which are behind the section; if, after having ascertained this fact, the section of a lateral half is completed where the posterior columns have been divided (see Fig. 10, *s s'*), we find that the hyperæsthesia seems to increase on the side of the second operation, while, on the opposite side, not only the hyperæsthesia, but sensibility entirely disappears.

4th. There is another mode of proving that the conductors of the sensitive impressions decussate in the spinal cord. In several points of view this mode of demonstration is superior to the preceding. It consists in a longitudinal section of the spinal cord, an experiment already made by Galen, but the results of which, as regards sensibility, have been overlooked by him.

The spinal cord is laid bare in the whole lumbar region, and a careful division of the entire extent of the part of the organ giving origin to the nerves of the posterior limbs, is made so as to separate the two lateral halves of the organ, one from the other. If this experiment could be executed perfectly well, nothing would be divided in the cord except the commissures, which unite the right side with the left side of the cord, and all the longitudinal elements of this nervous centre would be left uninjured; but it is impossible not to cut more or less on either side. However, when the operation has succeeded well—*i. e.*, when the two separated halves have been very little injured, a striking result is obtained. The voluntary movements still exist in the posterior limbs (though diminished on account of the injury to the muscles of the lumbar region), but *sensibility is entirely lost* in them. To those who know that injuries to the spinal cord, which cause a diminution of sensibility, always produce a greater diminution of voluntary movements, this fact will not be explained by the supposition that some injury has, then, been made to the two halves of the cord, and that it is, in consequence of this supposed injury, that the loss of sensibility is due. At least it will, I think, be easily admitted that if the two lateral halves of the cord had been injured enough to produce a complete and a lasting anæsthesia, there would be a notable degree of paralysis of voluntary movements. We repeat that such is not the case: the animal has the use of his two limbs; he moves about pretty freely, as Galen had already said. The loss of sensibility, therefore, must depend on the section of the commissures of the spinal cord, or, in other words, on elements of this organ which cross each other in the median line, or, rather, the median plane.

If now we compare the results of this experiment with those of a transversal section of a lateral half of the spinal cord, we find that they agree perfectly in showing that the conductors of the sensitive impressions decussate in this organ. It is useless to stop to show that the longitudinal separation of the lumbar enlargement of the spinal cord would not produce anæsthesia, if the German physiologists were right in admitting that the gray matter has the power of transmission in every direction. It would be useless, also, to insist upon the disagreement between the results of a longitudinal section of the spinal cord, and the views of the physiologists who admit that the posterior columns are composed of sensitive fibres, coming from the posterior roots, and going up to the encephalon. These columns are left almost entire and uninjured, and, nevertheless, sensibility is lost.

5th. Another experiment, which is a combination of two of the preceding, gives a still better proof of the decussation of the conductors of sensitive impressions in the spinal cord. A longitudinal section is made on the cervico-brachial enlargement of the spinal cord, so as to separate it in two lateral halves. I ascertain then that sensibility is lost in the two anterior limbs, while it remains, and even seems to be increased, in the two posterior limbs. Of course, if the loss of sensibility in the two anterior limbs depended upon an injury to the two sides of the cord, and not upon a section of the decussating conductors of sensitive impressions, there would be a loss of sensibility, or, at least, a diminution of it in the posterior limbs. The admission of a decussation explains the two facts: loss of sensibility in one set of limbs, and conservation in the other set. (See Fig. 11.) If we divide transversely, in the same animal, the right lateral half of the spinal cord (see Fig. 11, *s*), we find then that the posterior limb on the same side becomes more evidently hyperæsthetic than before, and that the left posterior limb loses its sensibility. The transmission for this last limb therefore took place by the right half of the cord, while that for the right posterior limb continues to take place by the left half of the cord.

I think that the facts I have mentioned sufficiently show that there is a decussation of the conductors of sensitive impressions in the spinal cord. But several questions remain to be solved concerning this decussation. The first one we intend examining is, whether the decussation is complete or not.

The fact that the loss of sensibility seems to be absolutely complete, after a longitudinal section of the whole length of the lumbar enlargement of the spinal cord seems to show that all the conductors of sensitive impressions which reach the cord, coming from the posterior limbs, make their decussation in this enlargement. But if we admit that the decussation is complete, how do we explain that there is an appearance of sensibility, and sometimes a well-marked degree of it, in a limb on the opposite side to that of a section of a lateral half of the spinal cord? In the first place, I must say that very often when we try to divide transversely such a part of the cord, being afraid of cutting too much, we leave undivided a part of the gray matter and of the anterior column, so that the persistence of sensibility in the opposite side of the body is very natural, and not in opposition to our views. Very likely this is what has occurred in many of the experiments of Mr. Chauveau, who says that sensibility always persists in such a limb. If there is no notable diminution of sensibility anywhere, after an attempt to divide the lateral half of the cord, it is certain that the operation is not complete, and that a part has escaped division. It is wonderful how small is the quantity of gray matter which, being left undivided, may transmit sensitive impressions!

But even when the operation has been perfectly performed in certain animals, and especially guinea-pigs, in some cases, there seems to be a notable degree of sensibility remaining in the parts of the body which are behind the section, on the opposite side. I have ascertained that this appearance of sensibility is due to a very interesting cause. I suppose that the section has been made on the right side of the cord, above the origin of the nerves of the inferior limbs; when the left inferior limb is irritated, the impression is brought to the spinal cord by the posterior roots (see Fig. 4, P), and, by a reflex action, the muscles of the right inferior limb have a spasmodic contraction, just as if the anterior roots of their nerves had been irritated, and in consequence there is a pain produced which is of the same kind as that which Magendie has attributed to a *recurrent sensibility* (see Lect. I.). The proof that the irritation travels, as we believe, is given by the facts, that if either the anterior or the posterior roots of nerves are divided on the right side, behind the hemisection of the cord, the appearances of sensibility disappear in the left inferior limb. Starting from the left limb, the irritation goes to the spinal cord; it is reflected to the muscles of the right inferior limb, along the motor nerve-fibres; it comes back again to the spinal cord, and then, following the normal channel of a sensitive impression, it passes from the right half of the spinal cord into the left side, in which it goes to the encephalon. Although the spasmodic reflex contraction in the right inferior limb is not very strong, it is able to give a painful sensation, on account of the hyperæsthesia which exists in this limb. (See Fig. 4, and Lect. I.)

As far as experiments go, it is very difficult to decide whether the decussation of the conductors of sensitive impressions is absolutely complete or not, but it seems to be very nearly, if not absolutely, complete. We shall see, by and by, that pathological cases seem to show that the decussation, in man, is complete.

What is the place of decussation of the various posterior roots of a pair of nerves? I have said, in the preceding lecture, that the fibres which enter the spinal cord, from the posterior roots, are distributed, in this nervous centre, in such a way that some are going upwards, some downwards, and some transversely. There are, therefore, ascending, descending, and transversal fibres. Now, all these fibres reach the central gray matter, after a short way, above or below their place of entrance, and almost at once they decussate. A great many experiments show that this must be the arrangement of the conductors of sensitive impressions.

If we divide transversely a lateral half of the spinal cord in two places, so as to have three pairs of nerves between the two sections, we find that the middle pair has almost the same degree of sensibility as if nothing had been done to the spinal cord, while the two other pairs have a diminished sensibility, the upper one particularly in its upper roots, and the lower one in its lower roots: which facts seem to show that the ascending fibres of the upper pair, and the descending fibres of the lower one, have been divided before they had made their decussation.

If there is only one pair of nerves between two sections, its sensibility is almost entirely lost, as then the transversal fibres are almost alone uninjured (most of the ascending and deseending being divided), which fibres are employed for reflex action, and hardly for the transmission of sensitive impressions.

After having divided transversely a lateral half of the spinal cord in the dorsal region, if we divide longitudinally this organ, so as to separate its two lateral halves one from the other, and at a right angle with the transversal section (see Fig. 12), we find that sensibility persists in the segment partly separated from the rest of the cord, if it is not more than two inches long, in a large mammal, whether the longitudinal section has been made below or behind the transversal one, as is the case in Fig. 12, or above or before this transversal division. If the longitudinal section is more than two inches long, it is not sensitive in all its length. When there are three pairs of nerves attached to it, the one nearest to the transversal section (see Fig. 12, 1), is hardly able to give slight sensations; the next (2) is a little more sensitive, but much less than in a normal condition; and the third is very sensitive, though not so much as the others on the same side and behind it. With a segment attached to the cord by its upper extremity, similar results are obtained, and it seems certain, both from these facts and from many others which it is not necessary to mention, that the decussation of the conductors of the sensitive impressions in the spinal cord, whether they are, at first, descending or ascending, takes place at a short distance from the point of insertion of the posterior roots.

Experiments upon the medulla oblongata, to decide if the crossing of the conductors of sensitive impressions, coming from the trunk and limbs, has taken place before they reach this organ or not, cannot give positive results, because the reflex movements are so energetic after a section of a lateral half of this nervous centre, that it is very difficult to know the degree of sensibility. But pathological facts, observed in man, will settle the question, as we shall show in another lecture. We have not, however, to regret that experiments on the medulla oblongata are useless, as it seems that the question of the decussation of the conductors of sensitive impressions, as far as the trunk and limbs are concerned, is clearly solved by the experiments on the spinal cord, mentioned in this lecture.

There are some animals in which the decussation in the spinal cord is not so complete and so immediate as it is in mammals; such are reptiles and birds. This is one of the causes of some mistakes recently made by an able experimenter, Mr. Chauveau, of Lyons. He operated upon pigeons, and found that after a section of a lateral half of the spinal cord, sensibility seemed to be much diminished on the same side, and not at all on the opposite side. He concluded, therefore, that there is no decussation. I have ascertained that the results of the experiments vary with the place of the section. If it be made just above the lumbar enlargement, where Mr. Chauveau makes it, the decussation having hardly begun below this place, the results are as he says; but if the section be made two inches higher, in the dorsal region, there is, as in mammals, though less marked, an increased sensibility in the posterior limb on the side of the section, and a diminution of sensibility in the opposite limb. The loss of sensibility is never complete, showing that the decussation is not complete. The same results are obtained in reptiles.

As regards some other objections addressed to my theories by Mr. Chauveau, I do not think it worth while to mention them here. I have tried recently to show how little grounded they are,[1] and more decisive arguments than those founded upon vivisections will be given in my lectures on the pathological cases which prove the decussation in the spinal cord, and the power of transmission of the gray matter.

In the preceding lecture, and in this one, I have tried to show

[1] See my Journal de la Physiologie de l'Homme et des Animaux, Janvier, 1858, pp. 176–189.

that the sensitive impressions follow, in the spinal cord, quite a determinate course, and I think that the facts I have mentioned to establish what this course is, are positive evidences that there are fixed channels, and that some of them cannot compensate for the absence of others. It is, therefore, useless to show the untenableness of the theory of the Germans (Schiff and Stilling), that the gray matter has the power of transmission in any direction, and that any small part of it may act for the whole, without any diminution of intensity.

It may be thought that experiments on animals can show only what relates to painful impressions, and not to impressions of touch, of cold, of warmth, &c. I will try to show, in the next lecture, that the channel for impressions of touch, at least, seems to be the same as that of painful impressions, in the spinal cord.

LECTURE IV.

ON VARIOUS QUESTIONS RELATING TO THE TRANSMISSION OF SENSITIVE IMPRESSIONS AND OF THE ORDERS OF THE WILL TO MUSCLES, THROUGH THE SPINAL CORD AND THE MEDULLA OBLONGATA.

Most of the elements which are employed as conductors of the purely tactile impressions seem to pass by the same parts of the spinal cord as those which transmit the impressions which give pain.—The disposition of the conductors of the various sensitive impressions in the spinal cord is such that very deep alterations of this organ may not entirely destroy sensibility.—The gray matter of the spinal cord seems to have an important share in the transmission of the orders of the will to muscles.—The anterior columns of the spinal cord in the upper part of the cervical region have but a slight participation in voluntary movements, and the lateral columns, with the surrounding gray matter, in that part of the cord, are almost the only channels between the will and muscles.

Mr. President and Gentlemen: I hope I shall be able to show, in one of the succeeding lectures, that the various sensitive impressions—of *touch*, of *pain*, of *temperature*, of *muscular contractions*, etc. —are transmitted by conductors which are quite distinct from one another, and so much so that the conductors of painful impressions, for instance, are not more able to convey other kinds of impressions than to transmit the orders of the will to muscles. This view appears to be positively established by pathological cases observed in man. I hope I shall now be allowed to make use of this view as if it were proved, and I will examine if the conductors of tactile impressions follow the same course in the spinal cord as those of painful impressions. I will, at first, relate experiments which seem to solve the following question: *Do the conductors of tactile impressions proceed to the encephalon along the posterior columns, or do they pass into the gray matter as the conductors of impressions of pain?*

After having divided transversely the two posterior columns of the spinal cord in the dorsal region, in a dog, we cover its eyes and wait until it has lain down in a state of quietness. When it seems to be perfectly quiet, we find, if we gently touch the skin of one of its hind toes, that it lifts up its head and tries to see what is the cause of the irritation. It is certainly difficult to decide what kind of sensation this dog has felt, but I think I may show that it is a tactile sensation. Before discussing this point, however, I must say that it is not in consequence of a local reflex movement, shaking the whole body, that the animal looks anxiously around it. If it were so, the movement of the head would not take place immediately after the irritation and at the very same time that the irritated leg is withdrawn. Besides, after a complete transversal section of the spinal cord, when reflex movements are much stronger than after a section of the posterior columns, the head of the animal does not move at the time we touch the under part of its hind toes. Therefore the dog, in our experiment, moves its head because the touching of its toes has directly given a sensation. When we think that there is a real hyperæsthesia in these toes, it seems possible that the simple touching of the toes is painful; but the hyperæsthesia, I think, is not of a sufficient degree for the production of pain from such a trifling cause. Still more, the touching of other parts of the skin of the posterior limbs, which are endowed with the same morbid power of causing pain as the skin of the toes, is not followed by a movement of the head; so that it becomes very probable that the effect following the touching of the toes depends upon the propagation of a tactile impression to the encephalon, the skin of the toes being endowed with more tactile sensibility than that of the legs. The posterior columns, therefore, seem not to be the only channels of the tactile impressions.

Another experiment goes farther, and seems to prove positively that the posterior columns do not transmit directly any part of the tactile impressions to the sensorium. If we divide transversely, in the dorsal region, the whole of the spinal cord, except the posterior columns, the touching of the sole of the foot is not followed by any sign of feeling, and the head, if the eyes are covered, remains quiet. At times, however, it happens that the animal moves its head and its anterior limbs, because it has been shaken by the strong reflex movements which are produced in the paralyzed limbs. In this case reflex movements are always more energetic than after a complete section of the cord, and very much more than after the section of the posterior columns.

From the above facts it seems to result that the transmission of tactile impressions to the encephalon does not take place along the posterior columns. Other experiments, useless to be mentioned, show that the gray matter of the spinal and probably also the anterior columns are the channels of conveyance of the tactile impressions to the encephalon. We shall not insist upon the demonstration of these conclusions now, as we shall again have to examine their value when we compare the results of experiments with the results of pathological alterations of the spinal cord in man. We will then try to show the disagreement between these results and a theory recently proposed by Mr. Moritz Schiff, according to which the posterior columns of the spinal cord are the channels for tactile impressions, and the gray matter the conductor of painful impressions.[1]

We will now say a few words on the decussation of the conductors of tactile impressions. If a lateral half of the spinal cord has been divided transversely in the dorsal region, we find that when we touch the sole of the foot of the posterior limb on the side operated upon, the animal raises its head and tries to look at the place irritated (in which attempt it cannot succeed, as its eyes are covered). On the opposite side the touching of the skin of the toes does not produce the least effect. It seems therefore that *the conductors of the tactile impressions decussate in the spinal cord*, as well as that of painful impressions, so that the right side of this organ transmits to the sensorium the impressions which come from the left side of the body, and *vice versâ*. We will add that the experiments which show that the conductors of these two kinds of sensitive impressions decussate in the spinal cord are in opposition to the view that the posterior columns are the channels for both these kinds or for either of them, as it is well known that these two columns have no communication one with the other unless it be through the other parts of the cord.

The question relative to the place of passage in the spinal cord, of the impressions of temperature, and of some other kinds of impressions, cannot be solved positively by vivisections. We can say, however, that after a transverse section of the whole spinal cord, except the posterior columns, in the dorsal region, the application of ice or of fire to the toes, seems not to be felt, and that also spasms may be induced in the muscles of the paralyzed legs without causing a sensation. It seems, therefore, that the posterior columns are not the channels of transmission of these impressions.

[1] Untersuchungen zur Naturlehre des Menschen und der Thiere. Von J. Moleschott. Vol. iv. pp. 84–87. 1858.

Some experiments also seem to show that the conductors of these impressions decussate in the spinal cord. But pathological facts observed in man will teach us much more concerning all the sensitive impressions which are not purely painful, than experiments upon animals. In consequence, we shall postpone also, till we come to pathological facts, what relates to this question: Is it possible to recognize the place upon which an impression is made, when the posterior columns of the spinal cord are divided or altered? We will merely say, at present, that animals, after a section of the posterior columns or of a lateral half of the spinal cord, seem to discover the point irritated, as, although their eyes are covered, they try to bite near the place upon which a painful irritation has been produced.

I pass now to another and capital question, the solution of which will explain a great many mysterious pathological cases observed in man: How is it that sensibility is not lost and is only more or less diminished, although the spinal cord is deeply altered? This question seems to be solved by the following experiments: If we divide transversely the posterior columns in the upper part of the lumbar region in a mammal, we find that there is hyperæsthesia *everywhere* behind the section; if, then, we divide the posterior parts of the lateral columns and the posterior gray horns, we find that the hyperæsthesia increases also *everywhere* behind the section. If the section is carried farther, so that the whole posterior half be divided transversely, the posterior part of the gray matter, behind the central canal, being cut, the hyperæsthesia remains excessive *everywhere* behind the section. When another section is made, cutting a little more of the central gray matter, the hyperæsthesia disappears from *everywhere* at once, and a certain degree of anæsthesia appears also *everywhere* behind the section. At last, if the whole of the central gray matter be divided, with also a good part of the basis of the anterior horns, sensibility is very much diminished *everywhere* behind the division, and it disappears entirely *everywhere* at the same time when the section has left only the anterior parts of the anterior columns.[1] The general result of this experiment is,

[1] I must say that it is absolutely impossible to know, *while* we make a section of parts of the spinal cord, what is the precise depth of the injury; it is mere guesswork. But if we study well the phenomena, and then, after having killed the animal, if we put the spinal cord in alcohol, we render it hard, and we can ascertain exactly what is the extent of the incision. This is the means that I always

that any change that takes place in the state of sensibility—either an increase or a diminution—shows itself *everywhere*, at the same time, behind the section.

If we now examine what might be the disposition of the conductors of sensitive impressions, in the spinal cord, we find that either they might be scattered without any order at all, or they might have one or the other of these two kinds of arrangements: 1st. They might be disposed in such a manner that the anterior parts of the body, the middle parts and the posterior parts, would each have a peculiar place in the cord. 2d. They might be arranged so that each small portion of the conducting part of the cord would contain conducting elements from the anterior, the middle, and the posterior parts of the body. Now, if we take the results of the above experiments, we find that they agree with this last supposition, and not with the others. If there was no order in the disposition of the elements conducting sensitive impressions, in the spinal cord, we should not have found changes taking place exactly in the same measure in all the parts of the body behind the section—*i. e.*, in the skin, in the trunks of nerves, in muscles, and in the viscera of the abdomen. If the anterior parts of the body had their conductors of sensitive impressions crowded together, as well as the posterior and middle parts also, we should have found that certain sections produced anæsthesia in certain parts, and not in others, while on the contrary we find anæsthesia, when it first appears, beginning everywhere at the same time, and when it increases, and also when it becomes complete, we find that it is so everywhere. We must, therefore, admit that elements representing the various parts of the body exist in the various portions of the spinal cord from behind forwards in the conducting zone of this organ. This explains clearly why a complete loss of sensibility is so rare in diseases of the spinal cord.

What we have said of the various parts of the body considered from the posterior to the anterior surface, we can say also of the various parts of the body considered transversely. We have shown that the left side of the spinal cord is the conductor of sensitive impressions coming from the right side of the body, and *vice versâ*. Let us now examine what takes place in the right posterior limb

employ in my experiments, and it is also the means employed by the Committee appointed by the Société de Biologie, in 1855, for the investigation of my researches on the spinal cord.

when we divide the left side of the spinal cord. We find that, after a division of a part of the left lateral column, there is no diminution of sensibility anywhere in the right limb; if the section is deeper, and involves a part of the gray matter, with the whole of the left lateral column, sensibility is diminished *everywhere* in the right posterior limb; if the section is still deeper, so that there remains only a very slight part of the central gray matter, or of the anterior column on the left side, sensibility is then much more diminished everywhere in the right posterior limb, and, as in the preceding case, the same degree of diminution exists in all the parts of this limb. At last, when the whole of the left side of the cord has been divided, there is only in the right limb the false appearance of sensibility which has been explained in the preceding lecture. It results from these facts, that the various parts of this limb, the outside parts, the inside parts, and the middle parts, are not represented in the left side of the spinal cord by conductors of sensitive impressions disposed in distinct layers; because, had it been so, the diminution of sensibility, instead of being gradual everywhere, and appearing in all the parts at the same degree, would have taken place in one part more than in another, after some of the sections. It seems, therefore, that transversely, as well as in the direction from behind forwards, the spinal cord, in the various parts of the conducting zone, contains fibres or other elements, conductors of sensitive impressions coming from the various parts of the body, one lateral half of the cord, however, being the agent of transmission for the opposite lateral half of the body.

If, for instance, we imagine that there are a thousand conducting elements coming from a small part of the right side of the body, in the left half of the spinal cord, they are scattered in all the parts of the conducting zone of this half, so that to divide them all, a section must divide the whole of this zone. In other words, we can say, that *every small portion of the conducting zone in a lateral half of the spinal cord contains conductors of sensitive impressions coming from all the points of the body on the opposite side, which are behind the place of this small portion.* We can say, also, that *the sensitive impressions made on any point of a lateral half of the body are transmitted to the sensorium by conducting elements, distributed in all the parts of the lateral half of the spinal cord on the opposite side.*

This view, which explains the so frequent persistence of sensibility in cases of disease of the spinal cord, is entirely different from that of Stilling and others who admit that a part of gray matter in one half of the cord is sufficient for the transmission of sensitive impressions from both sides of the body.

We pass now to the transmission of the orders of the will to muscles through the spinal cord. It is by far very much more difficult to determine what are the parts of this organ employed in voluntary movements than to find out what are those through which the sensitive impressions are transmitted. I have long been in doubt in this respect, and even now, after having carefully watched a great many animals, on the spinal cord of which certain alterations had been made, and after having read a great many pathological cases, I still hesitate as regards various points. I will try in this lecture to show what seems to be positive, and I will also point out some of the questions that seem not to have yet been solved.

It is very well known that Sir Charles Bell did not give any proof of the idea that he seems to have entertained all his life, that the anterior columns of the spinal cord are the only channels by which the will exercises its power on muscles. Most of the physiologists who have experimented on this subject admit that a transversal section of the anterior columns is a cause of paralysis. Stilling alone does not admit the exactitude of this assertion. Various experiments which I will relate show how difficult it is to decide most of the questions on this subject.

If we divide transversely, in the dorsal region, the two posterior columns of the spinal cord in a mammal, we find that its voluntary movements seem not to be at all disturbed or diminished. If in another mammal we divide transversely the whole of the spinal cord, except the posterior columns, we do not find the least appearance of a voluntary movement in the muscles which receive their nerves from the parts of the spinal cord which are behind the section. So far, therefore, as the posterior columns alone are concerned, we arrive at a positive, and, I think, undeniable conclusion, which is, that *the posterior columns of the spinal cord are not directly employed in the conveyance of the orders of the will to muscles.*

If we compare this conclusion with this well-known fact, that there are several, I may even say many, pathological cases, showing that in man an alteration of the posterior columns has caused nothing but a loss or a diminution of voluntary and reflex movements, we find an appearance of contradiction which in reality, however, does not exist, as I will show in another lecture.

After having divided transversely the two posterior columns as in the preceding experiment, if we divide a part of the lateral columns and the posterior gray horns (see 1, Fig. 13), we find that there is an evident, although very slight diminution of voluntary movements. But now, if instead of dividing this part of the spinal cord, we divide the whole of this organ, except this part, we find that voluntary movements are completely lost. It seems, therefore, that there are some conductors for voluntary movements in either the posterior horns or the posterior part of the lateral columns, or in both; but it appears also that there is but a small number of such conductors in either of these parts.

If we divide transversely, in the dorsal region, the whole posterior half of the gray matter, and a part of the lateral columns, besides the posterior columns (see 2, Fig. 13), we find that the voluntary movements are much diminished in the abdominal limbs. If the division is carried farther, so that the whole of the central gray matter be divided (see 3, Fig. 13), the animal can hardly move its abdominal limbs; and if we add to this section that of the anterior horns of gray matter, the loss of voluntary movements seems to be complete.

These experiments seem to lead to the conclusion that the anterior columns of the spinal cord are not at all employed in voluntary movements; but now, on the other side, if we divide only the anterior columns in the dorsal region, we find voluntary movements almost entirely lost, in the abdominal limbs—a fact which seems to prove that the anterior columns are the principal channels for the orders of the will to muscles. Besides, if we compare the results of the two experiments represented in Fig. 13, at 3 and 4, we find in the case of a section of little more than the posterior half of the spinal cord, that voluntary movements are almost entirely lost; while, in the case of a section of less than the anterior half (see 4, Fig. 13), voluntary movements seem to be entirely lost. We do not see any other way of explaining these various results except in admitting, what seems to be proved by thousands of pathological cases and vivisections, that voluntary movements require very powerful excitations from the nervous system upon muscles, and that when one-half or one-third of the normal amount of excitation is missing, what remains is insufficient.

If we add to the preceding experiments that any injury to the central gray matter, and that a deep injury to the lateral columns, in the dorsal region, always produce a diminution of the voluntary movements, we are led, by all the facts we have mentioned, to the conclusion that, *in the dorsal region, the various parts of the spinal cord, except the posterior columns, seem to be employed in the conveyance of the orders of the will to muscles.*

Now, as regards the question, which of these parts of the spinal cord is the principal channel for the orders of the will? we cannot give a very positive opinion. We can, however, state that of these three parts—the lateral columns, the anterior columns, and the gray matter—each of the last two seems to have a greater share in this function than the first. Besides, the gray matter appears to have as great a share as the anterior columns, and in the gray matter the most important parts seem to be those in the anterior half of the cord.

In the upper part of the cervical region of the spinal cord, near the crossing of the anterior pyramids, the results of experiments on the various parts of the spinal cord are very different from those of the same experiments in the dorsal region. In that part of the cervical region it is the section of the lateral columns, and of the part of the gray matter placed between the anterior and the lateral columns, which produces the most decided effect on voluntary movements—viz., a complete paralysis. The section of the anterior columns alone, when it has been made without a notable injury of the neighboring parts, causes a diminution of voluntary movements, which is by far not so considerable as after a section of these columns in the dorsal region. The section of the posterior columns and of the posterior parts of the gray matter in the cervical region hardly causes a diminution in the energy of the voluntary movements. From these results we conclude that *in the upper part of the cervical region of the spinal cord, near the medulla oblongata, most of the conductors of the orders of the will to muscles are in the lateral columns and in the gray matter between these and the anterior columns.*

Is there any decussation of the voluntary motor conductors in the spinal cord? The celebrated experiments of Galen, which we have already mentioned, seem to answer positively that there is no such decussation. Haller (*Elem. Phys.*, vol. iv. p. 326) says: "Alterius demum lateris musculi resolvuntur, si dimidiam medullam spinalem dissecueris." It is probable that his assertion in this case was not grounded upon any experiment made by himself. He quotes as his authority Galen, who had said the reverse, and Oribase, who seems to have copied Galen. In the same volume of his great work (*loco cit.*, p. 334), Haller gives the very opposite assertion. He says: "Id latus corporis resolvitur in quo ea medulla vulnus passa est aut pressionem." In the experiment already quoted, which was made by Sir Astley Cooper on the cervical part of the spinal cord of a dog, the section of a lateral half of this organ produced a loss of voluntary movements in the corresponding side of the body. Most of the living experimenters agree upon this fact that such a section causes paralysis only on the side injured. I have ascertained, a great many times, that this is not entirely right. There is always, even in mammals, after a transversal section of the whole of a lateral half of the spinal cord, at least some appearance of voluntary movements in the side of the injury, and always also a diminution of voluntary movements in the opposite side; so that, in animals, there seems to be in the spinal cord a decussation of a few of the voluntary motor conductors. As there seems to be no such decussation in man, at least according to several pathological facts, we shall not insist on its existence in animals.

We have now to say a few words on a theory which was first proposed by Bellingeri,[1] and had the good fortune of being accepted by an eminent physiologist, Professor Valentin, of Bern.[2] According to these experiments, the motor nerve-fibres which go to the extensor muscles pass in the posterior columns, while those which go to the flexor muscles pass in the anterior columns. We have already said that a section of the posterior columns does not produce any kind of paralysis, so that they are not more for extension than for flexion. But the question remains whether the other posterior parts of the spinal cord are, or are not employed for one of these kinds of movements more than for the other. To solve this question, we divide, in the dorsal region, the posterior half of the spinal cord (see 2 and 3, Fig. 13) in a mammal, and nearly the whole of the anterior half of this organ in another (see 4, Fig. 13); and we find that all the muscles seem to be almost completely paralyzed in the abdominal limbs, the flexors as much as the extensors, in the two animals. If some pathological facts observed in man, and of which we will speak in another lecture, appear to be different from these facts, we will show that there was in them an irritation, and not a destruction or a section, of certain parts of the spinal cord or of its nerves.

As regards the place of passage of the voluntary motor conductors in the medulla oblongata, I will now say only a few words.

[1] De Medulla Spinali Nervisque ex ea Prodeuntibus, &c. Torino, 1823.

[2] De Functionibus Nervorum Cerebralium, &c. 1839.

The crossing of the anterior pyramids I shall try to prove by and by to be very nearly the only one for the conductors for voluntary movements. I will merely state now that if a section is made longitudinally just at the place of the decussation of the anterior pyramids, so as to divide entirely all the decussating elements, we find that, although the animal lives some time after the operation, it has no voluntary movement at all in any of its limbs, which are almost always the seat of convulsions. A section of the two anterior pyramids is followed by the same results, while a section of the olivary columns, which are chiefly the continuation of the anterior columns of the spinal cord, does not seem to produce a notable paralysis; so that the greatest difference exists between the spinal cord and the medulla oblongata, as to the place of passage of the voluntary motor conductors.

From the facts we have related, concerning voluntary movements, we think it may be concluded that the idea that there are two columns of the spinal cord (the anterior) alone employed in the production of these movements, must be completely abandoned. It is extremely probable that the voluntary motor conductors pass in the anterior pyramids, and, after having made their decussation, pass chiefly in the lateral columns of the spinal cord and in the gray matter near these columns, and, at last, that, after a short distance, a number of these conductors leave the lateral columns to pass into the gray matter and into the anterior columns.

As regards the practical deductions from the various facts we have related, concerning the channels of sensitive impressions, and of the orders of the will to muscles, they will be discussed in the future lectures.

LECTURE V.

CONCLUSIONS FROM THE FACTS MENTIONED IN THE PRECEDING LECTURES, AND PATHOLOGICAL CASES SHOWING THAT THE TRANSMISSION OF SENSITIVE IMPRESSIONS SEEMS NOT TO TAKE PLACE THROUGH THE POSTERIOR COLUMNS OF THE SPINAL CORD.

Conclusions from the results of the Lecturer's experiments concerning the transmission of sensitive impressions and of the orders of the will to muscles, in the cerebro-spinal axis.—Agreement between the three principal sources of our knowledge concerning the spinal cord considered as a conductor of sensitive impressions and voluntary movements: *i. e.*, anatomy, experimentation upon animals, and pathological cases observed in man.—Hyperæsthesia or conservation of sensibility after injury to the posterior columns.

Mr. President and Gentlemen: In the preceding lectures I have related a great many experiments which have given results, or which may lead to conclusions, some of which I have already mentioned, while there are others of which I have hardly spoken. It will be useful now to give, together, most of these conclusions or results, before I relate the pathological cases which seem to concur with my experiments in proving the exactitude of these facts or deductions. I will mention most of them without discussion, and say only a few words in the way of explanation about two or three of them.

1st. The laying bare of the spinal cord, and its free exposure to the action of the atmosphere, instead of being a cause of loss or diminution of sensibility, as has been said, seems to be followed by a marked increase of sensibility in the parts of the body which are behind the point where the cord is exposed.

2d. The laying bare of the spinal cord, even in mammals, is very rarely followed, even after a number of days, by any kind of accident (meningitis, myelitis, &c.) producing a diminution of sensibility.

3d. The posterior columns of the spinal cord are not, as has been imagined, a bundle of fibres, from the posterior roots of the spinal nerves, going up to the encephalon.

4th. The restiform bodies are not a collection of fibres, chiefly from the sensitive nerves of the various parts of the body, going up to the encephalon, and, therefore, the cerebellum is not the recipient, through the restiform bodies, of most of the sensitive fibres of the trunk and limbs.

5th. The hyperæsthesia which appears in all parts of the body, behind deep injuries to the posterior columns of the spinal cord, is always more marked than that which is due to the mere laying bare of this nervous centre.

6th. All parts of the encephalon which are situated in its posterior or superior side are like the posterior columns of the spinal cord, in this respect—that a marked degree of hyperæsthesia always follows a transverse section upon any of them.

(If a complete transverse section is made upon any part of the restiform bodies, sensibility becomes very much increased in every part of the trunk and limbs. Hyperæsthesia is also, but in a less degree, one of the results of a transversal incision in the cerebellum, in the processus cerebelli ad testes, and in the tubercula quadrigemina.)

7th. A section of either the anterior or the lateral columns is followed by a certain degree of hyperæsthesia.

8th. The hyperæsthesia is greater after a section of the posterior columns and the posterior horns of gray matter and the neighboring parts of the lateral columns and central gray matter, than after a section of any other part of the spinal cord.

9th. The power of transmission of a nervous excitation, for either sensation or movement, may exist in parts of the nervous system which are not excitable.

10th. The posterior columns of the spinal cord are much less sensitive than they are said to be, and it even seems that their apparent sensibility depends upon the fact, that when they are irritated, the posterior roots, which are very sensitive, are also more or less irritated.

11th. The restiform bodies seem to be deprived of sensibility to mechanical excitation.

12th. Of the fibres sent to the spinal cord by the posterior roots, some go transversely, which do not seem to be employed for the transmission of sensitive impressions. Others go upwards and others downwards, both of which are conductors of sensitive impressions. These two sets of conductors, the ascending and the descending, seem to go ultimately into the central gray matter of the cord or into the anterior columns, after having, for a short distance, passed through the posterior columns, and most likely also through the lateral columns and the posterior gray horns.

13th. The transmission of sensitive impressions to the encephalon takes place chiefly in the central gray matter of the spinal cord, and for a small part in the anterior columns.

14th. The decussation of the conductors of sensitive impressions, coming from the various parts of the trunk and limbs, does not take place in the upper part of the pons Varolii nor beneath the tubercula quadrigemina, nor in the medulla oblongata, as it has been imagined. It takes place in the spinal cord in the case of sensitive impressions conveyed by the posterior roots of the spinal nerves.

15th. The decussation of the conductors of sensitive impressions in the spinal cord takes place very near their place of entrance into this organ, some above and others below this place.

16th. The transmission of sensitive impressions through the spinal cord takes place in certain definite directions, and not, as several German physiologists have thought, in almost every direction.

17th. Every small portion of a transverse section of the conducting zone, in a lateral half of the spinal cord, contains conductors of sensitive impressions coming from all the points of the body, on the opposite side, which are behind the place of this small portion.

18th. The sensitive impressions made on any point of a lateral half of the body are transmitted to the sensorium by conducting elements, distributed in all the parts of the lateral half of the spinal cord on the opposite side.

(This conclusion and the preceding explain why the transmission of sensitive impressions is so rarely lost in pathological alterations of the spinal cord, and also why the degree of diminution of sensibility in those cases is nearly in the same degree in almost all the parts where it exists.)

19th. Most of the elements which are employed as conductors of the purely tactile impressions, seem to pass by the same parts of the spinal cord as those which transmit the impressions which produce pain.

20th. The posterior columns of the spinal cord are not directly employed in the conveyance of the orders of the will to muscles.

21st. The gray matter of the spinal cord seems to have an important share in the conveyance of the orders of the will to muscles.

22d. The lateral columns of the spinal cord have a notably greater share in the conveyance of the orders of the will to muscles in the upper parts of the cervical region than in the dorsal and lumbar regions.

23d. The anterior columns of the spinal cord everywhere except in the upper part of the cervical region have a great share in voluntary movements.

24th. The decussation of the conductors for voluntary movements in animals seems to take place chiefly, but not entirely, where the anterior pyramids cross each other.

When we compare the conclusions above mentioned with the results of recent microscopical researches on the structure of the spinal cord, we find that they agree very well as regards several of the main points. We shall not insist upon this subject here, but we must say a few words on the *descending* fibres which enter the cord with the posterior roots, and we must also speak of the decussation of the conductors of sensitive impressions.

As regards the descending fibres, the existence of which we had been led to admit nearly six years ago,[1] we will refer our hearers to the second of the important papers of Mr. J. Lockhart Clarke,[2] in which these fibres are described and represented (Plates XXIII. and XXIV.).

Vivisections show that there is but a slight decussation of the conductors for voluntary movements in the spinal cord in animals, while pathological cases seem to show that there is no decussation in man of these conductors in this organ at all. Anatomy, however, teaches that the anterior roots send a large part of their fibres transversely across the cord, so that many fibres of the anterior roots of the left side decussate with as many fibres of the anterior roots of the right side. The teachings of experimentation and of pathology are both opposed to our admitting that these decussating fibres are all voluntary motor conductors. It seems extremely probable that many of these fibres are employed for reflex movements.

How is it that there is not an evident decussation of many, if not all, the fibres of the posterior roots in the spinal cord? Vivisections, and, as we shall show, pathological cases establishing positively the necessity of admitting the existence of such a decussation, it seems certainly strange that we do not see a manifest and con-

[1] See Boston Med. and Surg. Journal, Nov. 1852.

[2] Transactions of the Royal Society, 1853. See also my Journal de Physiologie, No. I., Janvier, 1858, Plate I.

siderable decussation between the continuations of the fibres of the posterior roots in the spinal cord. It may be that some of the fibres which cross each other in front of the central canal of the cord are not, as now admitted, fibres of the anterior roots, but fibres of the posterior ones, which, after having passed obliquely from the posterior parts of the cord into the anterior, become transversal there, and pass horizontally into the other lateral half of the cord. But, whatever may be true in this respect, there are conductors connected by means of cells with the fibres of the posterior roots, and they pass from one lateral half of the cord into the other one. They have been seen and described, and represented more or less clearly, by most of the micrographers who have recently published papers and plates on the organization of the spinal cord. We will name only R. Wagner, Lenhossek, Schrœder Van der Kolk, Bidder and his pupils (Kupfer, Owsjannikow, Metzler) Stilling, and Gratiolet. According to the actual teachings of microscopical examinations of the spinal cord, many of the fibres of the posterior roots reach the cells of the gray matter on their own side, and these cells send fibrils to cells which are in the other half of the spinal cord, and these last cells send fibrils upwards towards the encephalon. This organization is assuredly sufficient to explain the crossed transmission of sensitive impressions.

Omitting the representation of the cells, we give a diagramatic view of a transversal section of the spinal cord. (See Fig. 14.) The fibres of the posterior roots are seen to pass through the gray matter into the posterior and the lateral columns. It is necessary to understand that most of them do so only after having been in communication with cells, or, rather, that we consider the fibrils emanating from cells as the continuations of the fibres of the posterior roots in connection with them.

Pathological cases, as I will now begin to show, bear out almost all the conclusions I have just related, and they are not in opposition to those few conclusions which they do not prove. Experiments on animals could not lead to certain conclusions which I shall be able to draw from some of the pathological cases I intend relating.

I shall first examine what are the effects of alterations or injuries to the posterior columns of the spinal cord. It is necessary, in the first place, when discussing the principal circumstances of these cases, to take notice of the extent of the injury. In the experiments I have mentioned, after a transversal section of the posterior columns there is hyperæsthesia in the parts of the body which are behind the section; the same thing exists in man, after either a section of the posterior columns, or pressure by a tumor, a piece of bone, &c. But there is much less hyperæsthesia when the posterior columns are altered in a great part of their length, even when the posterior roots and the gray matter remain normal, and this is explained by the fact that many conductors of sensitive impressions, which pass for a short distance in these columns, are injured, and, although the same causes of hyperæsthesia exist then, as after a simple section, this excess of sensibility does not show itself, on account of the diminution of sensibility due to the alteration of the posterior columns. There is, then, a kind of compensation between the causes of hyperæsthesia and those of anæsthesia, so that the degree of sensibility remains nearly normal.

In cases of alteration occupying a great length of the posterior columns, there is a notable diminution in the power of standing and of walking, and when the affection has lasted long, there may be a complete loss of these powers. The causes of this weakness are: 1st. That the posterior columns, as we shall show hereafter, are the principal channels for the excitations which produce reflex movements, so that when they are altered there is a great diminution of these movements, and as they are absolutely necessary for the actions of standing up or walking, it seems very plain that these actions become lessened when the posterior columns are altered. 2d. That after a time, when an alteration exists in these columns, the amount of power of action in the other parts of the spinal cord diminishes.

Besides these two causes of weakness of the lower limbs, there are others, when, with the posterior columns, the posterior roots of nerves and some parts of the gray matter and of the lateral columns are altered. This was the case in the pathological facts which Longet has collected to establish his view, that the posterior columns are the only channels of sensitive impressions in the spinal cord. We will show that the case he relates cannot give such a proof; and, still more, that in some respects there is a disagreement between the views he held and the facts he mentions.

CASE 1.—L—— was admitted in December, 1823, at Bicêtre, for an *extreme weakness* of the lower limbs, which could hardly bear the weight of the body. In 1825, his limbs, which were atrophied, when not prevented doing so, had automatic and irregular movements, which the patient could not control. Sensibility was absolutely lost everywhere except in the face. He did not feel the coldest objects.

Autopsy.—The whole encephalon without alteration. From the origin of the spinal cord to its termination, its posterior half, inclusive of the gray matter, as far as the central commissure, was converted into a yellow, transparent substance, shining like a solution of gum, and resembling gelatin or softened horn, without any appearance of organization. The rest of the cord was perhaps harder than the pons Varolii is normally, but it had no other alteration. The anterior roots were normal. *The posterior roots were of a yellow-grayish color; they shared the alteration of the corresponding part of the cord.* (Hutin, cited by Longet, *Traité d'Anat. et de Physiol. du Syst. Nerv.*, 1843, vol. i. p. 346.)

This fact is certainly in opposition to the views of Longet and of those who contend that the antero-lateral columns of the spinal cord are the only channels for the orders of the will. Before the appearance of choreic movements in this case, there was an extreme weakness in the lower limbs, and the antero-lateral columns were not altered, except that they were a little harder than in a perfectly normal condition. The loss of sensibility cannot account for this *weakness.* In cases of complete anæsthesia without paralysis of movements, as we shall show hereafter, there is no *weakness*, but a difficulty or a complete impossibility of guiding the voluntary movements, unless the patient looks at the limbs, in which case he can execute any movement. In the above case the lower limbs could hardly bear the weight of the body; it is not so with patients who have lost only sensibility.

As regards the value of the case for the question at issue in relation to the transmission of sensitive impressions, the posterior roots being altered, the case cannot prove anything concerning the posterior columns. Dr. R. B. Todd[1] has already, with great propriety, stated that in cases capable of proving anything in this respect the posterior columns must be altered, while the posterior roots and the antero-lateral columns are not. To this we will add that the gray matter also must not be altered.

CASE 2.—A woman, partially paralyzed of sensibility and motion, dies from a disease having no relation to the paralysis.

[1] Cyclopædia of Anatomy and Physiology, vol. iii. p. 721, P.

Several times I had endeavored to make her walk; but her inferior limbs gave way, and were entirely unable to support her.

Autopsy.—The two posterior columns are converted into a soft gray-pinkish pulp, rich in bloodvessels. The alteration diminished gradually from the lower to the upper regions of the spinal cord, and it stopped at about an inch from the nib of the calamus. In the lower part of the cord the alteration had begun to invade the lateral columns in the neighborhood of the posterior ones. *The posterior roots of nerves were very thin*, particularly in the lower part. The rest of the spinal cord was perfectly healthy. The whole encephalon was in the most perfect condition. (Cruveilhier, cited by Longet, *loco cit.*, vol. i. p. 347.)

In this case, also, we find the posterior roots altered, and, therefore, the diminution of sensibility cannot be attributed to the state of the posterior columns. As regards movements, we see here that the lower limbs were not able to bear the weight of the body, although the alteration had attacked only a very small part of the lateral columns besides the posterior.

CASE 3.—M——, for two years paralyzed. In the beginning, numbness in the lower limbs. Afterwards, a numbness and half-paralysis appeared in the upper limbs. To keep a needle between her fingers she must look at them. Motion is diminished; all the movements are executed, but they are weak, and cannot accomplish the functions for which they are designed. The lower limbs, which she can move when in bed, are not at all able to serve for the vertical position.

Autopsy.—Spinal cord small; a pseudo-membrane on the hind part of the cord; gray degeneration of the posterior columns of the cord; *atrophy of the posterior roots of nerves.* (Cruveilhier, cited by Longet, *loco cit.*, vol. i. p. 349.)

Here, again, the posterior roots were altered. There was also such a weakness that the patient could not stand, although it is stated that the antero-lateral columns were no otherwise altered than is implied in the statement that the spinal cord was small. There were here all the circumstances which, in such cases, usually cause the impossibility of standing on the lower limbs.

CASE 4.—Miss G——, admitted at the Salpêtrière, in 1825, died in 1835, having never been out of bed during these ten years. After several years, during which there was numbness and difficulty of walking, the patient was confined to bed. When observed last, she had disordered involuntary movements, which she could not control. When not prevented by the bed sheets, the lower limbs were agitated by the most violent and irregular movements. These convulsions were produced when the patient attempted to move voluntarily. The upper limbs were less attacked than the lower. The muscles of the face, of the larynx, and those employed in deglutition and respiration, shared also in the disorder. Sensibility was very obtuse; pinching and pricking were perceived, but very slightly. To hold a pin between her fingers she must look at them. She did not feel an eschar on the sacrum.

Autopsy.—Red softening of the occipital circonvolutions of the left side of the brain. Brain otherwise healthy, as also the cerebellum and medulla oblongata. The spinal cord was atrophied, and reduced to two-thirds of its ordinary volume. The posterior *median* columns were transformed into a gray-yellowish, indurated strap all along the spinal cord, and extending into the middle of the cerebellum. In the spinal cord, the alteration is confined only to the *median* posterior columns, while the antero-lateral columns were perfectly healthy. *The posterior roots of the spinal nerves were completely atrophied; they were transparent, filiform*, and quite different from the anterior roots, which had their normal appearance and volume. (Cruveilhier, cited by Longet, *loco cit.*, vol. i. p. 355.)

In this case, the posterior roots were altered with only a part of the posterior columns—the *median columns.* It is strange, to say the least, that such a case has been presented, as proving that the posterior columns are the only channels for sensitive impressions! We will point out the atrophy of the spinal cord as being a sufficient cause, with the choreic movements and the alteration of the posterior roots, to prevent walking and standing.

CASE 5.—A woman had, at first, a numbness which rendered her walking similar to that of a drunken man. She had frequent falls, and in one of them she broke her leg. Three months afterwards she was paraplegic. The fracture had not been painful. On admission, she had a complete loss of sensibility in all the parts of the body below the epigastric region; but she felt pain in the bones and in the joints of the lower limbs. Frequently she had cramps, which were painful and made her shriek. Pinching and pricking were not at all perceived. *In bed she executed all the movements of exten-*

sion and flexion of the lower limbs; but when put on her feet and held up by two persons, she was hardly able to make use of her limbs to support herself. Hardly could she move these limbs to go forward; they gave way, crossing each other. In the upper limbs sensibility was diminished, not lost; voluntary movements were nearly perfect.

Autopsy.—Brain perfectly healthy. The alteration of the spinal cord was exactly limited to the posterior columns, and consisted in the transformation of the posterior columns into a gray-yellowish transparent substance. It occupied the whole extent of these columns in the lumbar and dorsal regions; but it became narrower and occupied only the *median* columns in the cervical region. The antero-lateral columns and the gray matter were perfectly healthy. (Cruveilhier, cited by Longet, *loco cit.*, vol. i. p. 351.)

In this case there is no mention at all of the state of the posterior roots. The case, therefore, cannot be of use. It would be if it had been stated that the posterior roots were healthy. Perhaps it will be urged that, had they been found in an abnormal condition, Cruveilhier would have stated the fact, and that his not having spoken of these roots is a proof that they were in a normal condition. This is no proof at all, as Cruveilhier usually speaks of the healthy parts as well as of the altered ones, and in the case we are examining, he states that the brain and certain parts of the spinal marrow were healthy. At any rate we shall bring forward so many facts showing that the posterior columns are not the channels for sensitive impressions, that it will become evident that, in this case, the posterior roots of nerves must have been altered.

The five cases above related are all those which Longet has published in proof of his views. It is pretty evident, from the examination of the circumstances of these cases, that they do not give the least support to these views; and we may safely state, that the pathological facts mentioned by Longet are not more able than his experiments to prove his views. Still more, as regards voluntary movements, these facts are certainly in positive opposition to the view that the antero-lateral columns are the only channels through which the will acts upon muscles.

We pass now to the exposition of other facts, which positively establish that the transmission of painful and purely tactile impressions may take place through other parts of the spinal cord than the posterior columns.

CASE 6.—A young man was admitted into the Charité on the 10th of June, 1839, under the care of M. Bouillaud. He complained of pain in the left shoulder and in the neck. The next day he could not turn his head. There was no paralysis anywhere, either of motion or sensibility; but the left upper limb was weak. Heat normal. On the 19th, headache; pulse 52–56. No paralysis, but the legs were weak. On the 22d, intelligence diminished; senses affected. No trace of paralysis. On the 25th, symptoms of meningitis; death.

Autopsy.—The lower part of the cervical region of the spinal cord was much enlarged, and contained a cancerous tumor of the size of a large olive, around which the nervous substance was notably softer than elsewhere. The seat of the tumor was in the posterior part of the cord. The development of the tumor had taken place from the surface of the sheath of the cord. The tumor being taken away, the white substance of the spinal cord was found to be composed of two large bands, of a soft consistence, without notable injection. The rest of the spinal cord was healthy. The roots of nerves were normal. Slight inflammatory alterations in the encephalon. (Henroz and Bouillaud, in the *Journal des Connaissances Médicales*, 1844, vol. xi. p. 40.)

This is a decisive case, although the description of the condition of the spinal cord is not clear. It is quite certain that very little if any part of the posterior columns remained, and, nevertheless, sensibility was not diminished. Had the patient been observed sooner, and at a time when he had, for three weeks, what he called rheumatismal pains, it would very likely have been ascertained that he had hyperæsthesia. When he was admitted the tumor had grown, and had produced more or less alteration in the gray matter, so that hyperæsthesia had ceased. This case is excellent, as it shows that a destruction of the posterior columns in a small part of their length does not cause a paralysis of voluntary movements.

CASE 7.—P. N——, a soldier, received a bayonet wound between the twelfth dorsal and the first lumbar vertebræ, injuring the spinal cord. After several bleedings the first pains diminished; but, on the second day, and till his death, he had the most excruciating pains and violent cramps in all the parts below the wound. The skin of the lower parts of the trunk and the surface of the abdominal limbs was so sensitive that one did not dare touch him, and he had to keep himself on his knees and hands. He died on the seventh day, without having had any paralysis.

Autopsy.—The existence of a wound of the spinal cord was ascertained. There was an inflammation of the spinal cord and its membranes, and also of the brain. (Gama, *Traité des Plaies de Tête et de l'Encéphalite*, 1830, p. 318.)

There is no doubt that, in this case, the hyperæsthesia was, in a certain measure, the result of the meningitis; but as this inflammation existed all along the cranio-spinal cavity, while the excessive hyperæsthesia was limited to the lower limbs and lower part of the trunk, we must admit that there was another cause to it. Probably the inflammation of some of the nerves originating from the cord, in the neighborhood of the wound, contributed to the hyperæsthesia; but the principal cause, most likely, was the injury to the spinal cord itself. I have ascertained, upon animals, that a wound, on the posterior surface of this organ, is followed by a greater hyperæsthesia, in the lower limbs, when it is made in the middle of the enlargement which gives nerves to those limbs than when it is made higher. It is to be regretted that Gama did not state what was the extent of the injury to the spinal cord, but it is evident that the posterior columns were the principal, if not the only parts wounded.

CASE 8.—A man fractured his spine in the cervical region; he was at first paralyzed in the lower and upper limbs, and he lost sensibility, almost entirely, in the left limbs, and had only a diminution of this property in the right limbs. Gradually he recovered sensibility and voluntary movements, and, after three months, being completely cured, though weak when walking, he left the hospital. The same day he went on foot to a distance of nine miles from Paris, and, on his return, he fell, and became again paralyzed both in motion and sensibility. Nearly two weeks after he died.

Autopsy.—The fracture which had first caused a paralysis had produced a displacement of a part of the posterior arch of the fourth cervical vertebra, in consequence of which the posterior columns had been divided. (See Fig. 15.) There was in the centre of the cord, where the pressure had taken place, a fibro-cellular nucleus, chiefly formed by the pia mater. The anterior columns of the cord evidently existed, but the posterior seemed to be interrupted at the place of the fibro-cellular nucleus. The gray matter, from above and from below the injured part, extended to this nucleus. (Ollivier d'Angers, *Traité des Maladies de la Moëlle Epinière*, 3d edit., 1837, vol. i. p. 294.)

We give here (see Fig. 15) a reproduction of a figure, published by Ollivier, representing the extent of injury in this case. It seems evident, from the description and from the figure, although both are obscure, that the continuity of, at least, a part of the gray matter and that of the anterior columns was preserved; but the posterior columns entirely, and, probably, a part of the lateral columns and the gray horns, had been severed. However, sensibility and voluntary movements had returned, after a period of great diminution. This case is, undoubtedly, an excellent one to show that the posterior columns are not the channels for voluntary movements nor for sensitive impressions. We must remark, that this condition of the spinal cord had not been produced when the man fell down and became paralyzed a second time. He had then a fracture of the callus, which had united the broken parts of the first fracture, and paralysis was probably due to a pressure near the divided portion of the cord.

Case 9.—G——, aged fourteen, admitted into the *Charité*, under the care of M. Rayer. From his childhood, after having been very ill, the four limbs of this patient have been drawn convulsively, and kept in the position of those of a fœtus in the uterus. He seems to be completely paralyzed. Some muscles of the shoulders, however, appear to have voluntary movements, and the head, eyes, larynx, and tongue obey the orders of the will, as also most of the respiratory muscles. Energetic spontaneous or reflex convulsions take place in the four limbs. There is hyperæsthesia everywhere in the limbs and in the trunk. He shrieks every time he is touched. Lately convulsions have increased, delirium has appeared, and death has taken place eight hours after the state of exquisite sensibility has shown itself.

Autopsy.—There were various alterations belonging to a very old spinal meningitis, and an acute cerebral meningitis. Tubercles upon the left cerebral lobes. There is softening of the posterior columns of the spinal cord principally at the level of the sixth and seventh cervical vertebræ; the softening diminishes gradually from this point, and ceases at the level of the third or fourth dorsal vertebra, and at the medulla oblongata.

This case, which I witnessed at the Charité, in 1849, is a valuable one, as regards the question we examine, in this respect, that sensibility was not lost nor diminished, although the posterior columns were softened. As to the loss of movements and the morbid increase of sensibility, there were too many alterations sufficient to produce them for us to try to show what relation they had with the softening of the posterior columns. The following case is very much like the preceding, but it is, in some respects, more important.

CASE 10.—Mr. F. F—— had been in good health until 1837, when he had an attack resembling congestive fever. The next year he had a similar attack, with a more lasting delirium. His strength did not return, although his appetite became very good. His walk was peculiarly unsteady and tottering. Pulse slow; temperature of skin low. Gradually paralysis came on in both the upper and the lower extremities. Violent counter-irritation was employed, and he got better, but soon became worse again. In May, 1839, he began to complain of pain in the joints, and soon after the pains came on with paroxysms attended with spasmodic contractions of the limbs. Any forcible attempt to extend the limbs caused immediate spasmodic contraction, with excruciating pain. The upper and lower extremities became permanently contracted, the lower more than the upper, in which the spasms were attended with less pain. He could use his fingers to a certain extent, but had little power over the larger joints. The knees were drawn up towards the abdomen, the legs bent upon the thighs, so that the heel rested firmly upon the soft parts covering the tuber ischii. The surface of the body during the early stages of the contractions of the limbs was morbidly sensitive, so that the approach of a person caused him to cry out, lest he should be hurt. He remained in this state for several months, with little amendment, except a gradual diminution of pain. Hectic fever set in, and he died.

Autopsy.—Various alterations of the cranium, the dura mater, the arachnoid, &c. Hardly any morbid appearance in either the pia mater, the brain, or the cerebellum. Tuber annulare and medulla oblongata firmer than usual. From the foramen magnum to the first or second dorsal vertebræ all the membranes of the spinal marrow were firmly united. The spinal cord in the cervical region very soft; *on its back part semi-fluid.* The lower end of the spinal marrow firmer than usual. (McNaughton in *American Journal of the Medical Sciences*, July, 1842, pp. 57–63.)

We are very willing to admit that at least a good part of the morbid excess of sensibility in this case was due to the meningitis, but whatever be the exact truth in this respect, it remains certain that sensitive impressions were freely transmitted, and the autopsy showed that the back part of the spinal cord—*i. e.*, its posterior columns—was *semi-fluid.*

CASE 11.—A woman, for many months, complained of headache. Four or five months before admission into a hospital she felt weak, and had numbness in the four limbs, with vertigo, and diminution of sight. All the senses were somewhat impaired. No facial palsy. Very violent headache; paralysis not very marked; diminution of the general sensibility; the muscles of the neck in a tetanic spasm; respiration embarrassed, interrupted. She died five or six hours after admission.

Autopsy.—Encephaloid tumor, of the size of a small walnut, in the triangular space formed by the left processus cerebelli ad pontem, the pons Varolii, and the restiform body. The medulla oblongata was at least four or five lines larger than usual; between the medulla oblongata and the processus cerebelli ad pontem there was a notable quantity of softened and yellowish nervous matter, chiefly from the left restiform body, which was entirely destroyed. The fourth ventricle was considerably dilated by a yellowish serosity. (Cartier, in *Bulletins de la Société Anatom.*, 1840, pp. 85–87.)

This case is extremely important; here is a complete destruction of the assumed sole channel for the sensitive impressions on one side, and yet sensibility persists! It is true sensibility was diminished, but the diminution existed on both sides, and, therefore, could not depend upon the destruction of one of the posterior columns of the medulla oblongata, and there were alterations enough to produce this diminution (notable enlargement of the medulla oblongata, dilatation of the fourth ventricle, &c.).

CASE 12.—A woman, aged fifty-five, began in 1831 to feel great weakness, with extreme pain in her lower limbs, and, from time to time, spasms. The weakness increased gradually, and, after a few months, the patient was unable to stand on her feet, the lower limbs losing all voluntary movement, while their sensibility remained entire. In January, 1832, she recovered some power of motion, but after two months the paraplegia returned, and with it acute pain in the lower limbs and abdomen. In October, 1833, she was admitted into St. Louis; her lower limbs had lost all movement; they were atrophied; a slight "contracture" existed. These limbs retained all their sensibility; feelings of pricking and painful sensations seemed to originate in them. The bladder and rectum were paralyzed. Pain became so violent, that it prevented sleep. The "contracture" increased, and the heels came almost in contact with the thighs. It was impossible to extend the legs. No new symptom appeared, and death occurred on the 26th of October, 1833. During the last days, however, sensibility seemed to be slightly diminished (*émoussée*) in the paralyzed limbs.

Autopsy.—Brain and cerebellum healthy. At the level of the second dorsal vertebra, against the left and posterior part of the spinal cord, there was a tumor, two inches long, six lines wide, nearly oval, lying longitudinally between the two sheaths of the arachnoid. The part of the spinal cord upon which the tumor had pressed was reduced nearly to two-thirds of its normal volume. It seemed, with the part below it, to be softer than usual. (Hardy, in *Archives de Médecine*, &c., 1834, vol. v. pp. 229–233.)

The author of this important case observes, that sensibility was slightly diminished, only during the last hours of life, and that the conservation of this property is "the more remarkable as the tumor, situated behind the cord, compressed principally its posterior part, which, according to modern physiologists, is especially used for sensation."

It is to be regretted that the author has not described with more precision the alteration of the spinal cord; but as it is, however, this case shows that, although the posterior columns, and one of them particularly, were much altered, if not destroyed, the transmission of sensitive impressions continued to take place. Other parts of the spinal cord must also have been altered, and to this fact we attribute the loss of voluntary movements. We will try, by and by, to explain why any alteration of the spinal cord, and particularly that which is due to pressure, so often produces a paralysis of voluntary movement, and allows the transmission of sensitive impressions to continue. We will merely state now that this difference between voluntary movements and sensibility is very well known. In an important work of one of my most eminent hearers, I read, that "occasionally the loss of voluntary power over the muscles is a total loss of sensibility (in cases of caries of the spine); but more frequently, while the former function of the nerves is destroyed, the latter remains but little or not at all impaired."

(Sir B. C. Brodie, *Patholog. and Surg. Observ. on Diseases of the Joints*, p. 332.) A very able observer, Dr. W. W. Gull, has collected many facts establishing the truth of this statement. (*Gulstonian Lectures on the Nervous System.—Medical Times*, 1849.)

The following case is very important, and it has more value than most of those we have related, on account of the microscopical examination of the altered parts of the spinal cord.

CASE 13.—A woman, aged forty-seven, on admission at the Salpêtrière, on the 11th of July, 1855, gave the following account: Three years ago, after a violent emotion, she had a feeling of numbness and formication in the upper limbs, more in the left, and afterwards in the lower limbs. Gradually weakness came in all the left side, and, after eight months, the left arm could not hold anything unless she looked at it, while the right was only weakened; she also had violent pains in the spine and chest with a feeling of burning. The sensibility of the skin was then so great that she dreaded the presence of any one by her. Galvanism produced an amelioration in her condition, but a vicarious menstruation by the anus weakened her, and then she came under my observation. There was violent spontaneous pain and an extreme sensibility in all the left arm, and between it and the spine; touching these parts made her cry out. The degree of morbid sensibility was not so great in the right arm. Although so sensitive for painful impressions, these parts, and particularly the left arm, or at least the fingers, had lost the *tactile* sensibility. Hyperæsthesia was as great in the lower as in the upper limbs, and particularly on the left side; the feet, however, felt numb. The skin of the face was the seat of formication.

Movements of the left arm were easy, but, if she did not look at it, she would drop what might be between her fingers. The movements of the right arm were perfectly free. It was so with the lower limbs; they were moved easily in bed, but walking was possible only with the help of an assistant, as there were weakness and vacillation in the lower limbs. The pain went on increasing, and diarrhœa caused death.

Autopsy.—Brain and cerebellum, carefully examined, were found healthy. No alteration of the membranes of the cord. The posterior columns were altered in all their length, from about one inch above the cervico-brachial enlargement to the lower extremity of the organ. They were yellow, and infiltrated with serosity. On transversal sections it was ascertained that the whole thickness of the posterior columns was altered. A microscopical examination of these columns made by me (Dr. Luys) and by Dr. Charles Robin showed: 1st, a considerable amount of yellow, spherical, granular bodies, mixed with broken nerve-fibres, and a small number of longer nerve-fibres; 2d, an amorphous matter containing many granulations, amongst which several were fatty; 3d, the blood-vessels were in a state of fatty degeneration. The gray matter was normal, except that there was more fat than usual both in the cells and in the amorphous substance. The anterior and lateral columns, and also the anterior and posterior roots of the spinal nerves, were healthy. (Luys in *Comptes rendus de la Société de Biologie, pour* 1856, pp. 94–97.)

This case is important in many respects. In the first place, it shows that the posterior columns are not directly employed in voluntary movements, as we see that the movements existed when guided by sight (tactile sensations and reflex actions missing). In the second place, this case shows hyperæsthesia (for painful impressions), and therefore the transmission of painful excitations, continuing to exist, although the posterior columns were hardly able to have a share in this function. And lastly, this case would *seem* to show that the tactile impressions are transmitted to the sensorium by the posterior columns. In this respect the case is in opposition to several others that I have mentioned, and still more to a few that I have yet to relate. In the long and detailed account given by M. Luys there are some facts of which I have not spoken, which prove that there were some cerebral alterations which have not been detected at the autopsy. It may be that these alterations have caused the tactile anæsthesia. The facts I allude to were, a paralysis of the motor branch of the trigeminal and of the facial nerve on the two sides (more on the left), and a notable diminution of sight, with an acoustic hyperæsthesia.

I do not think, however, that an alteration of the posterior columns occupying such a length as in this case could exist without impairing the transmission of sensitive impressions; as my experiments, as well as anatomy, establish that a number of fibres of the posterior roots pass into the posterior columns. There may be a certain number of these fibres transmitting tactile impressions, and others transmitting painful impressions; and, therefore, an alteration of the whole of the posterior columns in the length of the dorso-lumbar enlargement, for instance, ought to diminish tactile and painful sensibility in the lower limbs. If we see that there is no appearance of diminution, this depends upon the fact that there is a cause of increased sensibility which gives more than what is lost.

In the justly celebrated cases of Mr. Stanley, of Dr. Webster, and of Dr. Budd, of which I will now give a short summary, it is very probable that *tactile* sensibility persisted as well as *painful* sensibility.

CASE 14.—J. C——, aged forty-four, admitted into St. Bartholomew's Hospital for paraplegia. The patient was lifted into a chair, and when thus sitting, he did succeed, by a great effort, in raising his legs from the ground; but afterwards the inability of motion became complete through each lower limb in its entire extent. There was no discoverable impairment of sensation in any part of the limbs; on *scratching, pricking and pinching the skin*, nowhere was any defect of feeling acknowledged by the patient. In the upper limbs there existed no defect either of motion or sensation.

Autopsy.—The spinal cord was the only seat of disease; membranes healthy. The posterior half, or columns of the cord, throughout the entire length, from the pons to the other end, was of a dark-brown color, extremely soft and tenacious. The anterior half exhibited its natural whiteness and firm consistence. The roots of the spinal nerves were unaltered; the brain was healthy. (Mr. Edward Stanley, in *Medico-Chirurgical Transactions*, 1840, vol. xxiii. pp. 80–83.)

This case is undoubtedly one of the principal that I have to mention against the view that the posterior columns are the only channels for the sensitive impressions. Many things are united here to give value to the case. In the first place, the name of the observer is a perfect guarantee of exactitude in the observation of symptoms, and the description of the condition of the nervous centres. In the second place, the color of the softening shows that it was not a recent one. In the third place, the patient seems to have had sensations of touch (scratching) as well as sensations of pain (pricking and pinching.) "Throughout the progress of the case," says Mr. Stanley, "the opinion had been freely expressed, that it was one of disease of the anterior half, or columns of the spinal cord." So that, were this not entirely unnecessary, we should have in this expectation another guarantee of correctness. But we must say that there are details which we should have liked to see mentioned, and that there are circumstances in this case which render it probable that certain alterations have escaped notice.

We are not told when the last examination was made as regards the state of sensibility. The loss of movement was so absolutely complete that there was certainly some other alteration, besides that of the posterior columns, producing it, and to which was due the difference between the upper and the lower limbs. However, one clear and positive fact remains; there was a notable alteration (and one of long standing) of the posterior columns, and sensibility was not lost. We shall find the same fact in the following case:—

CASE 15.—R. H——, a sailor; on admission at the Seamen's Hospital, his lower extremities were extended, and very rigid, with sensation unimpaired, except slight numbness of the thighs. Voluntary movements completely impossible in the lower limbs; reflex convulsive movements very powerful; slight convulsions (much more feeble than before) could be excited to the last; his intellect remained unimpaired, and sensation in the lower limbs, and elsewhere, unaffected.

Autopsy.—There was a curvature of the spine formed by prominence of the dorsal vertebræ, from the fourth to the ninth inclusive. The posterior columns of the cord, for the extent of about two inches in the portion corresponding to the curvature, were softened. The tissue was not diffluent, but became flaky and partially dissolved when a small and gentle current of water was poured on it. The anterior columns were scarcely, if at all, softened, and resisted considerable traction. The cord above and below the affected part was perfectly healthy, and so were the nerves, even those arising from the softened part. (Dr. W. Budd, *Medico-Chirurgical Transactions*, 1839, vol. xxii. pp. 162–165.)

The condition of the gray matter is not mentioned. However, this is an important case, showing that although the posterior columns were deeply altered, the transmission of sensitive impressions continued to take place. There was in this case complete loss of voluntary movements, for the explanation of which we refer to our remarks on the succeeding case; but we must say that there was here, for a long period, a cause of difficulty and even of impossibility of voluntary movement—I mean, the spasmodic state of the muscles. In two ways the spasms act to prevent the will from producing movements: whilst they exist, they oppose a direct resistance to the will; and after they have ceased to exist, the muscular irritability is for a time too much exhausted to allow voluntary contractions to occur.

We regret that we have not time to speak of various important circumstances of this and other cases observed by Dr. Budd or by Prof. Busk, which cases are recorded in the very interesting paper of Dr. Budd which we have quoted.

CASE 16.—W. H. G——, aged thirty-six. After various accidents and epileptic fits, he became unable to walk steadily without support. He became better, but soon had a relapse, and then was entirely deprived of the use of both legs and arms. Ultimately the muscles of the abdomen and chest were also affected. Notwithstanding the total loss of power over all the muscles situated below the neck, the *sense of touch* still continued as acute as ever throughout the entire frame; indeed, the cutaneous surface appeared occasionally to be even more sensitive to external impressions than in the patient's previous good health, since he could, for instance, feel most acutely the slightest change in the temperature of the surrounding atmosphere. His sense of feeling was so accurate that he could distinctly tell the particular part of his body to which the attendant's finger was applied. He had spasmodic twitchings of the legs attended with great suffering.

Autopsy—about eighteen hours after death. Slight and unimportant alterations of the brain and its membranes. The part of the spinal cord corresponding to the three or four lower cervical vertebræ appeared larger than usual, felt soft and pulpy, and, on being divided, its substance seemed to be in an almost diffluent state, infiltrated with serum, but of a normal color; in the anterior and posterior columns not much difference was observed at the first superficial examination of the cord; both divisions seemed considerably softened, infiltrated, and disorganized, particularly the posterior columns. Above and below the affected part, the medulla spinalis was healthy and quite natural in appearance. Dr. Todd made a microscopical examination: he found great destruction of the posterior columns, and did not find any loss of substance in the antero-lateral columns. He says that he was unable to detect any trace of gray matter. (Dr. J. Webster, in *Med.-Chir. Trans.*, 1843, vol. xxiv. pp. 1–18.)

This case differs from the preceding by the extent of the injury to the posterior columns, and here we find hyperæsthesia, as in cases of tumors upon these columns, or after their transversal section in animals. There was, however, a cause of diminution of sensibility here, otherwise the hyperæsthesia would have been much greater. If we were to take for granted, as it might be concluded from a few words of Dr. Todd, that the gray matter was destroyed, we should have to admit that the antero-lateral columns, even somewhat altered, are sufficient for such a notable degree of transmission of sensitive impressions as that which existed in this case. But I will remark that when this eminent biologist made his examination the gray matter had been divided, and then exposed for some time to the action of the atmosphere on a July day, and then the specimen had been put in spirits and kept some time longer, before it came into the hands of Dr. Todd. Although it is probable that the gray matter was more or less altered in this case, it seems certain, from what is shown by other pathological cases and by experiments, that it had not entirely lost its share in the transmission of sensitive impressions. A striking fact, well made out by Dr. Todd, is that the antero-lateral columns, although softened, had not lost their structure. The loss of movement in this case, in the lower limbs, did not depend in any way, upon the same cause, as in Cases 1, 2, 3, 4, 5, 14, &c., and the alterations in the posterior columns in the cervical region cannot have produced the loss of voluntary movement in the lower limbs, as will be shown in a moment by a case I will relate. The real cause of loss of movement probably, therefore, resided in alterations in the antero-lateral columns and in the gray matter. The question, How could these alterations have destroyed the power of action of the will on muscles without rendering impossible the transmission of sensitive impressions? we cannot answer, otherwise than by stating, as we have already done, that any cause acting on the whole circumference of the spinal cord or of a nerve produces very much more easily a diminution or a loss of motor transmission than of sensitive transmission, and that in a great measure this difference is due to the difference in the reagents at the extremities of the conductors: for one kind, the sensorium, so easily acted upon; for the other kind, muscles and bones, so difficult to move.

Case 17.—A soldier was paralyzed of voluntary movement in the upper limbs only. He had not lost sensibility anywhere.

Autopsy.—The posterior columns of the spinal cord were altered in structure between the fifth cervical and the third dorsal vertebræ. They were softened, and this alteration gradually diminished from the surface to the centre of the cord. The posterior roots also were altered. (Malle, in *Clinique Chirurgicale de l'Hôpital de Strasbourg.* 1838.)

This case is unfortunately without details, and, for instance, it is not stated when sensibility was ascertained to exist. But, at any rate, we find here an alteration of the posterior half of the spinal cord, with a loss of voluntary movements in the limbs alone that correspond with the part altered. The action of the will on the muscles of the lower limbs had continued to take place through a spinal cord altered enough to prevent voluntary movements in the upper limbs. As regards the posterior roots of the cervico-brachial nerves, which are said to have been in a state of *putrilage*, it is certain that they must have lost at least a part of their power of transmitting sensitive impressions; and this proves that the last examination of the patient, when sensibility was found existing in the upper limbs, must have been made a somewhat long time before death. But in this case, as well as in others, the loss of certain functions has more value than the conservation of others; and we find voluntary movements lost in the upper limbs, and nothing to explain this loss except the alteration of the posterior parts of the cord—an alteration which, for some time at least, had not destroyed sensibility.

Case 18.—A woman, aged forty, received a blow on her back. Six weeks after, she felt pain starting from the right foot. Gradually the pains extended to the various parts of the limb, and after a month they were accompanied with spasmodic contractions and a diminution of voluntary movements. She walked with great difficulty, even with the help of a stick. There was no alteration in sensibility nor in temperature in this limb. The convulsions extended to the other limbs and to the head, and the patient died.

Autopsy.—Brain normal; cerebellum a little softened; no meningitis; spinal cord healthy, except in the swelling for the lower limbs, which, for an extent of eighteen lines and a depth of one line in its posterior part, was softened, looking like cream somewhat rose-colored. (Genest, Clinique de Chomel, in *Gazette Médicale de Paris*, 1831, p. 34.)

We have no remark to present about this case, except that there was a considerable alteration of the posterior columns, and conservation of sensibility.

CASE 19.—A young girl died after having been paraplegic, and without having lost sensibility. The encephalon was in a normal condition, except that the *corpora geniculata* were of a gray color. The spinal cord in all its length had a gray-rose color column formed by the *median* posterior columns; the rest of this organ was healthy. (Cruveilhier, in *Anat. Pathol.*, 32d livraison, p. 21.)

It is quite certain that the loss of voluntary movement in this case cannot be attributed (at least only) to the alteration found in a small part of the cord; but we relate this fact (which Cruveilhier has published without any detail) because it shows that there may be an alteration of the little median posterior columns with preservation of sensibility.

We might relate a great many other cases showing that alterations of the posterior columns do not produce anæsthesia, and are often, on the contrary, attended with hyperæsthesia. For the sake of brevity, we will merely point out a few circumstances connected with some of these cases, and give the references of the others. In a paper by Dr. Ludwig Türck (*Beobachtungen über das Leitungsvermögen des Menschlichen Rückenmarkes*, 1855), there is a case of old alteration of a part of the right side of the spinal cord extending between the origins of the fourth and sixth cervical nerves. In certain sections the alteration occupied a part of the lateral column and a part of the posterior column (see Fig. 16, *al*); and, in another section (between the fifth and sixth cervical nerves), it occupied the whole of the right posterior column. The altered parts were indurated, of a reddish-gray color, and *did not contain a trace of nerve-fibre.* This alteration, therefore, had produced there just the same result as a transversal section of the posterior column and of a part of the lateral column on the right side. Numerous and careful examinations have shown that the hands and fingers had no anæsthesia. In this case the anterior parts of the spinal cord were also altered in the cervical region, so that the transmission of sensitive impressions must have taken place through the central gray matter. The last examination of the state of sensibility unfortunately was made long before death; but the alteration found is one that occurs very slowly. The same remarks might apply to another case observed by the same pathologist. The two internal segments of the posterior columns (see Fig. 17, *al*) were altered (and without any trace of nerve-fibre) between the fifth and sixth cervical nerves, and sensibility to touch in the parts animated by these nerves persisted.

Dr. R. B. Todd says, that in two cases which occurred in King's College Hospital, under his own care, the prominent symptom was impairment of the motor power, without injury to the sensitive; yet the seat of organic lesion in both was in the posterior columns of the cord. (*Cyclopædia of Anatomy and Physiol.*, vol. iii. p. 721, P.)

Serres speaks of a woman who had been paraplegic for two months, and had sensibility preserved in her lower limbs, although the posterior columns were alone altered, and in three places. (*Anat. Comparée du Cerveau*, vol. ii. p. 221.)

H. Nasse mentions a case, observed by Wittfeld, in which a tumor pressing upon the posterior columns in the lumbar region had produced a paralysis of movement, and not of sensibility. (*Untersuchungen zur Physiol. und Pathol.*, vol. i. p. 226.)

Sandras says, without any more detail, that he has seen two cases of alteration of the posterior columns, in one of which sensibility was lost, and, in the other, voluntary movements. (*Journal Général de Méd., &c.*, 1829, p. 360.)

M. Nichet relates a very important case, of which we shall have to speak elsewhere, in which sensibility had persisted, although the spinal cord had been reduced to a thickness of two lines near the medulla oblongata, the gray matter, almost alone, seeming to exist. (*Gaz. Méd. de Paris*, 1835, p. 534.)

We might cite many other cases by Hutin, Prus, Velpeau, Bellingeri, Liberali, Colin, Bourdon, Ollivier, Caron, Hersent, Fricault, Cruveilhier, Guyon, Goupil, J. W. Ogle, &c., in which sensibility has persisted, and, sometimes, has been much increased, although the posterior columns were the only, or principal seats of alteration.

I think that it is impossible, after such a mass of evidence, not to admit that if the posterior columns of the spinal cord convey sensitive impressions to the encephalon, their share in this function must be extremely slight.

In the next lecture, before speaking of the pathological facts which prove that the conductors of sensitive impressions decussate in the spinal cord, I will relate some facts concerning the transmission of these impressions through the gray matter, and discuss some important questions on the diagnostic value of anæsthesia and hyperæsthesia.

LECTURE VI.

SOLUTION, BY PATHOLOGICAL CASES, OF VARIOUS QUESTIONS RELATING TO THE TRANSMISSION OF SENSITIVE IMPRESSIONS THROUGH THE SPINAL CORD.

Value of the cases related in the preceding lecture, in opposition to the view that the posterior columns of the spinal cord are the only channels of sensitive impressions.—Cases opposed to the views that the cerebellum is either a channel of transmission of sensitive impressions, or a centre of perception of certain sensitive impressions.—Cases of alteration of the whole spinal cord, with conservation of sensibility.—Is an alteration of any part of the spinal cord able to produce anæsthesia alone?—General remarks on anæsthesia and hyperæsthesia.—Cases of alteration of the gray matter alone, with loss of sensibility and voluntary movements.—Cases which seem to be in opposition to the view that the gray matter is the principal channel of sensitive impressions.—Summing up of the evidence as regards the share of the gray matter in the transmission of sensitive impressions.

Mr. President and Gentlemen: In the preceding lecture I related a great many cases of alteration of the posterior columns of the spinal cord, in which sensibility was more or less completely preserved, and, sometimes, increased instead of being lost. It would be easy to add many other cases having the same meaning as those I have mentioned. But I think that it would be useless to do so, because what I wish to prove may be considered as more than sufficiently established by the facts already related. Besides, when I come to the subject of the transmission of the orders of the will to the muscles, I shall relate two or three of the most important facts concerning the posterior columns amongst those that I have not previously mentioned.

Several objections might be urged against the signification of the cases I have narrated, especially those in which there was a softening of the posterior columns. These last cases might be considered as valueless, for either one of the following reasons, or several of them at the same time—1st. That the softening may have been produced during the interval which has preceded the last examination of the patient and his death. 2d. That the softening, very slight before death, has become considerable after death, in consequence of a rapid putrefaction. 3d. That numerous cases of softening of the whole thickness of the spinal cord may be found in the bodies of individuals who have not presented any symptom of paralysis of either sensibility or motion; and that, therefore, if the softening had existed during life, and at the time the persistence of voluntary power and sensibility was ascertained, we must admit that the simple physical state of softening is not essentially capable of destroying the functions of the cord. Against the signification we give to cases of tumors pressing upon the posterior columns, it might be said—1st. That pressure may exist without destroying the structure of a number of the fibres of these columns. 2d. That a new organization of the cord may be produced, in cases of tumors slowly developed, and that this organization, of which we shall have to speak more at length hereafter, explains the persistence of sensibility.

These objections, and particularly those relating to softening, are of great importance, and they certainly may throw very well grounded doubts on the value of some of the cases I have related. But if we look at the details of most of them, we find that both the symptoms and the alterations may furnish evidences against these objections. In the first place, of the kinds of softening so well characterized by Professor Hughes Bennett (*Pathological and Histological Researches on Inflammation of Nervous Centres*, Edinburgh, 1843), the white, which alone can be a result of post-mortem decomposition, is not the one which has been seen in the cases which we have noted. In the second place, in none of those cases, except perhaps one, have the patients died from an acute and rapidly-mortal softening, neither have they had the symptoms of this affection, which has been so well described by Calmeil (in *Journal des Progrès des Sciences Médicales*, 1828, vol. xi. pp. 133–191). In the third place, most of these patients have had symptoms which really belong to alterations of the posterior columns, and not to diseases of other parts of the cord or the encephalon, as we shall show in another lecture. In the fourth place, a microscopical examination has been made in several of the cases (Cases 13, 16, and the two of Dr. L. Türck), and the posterior columns have been found in such a condition that the least part of their normal actions could scarcely persist.

As regards cases of pressure, the objections cannot be applied to most of them, especially to Cases 7, 8, 11, and to others which I have not time to relate, and which are recorded by Cruveilhier, Colin, Wittfeld, &c.

Certainly it seems quite evident, from the cases we have related, that the posterior columns are not, as they have been called, the *sensory tracts.* In other words, they are not, as has been generally admitted for about a quarter of a century, the reunion of the sensitive fibres of the posterior roots going up to the encephalon. Experiments upon animals and pathological cases agree in giving the most striking, the most decisive, proofs in this respect. But although decisive, according to my conception, these proofs perhaps might be considered as not having so great an importance, by those who, for so long a time, have held a contrary opinion. I will, therefore, give other arguments against this opinion.

It is positively and very well known that the restiform bodies, which are the continuations of the posterior columns, pass chiefly into the cerebellum. Now, if the restiform bodies contain, as is supposed, the whole of the conductors of sensitive impressions coming from the various parts of the trunk and limbs, most of these conductors must go into the cerebellum, and only a small number pass into the pons Varolii. (See Fig. 18, *f* and *f'*.) This is what "barred the progress" of Sir Charles Bell, and made him abandon the idea that the posterior columns of the spinal cord are the channels for sensitive impressions.[1] Other authors have not been arrested by this difficulty, and Longet[2] has imagined that the conductors of sensitive impressions pass through the cerebellum and go out of this organ in the processus cerebelli ad testes, under which they decussate. (See Fig. 18.) Foville[3] has admitted an opinion, which had been already held by Pourfour du Petit, Saucerotte, Sabouraut, &c., and which is, that the cerebellum is the centre for the perception of sensitive impressions. It would be easy to accumulate a great many facts against these views. We will merely mention a few, referring to Andral,[4] to Toulmouche,[5] and to W. Nasse,[6] for a number of others.

[1] The Nervous System of the Human Body, 3d edit., 1844, p. 239.

[2] Traité d'Anat. et de Physiol. du Syst. Nerveux, 1843, vol. i. pp. 420–21.

[3] Dictionn. de Méd. et de Chir. Pratiques, vol. ii.; art. "Encéphale," pp. 202–5.

[4] Clinique Médicale, 2d edit., vol. v. pp. 680, 700, and 708.

[5] Gaz. Méd. de Paris, 1845, p. 449.

[6] Comment. de Functionibus Sing. Partium ex Morborum perscrut. Indagatis, 1847, p. 52.

As regards the restiform bodies, we have already related a case (Lecture V., Case 9) of destruction of one of them, with conservation of sensibility, and we will merely mention now that there are several others on record, two of which (published by Velpeau and by Jobert) we shall give summarily in a subsequent lecture.

As regards the cerebellum, we find sensibility persisting in the celebrated case of *absence* of this organ, recorded by Combette.[1] There was also conservation of sensibility in two other cases in which the cerebellum had been *totally destroyed* by suppuration; at least it is stated that there was no paralysis and no other trouble in the functions of animal life. One of these cases having been considered as *impossible* by Bouillaud, who read a report about it, at the Académie de Médecine of Paris in 1834 (see *Gaz. Méd. de Paris*, 1834, p. 590), Marc, the learned physician of Louis Philippe, rose and said that it was possible, as he had seen an exactly similar case at the Charité.

I mention the above cases only because they offer instances of destruction of the whole of the cerebellum. Had I to give more proofs, I could relate a very large number of cases of alteration or destruction of either or both lateral lobes of the cerebellum or of its middle part, without loss of sensibility and, frequently, with hyperæsthesia, as after an injury to the posterior columns of the spinal cord.

Another and good method of proving that the cerebellum is neither a place of passage nor a centre for the perception of sensitive impressions, consists in showing that those writers who admit that this nervous centre has one or the other of these functions do not give facts in its favor, and, on the contrary, acknowledge that there are facts in opposition with it. Thus, Longet (*loco cit.*, pp. 748–54) adduces many cases to show that the cerebellum is not a centre of perception of sensitive impressions, and he does not perceive that these cases are as much opposed to his own view that the sensitive impressions pass through the cerebellum! Thus, again, Foville (*loco cit.*, p. 203) insists only upon one case to prove his view. It is a fact observed by Morgagni, in which a boy did not feel pain when his back was cupped, and felt pain when cupping was applied to his thigh. There was, in this case, two spoonfuls of blood effused; but where? Morgagni says: "At *sub* cerebello, cujus æquo mollior est visa substantia, in medio ferme, atrum concretum sanguinem

[1] Magendie's Journal de Physiol., vol. xi., 1831, pp. 27–45.

inveni ad duo circiter cochlearia."[1] It is unnecessary to show that a case of this kind cannot prove anything. Foville relates also a case of tubercle in the cerebellum, with hyperæsthesia, instead of anæsthesia (*loco cit.*, p. 202).

Of late, a much more rational view has been proposed concerning the relations of the cerebellum and sensibility. An eminent physiologist, Dr. Carpenter, at first suggested[2] that this organ is probably the special seat of the so-called muscular sense to which we owe the guidance of our movements. In the last edition of his *Human Physiology*, he explains that the cerebellum may only react, by reflex action, upon the impressions that reach it, without being itself the instrument of communicating such impressions to the consciousness. Recently Mr. R. Dunn, in an interesting work,[3] has adduced a case in proof of the view that the *corpora dentata* of the cerebellum are the seat of the muscular sense. In a child there was an imperfect paralysis of the right side, both of the arm and leg, but still they responded to the mandates of the will; she could move her arm about, and could grasp anything firmly enough in her right hand, when her eyes and attention were directed to it; but if they were diverted to something else, and the volitional power withdrawn, she would let the object that she had been holding fall from her hand, and *without being conscious of the fact.* At the autopsy, there was found in the lateral lobe of the cerebellum, on the left side, a mass of tubercular deposit a little to the outer side of the median line.

This case, certainly, seems to be a valuable one; but what can it prove, when we know that the movements have remained regular, and consequently well guided, in many cases in which tubercles or other morbid products, or various alterations, have existed at the same place where the deposit was found in Mr. Dunn's case? It is to explain the irregularity of movements in cases of injuries to the cerebellum that Foville and others after him have imagined that the guiding power of our movements has its seat in this organ; and of course if this irregularity exists only but very rarely, and still more if it often exists in cases of alteration of other parts of the encephalon, while the cerebellum remains normal, we must

[1] De Sedibus et Causis Morborum. Nona Ed. Curant. Chaussier et Adelon, vol. i. p. 187.

[2] Human Physiol., 5th Amer. edition, p. 735.

[3] An Essay on Physiological Psychology, 1858, p. 14, *note*.

reject this explanation. I have ascertained that it is by the irritation they produce on various parts of the basis of the encephalon that the diseases of the cerebellum, or its extirpation in animals, cause the disorder of movements which has been considered as depending upon the absence of a guiding power. In fact, the least irritation of several parts of the encephalon, with only the point of a needle, may generate very nearly the same disorder of movements that follows the extirpation of the cerebellum. I have thus been led to conclude that, after this extirpation, or after the destruction by disease of a large or small part of this nervous centre, it is not its *absence*, but some irritative influence upon *the parts of the encephalon that remain unaltered*, which causes the irregularity of movements. In birds I have found, long ago, that the mere exposure of the rhomboidal ventricle of the lumbar spinal cord is sufficient to produce in the posterior limbs the same trouble in the gait which exists after the extirpation of the cerebellum.[1]

I have seen a man in M. Rayer's wards at the Charité who had sensibility to touch, to pinching, to cold and heat, and also the peculiar feeling produced when muscles contract spasmodically under the influence of galvanism; and the autopsy showed that he had a tubercle the size of a small walnut in the cerebellum, near the median line, in the upper part of the right lobe. (See the particulars in this case, published by M. Tailhé, in the *Mémoires de la Soc. de Biologie*, 1849, pp. 147–52).

I regret not to be able to expose more thoroughly the facts and reasonings which are opposed to the views that some kinds of sensitive impressions reach the cerebellum or pass through it, but time urges me to go on, and I must now come to another question.

In a sceptical speech, delivered by Gerdy, at the Academy of Medicine of Paris, in 1839, he tried to show that there is no theory concerning the transmission of sensitive impressions in the spinal cord, which is not proved false by several pathological cases which he narrated. Besides these cases, there are several others in the most valuable work of Abercrombie,[2] and in a paper of F. Nasse[3] and elsewhere, most of them having the following characters: loss of voluntary movements; conservation of sensibility, with an

[1] See my work: Experimental Researches applied to Physiology and Pathology, 1853, p. 79.

[2] Pathological and Practical Researches on Diseases of the Brain, etc., fourth edition, 1845, pp. 338–53.

[3] Untersuchungen zur Physiol. und Pathol., vol. i. pp. 226–229.

apparent or real softening of the various parts of the spinal cord. We will briefly examine the principal features of these cases.

CASE 20.—A man fell from the second story of a house and broke his back. The next day, the two lower limbs were paralyzed, the left less than the right; sensibility seemed not to be lost. Twelve days after, sensibility, which had seemed to be limited to the calves of the legs (probably existing everywhere above, and not below), extended to the upper parts of the feet. On the twenty-third day, sensibility had extended to the extremities of the toes, but the paralysis was complete. Death ensued on the thirtieth day.

Autopsy.—Fracture of the twelfth dorsal vertebra, opposite which the spinal cord, which was healthy elsewhere, was softened and of a gray-yellowish color. (Ollivier, *Traité des Maladies de la Moëlle Epinière*, third edition, vol. i. p. 498.)

This case cannot prove much, because the last mentioned examination of the state of sensibility was made seven days before death, and also because the condition of the gray matter is not mentioned.

CASE 21.—A man broke his back, and was completely paralyzed of the lower limbs; until his death he had an obscure sensibility in all the paralyzed parts.

Autopsy.—The twelfth dorsal vertebra was displaced, and pressed upon the spinal cord, which was flattened and softened to the extent of an inch. (Ollivier, *loco cit.*, vol. i. p. 331.)

This case shows that a greater alteration of the spinal cord is necessary to destroy sensibility than to destroy motion, and that a softening does not necessarily prevent the passage of sensitive impressions.

Amongst the cases of softening of the spinal cord recorded by Abercrombie, there is one (Case 148) of a man who, from concussion of the spine, lost entirely the power of motion, without loss of feeling. About a month after, trismus and convulsions came on, and, some time after, death. There was most extensive ramollissement.

The cases of Abercrombie are interesting in showing that sensibility lasts much more than voluntary movements in cases of softening of the spinal cord, but they do not prove, as it has been assumed by some persons, that a softening is not a cause of loss of function of the spinal cord. In several of these cases (particularly Cases 143 and 146), there was loss of motion without loss of sensibility; the softening was much more marked in the anterior than the posterior columns. Unfortunately, nothing is said of the condition of the gray matter. Case 147 is that of a gentleman who, after a long illness, characterized by paralysis and various other symptoms, without loss of feeling, became comatose and died. The whole cord was of a pale-rose color, and in a state of complete ramollissement through its whole extent, being in every part entirely diffluent. I will remark that we do not know what was the real condition of the various parts of the spinal cord in this case, and that no conclusion, therefore, can be drawn from it.

The following extremely important case, carefully recorded by my learned friend Dr. Laboulbène, shows that what would have been considered, twenty years ago, or farther back, as a softening destroying the whole thickness of the spinal cord, may be only a destruction (and not a complete one) of the white substance of this organ.

CASE 22.—A man, aged forty-four, after having had cramps, formication, and weakness in the lower limbs, and paralysis of the upper limbs, for a long period, was admitted at *Charité*. Sensibility existed everywhere. On the evening of the 1st of November he was able to walk, but aided by some one. Sensibility continued everywhere to the last moment before his death, on the 3d of November, at three A. M.

Autopsy.—Encephalon normal. There was induration of the spinal cord from its upper extremity to the third dorsal vertebra, and from the sixth dorsal vertebra to the lower extremity. The tissue of the cord in these parts being cut, was shining, looking like porcelain, hard and difficult to be crushed. The gray matter was also a little harder than normally, but of its usual color. The anterior and posterior roots seemed normal. In the space between the third and sixth dorsal vertebræ the cord was softened, pultaceous, resembling a whitish, or rather slightly rose pulp (*bouillie*), punctated in some places. When placed in water, many parts became disintegrated, and formed a kind of emulsion. This alteration existed only in the white substance; the gray, on the contrary, seemed to have preserved its normal consistence. The microscope showed that the gray matter in both the softened and the indurated parts contained normal cells and fibres, and normal bloodvessels, while the white substance in the softened region contained but rare fibres, which were altered, containing an oily matter and granulations.

There was also a quantity of granulated corpuscles of inflammation, with many capillaries, oily drops, and amorphous matter. In the indurated white substance there was less alteration, and the fibres were more normal and numerous. (Laboulbène, in *Mémoires de la Société de Biologie, pour* 1855, pp. 233–45.)

The author of the report of this case adds, that he has ascertained that sensibility to pinching, pricking, touching, and tickling, and the feeling of cold, and that given by a muscular spasm due to galvanism, persisted in this patient, although the white matter, *i. e.*, the posterior and the antero-lateral columns had but few, and only altered fibres. A capital point in this case was the conservation of the gray matter with the persistence of sensibility.

In the following very important case, we find quite different features from those of the preceding:—

CASE 23.—A man became gradually paralytic. On his admission into St. Antoine, he was completely paralytic; sensibility (to pricking) at first lost, but after a time it returned everywhere. Tickling the soles of the feet is not felt, but induces reflex movements. Touching was not felt from the feet up to the middle of the thighs.

Autopsy.—Tubercular matter at the level of the fourth dorsal vertebra pressing upon the spinal cord, which is flattened, very thin, and diffluent, resembling cream, and perfectly white. This part of the spinal cord was washed away by a stream of water. Below this part the spinal cord is softened in an extent of eleven centimetres (three inches and a half); above this, the softening extends about four centimetres (an inch and a third); it is more marked in the posterior columns. M. Broca made a microscopical examination. He states that the gray matter, though very soft, seemed not to differ at all, as regards its structure, from its normal condition; and the same thing may be said of the white matter, except that the tubes, instead of being straight, presented flexuosities. (Guyon, in *Comptes Rendus de la Société de Biologie, pour* 1856, pp. 191–93.)

We must remark, that this was a case of white, and not inflammatory softening, as the preceding, and that the autopsy was made only thirty-five hours after death, in August, that is, in warm weather. The interest of the case lies in the fact, that although flattened and much reduced in size, the spinal cord was able to transmit *painful* impressions, while it was incapable of transmit-ing mere *tactile* impressions, at least from a part of the paralyzed limbs.

In the following case we find almost the reverse:—

CASE 24.—A young man had symptoms of myelitis. He became completely paraplegic, and he lost the faculty of feeling the contact of a foreign body, unless there was pressure, in which case he could, usually, say what place was touched. He did not feel when pinched or pricked, or when a very violent galvanic current was applied to the skin; *but the cold of a metallic vase, and also the least tickling were felt.* Spasms induced in muscles were not felt. During the last days of life tickling was no longer felt.

Autopsy.—A mass of tubercular substance had partly destroyed the right and posterior arch of the fourth and fifth dorsal vertebræ, and entered the spinal canal in which it pressed upon the posterior surface of the cord. This organ was flattened to the extent of about an inch, and there it seemed diffluent, and of a yellowish color. M. Verneuil made a microscopical examination of this softened part, and he found that there were but very few fibres, and they were so much altered that it was difficult to ascertain their presence. There were many inflammatory granular corpuscles.

This case was reported to the Société de Biologie in 1855, and it has not yet been published. I have now, all its history, written by M. Fournier, who has carefully studied the interesting features that it presents. It shows that certain kinds of impressions may still be transmitted to the sensorium, while others cannot be, through a very much altered spinal cord.

I shall not pursue farther the study of the softening of the entire thickness of the spinal cord. My object in speaking of the above facts will, I hope, be attained: it was to show—1st. That in cases where the cord is found extremely soft, the normal structure may be preserved (see Case 23). 2d. That when the whole thickness of the cord seems diffluent, the gray matter may be normal, the white substance having lost its structure, and that, therefore, the persistence of sensibility may be explained. 3d. That it would be wrong to say that sensibility does not persist if examinations have not been made to detect the various kinds of sensibility.

Although I intend to treat of the subjects of anæsthesia and hyperæsthesia in a future lecture, I will say a few words now of some peculiarities attached to these two symptoms. In the first place I will rapidly examine whether anæsthesia *alone* may be produced by alteration of some part of the spinal cord. I consider that such an effect is absolutely impossible, and just as much as it would be for an alteration of any part of a *compound* nerve (that is a nerve containing fibres for movement and for sensation mixed together) to cause anæsthesia alone. The cases of anæsthesia which have been admitted as depending upon alterations of the spinal cord—as is frequently the case in hysteria, and sometimes after a concussion of the spine—I will prove (or, at least, give arguments seeming to prove) to depend upon alterations of nutrition in the sensitive nerves of the skin and other parts, or of alterations from various causes (tearing in cases of concussion, &c.) in the posterior roots of nerves, or, at last, of encephalic diseases. There is only one case that I can conceive in which sensibility might be lost and movements preserved in a certain affection, or a peculiar injury of the spinal cord; but I hasten to say, that even in these cases, this organ, though divided longitudinally, must remain unaltered; I mean cases of spina bifida, and cases of longitudinal wounds on the median line.

Hyperæsthesia, contrary to anæsthesia, may exist alone, and this is the case when there is an alteration very little extended in the posterior columns of the spinal cord, or in the cerebellum, which we may consider as the representative of these columns for the pons Varolii. Most frequently, however, hyperæsthesia coexists with a loss of movements. I must remark that we must not confound the painful sensations that have existed in the cases of alteration of the posterior columns, which I have related in the preceding lecture, with pains sometimes extremely violent, which are due to the irritation of both or either the posterior roots of nerves or the spinal cord, in cases of a tumor pressing upon them, or of meningitis or myelitis. In patients who are completely deprived of sensibility, there may be the most violent pains, which are referred, or not, to the parts which are anæsthetic. The following case, which I owe to the kindness of Dr. Arthur Farre, is a good illustration of this kind of affection.

Case 25.—C. K——, aged thirty-six. After having suffered from pain in his back, he gradually lost the power of motion and the sensibility of his lower extremities. A constant pain in his back prevents him from sleeping. On one occasion, the patient shrieked with agony when he was turned upon the side for the purpose of examining the back. The loss of sensibility and of motion was complete in all parts below the pelvis.

Autopsy.—Outside of the spine there was a large tuberculous deposit. The vertebral canal being laid open, an oblong, yellowish mass was found on the posterior part of the sheath of the cord, extending over the third, fourth, and fifth dorsal vertebræ. The spinal marrow was much reduced in size for a length of three inches, in consequence of the pressure. (See Fig. 19, *a.*)

I have tried to prove, by a great many pathological cases, that the posterior columns are not the only channels for the transmission of sensitive impressions; I will now try to prove that the principal channel for these impressions is the gray matter.

Already I have related a case of the utmost importance for this demonstration; it is the case, so carefully recorded by M. Laboulbène, in which sensibility (every kind of sensibility) has been preserved, although the gray matter alone remained to establish the communication between the sensorium and many parts of the body. (See above, Case 22.)

I might relate several other cases more or less similar to this case of M. Laboulbène, but I hope the following will be found sufficient.

CASE 26.—A man, aged sixty-nine, after having felt some pain in the lumbar region and in his feet, suddenly lost the faculty of speech; left side of the face paralyzed; left upper limb moved with difficulty; the other limbs free; sensibility in the face and limbs unaltered. A few days after, breathing and deglutition difficult; two days after, the left arm had still a part of its voluntary movements; its sensibility persists. He passed into a state of coma, without any increase in the symptoms of paralysis.

Autopsy.—Several small holes, filled with a kind of coagulated albumen, in the encephalon, which is otherwise healthy. From about five centimetres (nearly two inches) below the line of separation between the pons Varolii and the medulla oblongata, there is a white softening, which descends forty-eight millimetres (nearly two inches) lower, and occupied the posterior, lateral, and anterior columns of the cord. A current of water broke the white matter into flaps, and more so its posterior than its anterior part. The gray matter is hardly altered. (Prus, in *Revue Médicale* vol. iv. 1840, p. 381.)

In another case, recorded by the same physician (*loco cit.*, p. 391), there was paraplegia and conservation of sensibility, and the autopsy showed a softening of the *circumference* of the spinal cord.

Many other cases, of which I shall have to speak when I treat of the functions of the medulla oblongata, have the same bearing as the preceding. They show that pressure all round this nervous centre, having destroyed much of it, but having left a good deal of its gray matter uninjured, has allowed the transmission of sensitive impressions to take place. I will then relate cases by Mr. Lawrence, Mr. E. Stanley, Dr. J. W. Ogle, and others.

In the cases I have just been speaking of, there was conservation of the central gray matter and alteration of the parts near the circumference of the cord; I will now say a few words on cases of alteration of the central gray matter, the rest of the spinal marrow remaining normal.

In cases of alteration of the central gray matter, sensibility, according to the extent of the disease, is diminished or lost. The following important case of this kind is reported by Mr. Curling:—

CASE 27.—A gentleman suddenly lost all sensation and power of motion in the lower half of the body. Twenty-four hours afterwards there was a feeling of numbness in the hands and imperfect power of using them. No reflex movements.

Autopsy.—Two small clots of blood, amounting together to about a drachm, were found in the interior of the medulla, occupying about an inch and a half in extent, and situated between the origins of the second and third pairs of dorsal nerves. The substance of the cord around the clots was somewhat soft; the medulla was more or less infiltrated and stained with blood from the site of the clots upwards as high as the third cervical vertebra, and downwards as low as the last dorsal. (*Report of the Pathol. Soc.* 1849, p. 28, cited by Messrs. Handfield Jones and Sieveking in their *Manual of Pathol. Anat.*, 1854, chap. xiii., American edition, p. 275.)

It is useless to insist on the value of this case. If we had time, I would relate also a case of hemorrhage in the centre of the cord, which, though more complicated than the preceding, leads to the same conclusion. (See Cruveilhier's work, *Anat. Pathol.*, 3d part, and Plate VI.) In another case of effusion of blood in the cord, the softening due to the pressure of the blood was central, and the anterior and posterior parts of the cord were not affected, and there was a loss of sensibility and movement. (Grisolle, in the *Journal Hebdom. des Progrès des Sci. Méd.*, 1836, p. 71.) In a case reported by Ollivier, there was a tubercle, olive-shaped, and ten lines long and from six to eight lines broad, in the middle of the spinal cord, at the level of the twelfth dorsal vertebra. Around this tubercle and elsewhere, the spinal marrow and its nerves were healthy. Sensibility was completely lost and movement almost entirely impossible in the lower limbs. (*Traité des Maladies de la Moëlle Epinière*, vol. ii. p. 522.)

There are some pathological cases which seem to be in opposition to the opinion that we held concerning the share of the gray matter in the transmission of sensitive impressions. We will try to show that in reality they have not a great value in this respect.

The following case, recorded by Maisonneuve, might particularly be advanced as a proof that the gray matter is not a channel of transmission of the sensitive impressions:—

CASE 28.—A woman, aged thirty, had been in good health till 1829. She then became suddenly exceedingly weak both in the upper and the lower limbs. Three weeks after the paralysis was completed. In 1831 she gradually lost the power of feeling in the upper limbs. Respiration, circulation, and digestion, with also the excretion of urine and feces, remained normal. In February, 1833, respiration became painful, symptoms of pneumonia appeared, and the patient died.

Autopsy.—Brain, cerebellum, pons Varolii, and medulla oblongata healthy. The spinal cord, in the dorsal region, is flattened from behind forwards; when rolled between the fingers it is found to have a central cavity. In blowing into this cavity, it is found to be nearly eight inches (nine English inches) long, and three lines in diameter. This canal seems to be formed in the place of the gray matter which is missing; numerous thin filaments are found in the canal, the walls of which are one line thick, and very firm and dense; below this canal the spinal cord is softened, pulpy, but the lumbar enlargement is almost normal. (Maisonneuve, in *Revue Médicale*, Juillet, 1833.)

The place occupied by the canal is not stated with precision; but the symptoms and also two or three sentences of the author, which we have not reproduced, point out that its beginning was pretty near the decussation of the anterior pyramids—*i. e.*, in the upper cervical region. The inferior limit was in the dorsal region, two inches above the lumbar enlargement, so that the canal, eight or nine inches long, occupied more than the whole length of the cervico-brachial enlargement. Now, if we try to explain the symptoms, we find that the upper limbs had lost their sensibility, which is certainly a fact in opposition to the view that the posterior white columns are the only channels of sensitive impressions, as these columns were still existing, and nearly normal. On the other hand it is stated that the lower limbs had preserved their sensibility, but it is not said how many days or weeks before death this has been ascertained, neither what its degree was, nor what *kinds* of sensibility remained. However, let us accept as a fact that the various kinds of sensibility at a notable degree persisted till the last hours of the life of this patient. By what channels were the sensitive impressions then transmitted? The author states that the walls of the canal were one line thick, so that we are entitled to conclude that some parts of the gray matter still existed in and along the posterior and anterior horns, and also lining the anterior surface of the posterior columns. Besides, my experiments (see Lecture II.) show that the anterior columns have a share in the transmission of sensitive impressions.

Experiments made by Magendie, by Sarlandière, and others, show that the passage of a stylet in the central part of the cord does not affect in a marked manner the sensibility and the movements of a dog. It is well known that the centre of this organ is occupied by a canal, lined with an epithelial membrane, around which is a good deal of areolar tissue (the *ependyma* of some anatomists). If now we admit an effusion of blood taking place slowly in this canal, voluntary movements will be affected more or less, because any pressure on the cord from inside or from outside affects them, while sensibility will remain. But if the effusion is much increased, there is a considerable pressure and, besides, a tearing of the parts of the gray matter round the ependyma—and, consequently, the loss of voluntary movements becomes complete, or nearly so, and sensibility diminishes or is destroyed in the parts receiving their nerves from the altered region of the cord. If the conductors of sensitive impressions decussate near the centre of the cord, as I will prove hereafter, those belonging to these parts are then torn away, and sensibility is consequently lost in these parts while it may persist in parts receiving their nerves from healthy regions of the cord, below the seat of the alteration, because the conductors of sensitive impressions after having decussated, in these healthy regions, pass in the altered region of the cord *further* from its centre than the conductors decussating in this altered part. This explanation of the above case receives value also from the results of one of our experiments, consisting in a section of the decussating conductors of sensitive impressions in the region of the cervico-brachial enlargement, after which, sensibility is lost in the upper limbs and not in the lower ones. (See Lecture III., and Fig. 11.) In the above case, therefore, I think that the loss of movement was due chiefly to the pressure, and the local loss of sensibility to the tearing of the crossing of the conductors of the sensitive impressions upon the upper limbs. Viewed in this light, this case is quite favorable to our views, instead of being opposed to some of them.

Wishing to find what is true, and not to try to establish a systematic view, which, if false, would sooner or later be put down, I have been hunting much more for cases that seem to be in opposition to the theories I propose, than for those which seem to support them. But, however extensive have been my researches in this respect, I have hardly found two or three cases that *seem* to show that the destruction of the gray matter of the spinal cord may allow sensibility to persist. In a paper of Prus, close by an interesting case in which sensibility persisted till the last hours, the white substance of the spinal cord being alone altered, there is another case in which there was paralysis of movement alone, and it was found that there were two places where the spinal cord was softened, in both of which the gray matter is said to have been *invisible*. (Prus, in *Revue Médicale*, 1840, vol. iv. p. 395.)

I will merely remark that the mere assertion that the gray matter was invisible, cannot be considered as a proof that this substance was missing, as a change of color may have rendered it invisible. Admitting, however, that its quantity had diminished, there is nothing, in the short details of the autopsy, showing that there was a total absence of this substance.

I shall not relate here cases in which not only the gray matter, but the rest of the spinal cord was destroyed, and in which, nevertheless, according to some writers, there was a conservation of voluntary movements and sensibility. I shall not try to explain how these functions and properties subsisted, as I think my hearers are too enlightened to content themselves with explanations like those of Magendie,[1] who admitted that nervous transmissions

[1] Journal de Physiol. Expér., vol. iii., 1823, pp. 187, 189.

took place through the membranes of the spinal cord, or of M. Hutin,[1] who imagined that the transmissions continued through the serous fluid which had replaced the spinal cord! Before trying an explanation, it would have been prudent in these cases, as in the celebrated case of the *gold tooth* in the last century, to ascertain that the pretended facts were positive. We are perfectly sure that no one knowing the effects of a transversal section of the spinal cord, will have any doubt about these cases: it is quite evident that the greatest part of the alteration found in this organ has taken place after the last examination of the patient.

If we sum up the evidence that the gray matter of the spinal cord is the principal channel of transmission of the sensitive impressions, we find—

1st. That there are many cases of alteration only, or almost only, limited to the gray matter, and in which both voluntary movements and sensibility have been lost. To the cases of this kind that we have already mentioned (see cases recorded by Mr. Curling, Cruveilhier, Grisolle, and Ollivier, in this lecture). We will add the following indications of similar cases which are eleven in number; one by Jeffreys, quoted by Ollivier,[2] one by Sir Everard Home,[3] one by Calmeil,[4] one by Portal,[5] and a most remarkable one by Ollivier,[6] which we shall have to relate by and by, for another and interesting feature that it has presented.

2d. That there are many cases of deep alteration of all the white substance of the spinal cord, the gray matter remaining normal, in which sensibility has persisted. In addition to the cases by M. Laboulbène, by Prus (Cases 22 and 26), and to others that I have related, and to several that I shall have to relate, I will merely mention one, recorded by Dr. J. Bostock, in which the whole circumference of the spinal cord had been pressed upon, so as to present a kind of circular gutter, and in which sensibility had been preserved.

From the cases I have adduced to prove my views concerning the transmission of sensitive impressions in the spinal cord, it may

[1] Nouv. Biblioth. Médicale, 1828, vol. i. p. 159, Obs. 13.

[2] Loco cit , vol. i. p. 333.

[3] Philosophical Transactions, 1814.

[4] De la Paralysie, Obs. xlix.

[5] Anatomie Médicale, vol. iv. pp. 117, 118. A canal, the size of a quill, was found in the spinal cord.

[6] Loco cit., vol. ii. p. 388.

certainly be concluded—1st. That the posterior columns of the spinal cord are not the principal channels for this transmission, and that they even seem not to convey any part of the sensitive impressions to the encephalon. 2d. That the gray matter of the spinal cord seems to be the principal channel of transmission of the sensitive impressions to the encephalon. These two principal conclusions are borne out also by the experiments related in my second and third lectures.

LECTURE VII.

PATHOLOGICAL CASES SHOWING THAT THE CONDUCTORS OF SENSITIVE IMPRESSIONS FROM THE TRUNK AND LIMBS DECUSSATE IN THE SPINAL CORD AND NOT IN THE ENCEPHALON, AND THAT THE CONDUCTORS OF THE ORDERS OF THE WILL TO MUSCLES DECUSSATE IN THE LOWER PART OF THE MEDULLA OBLONGATA AND NOT IN THE PONS VAROLII.

The decussation of the conductors of sensitive impressions, from the trunk and limbs, does not take place in the crura cerebri, neither in the pons Varolii, nor in the medulla oblongata.—Cases proving that this decussation takes place in the spinal cord.—Cases of loss of voluntary movements in one side of the body, and of loss of sensibility in the opposite side.—The decussation of the conductors, for voluntary movements does not take place, as has been imagined, all along the basis of the encephalon.—This decussation seems to take place almost entirely in the lower part of the medulla oblongata.—Symptoms of alteration in a lateral half of the spinal cord, the lower part of the medulla oblongata, and the rest of the encephalon, as regards voluntary movements and sensibility.

Mr. President and Gentlemen: We now come to the questions relating to the place of decussation of the conductors of sensitive impressions in the cerebro-spinal axis. In one of the preceding lectures, I have related the experiments by which we have been led to the idea that this decussation takes place in the spinal cord, for most, if not all, the conductors of sensitive impressions arising from the various parts of the trunk and limbs. (See Lecture III.) I will now try to show that the same view seems to be proved by pathological facts observed in man.

Anatomy teaches that there is a decussation of nerve-fibres all along the spinal cord, the medulla oblongata, the pons Varolii, and the crura cerebri. Let us see what would take place in cases of disease in a lateral half of one of these nervous centres, if the decussation of the conductors of sensitive impressions existed in the encephalon. Admitting that it is in the crura cerebri that these conductors decussate, as Longet has imagined, an alteration in one of these peduncles should produce a diminution of sensibility in the two sides of the body, because conductors belonging to these two sides should then be injured, those of the right side being in the right and in the left crura, and those of the left side being also in the left and in the right crura. This view does not agree with pathological cases, which show that an alteration in one of the crura, or above them in the two quadrigeminal bodies of one side, causes no diminution of sensibility in the corresponding side, and produces anæsthesia in the opposite side. So it was in cases recorded by Burnet,[1] Andral,[2] Mohr,[3] and Duplay.[4] These cases, as also several others, seem to show conclusively that the conductors of sensitive impressions, in their way to the brain proper, have already made their decussation before they reach the crura cerebri and the basis of the tubercula quadrigemina. Therefore the fibres, which really decussate beneath these tubercles, and which come chiefly from the cerebellum (see Fig. 18, *f*), cannot be considered as the conductors of sensitive impressions.

Is it in the pons Varolii that the decussation of these conductors takes place? If it were along the whole length of this organ, we should find a loss of sensibility in the two sides of the body, when one side only of the pons Varolii is altered, because, in each lateral half of the pons, there should be conductors belonging to the two sides of the body; *the right side of the pons*, for instance, containing the conductors which come from the right side of the body, *in their way to the left side of the pons*, and also the conductors from the left side of the body *after they have passed through the left side of the pons*. Clinical facts do not agree with this view, as they show that anæsthesia in one side of the body alone is the result of an alteration in one lateral half of the pons.

The same reasoning may be made as regards the medulla oblongata. When an alteration exists in one lateral half of this organ, there should be a loss of sensibility in the two sides of the body if the medulla oblongata were the seat of the decussation of the conductors for the sensitive impressions. Pathological facts do not leave room for doubt in this respect; they show that there is anæsthesia only in one-half of the body, and that this hemi-anæsthesia exists in the side of the body *opposite* to the side injured in the medulla oblongata.

Imagine an injury or an alteration anywhere you choose, near

[1] Journal Hebdomadaire, 1829, vol. v. p. 439.
[2] Clinique Médicale, 2d edit., vol. v. p. 326.
[3] In Casper's Wochenschrift, 1840, p. 479.
[4] Archives de Médecine, &c., Nov., 1834.

the median line and only in one lateral half, from the upper part of the crura cerebri and the tubercula quadrigemina down to the medulla oblongata; and if this injury produces anæsthesia, it is in one lateral half only, and this half is the opposite one. Now, to point out, another time, but in other words, the signification of these clinical facts, suppose that the injury is in the crura cerebri, the hemi-anæsthesia being in the opposite side of the body, it results that the decussation must take place in a part of the cerebro-spinal axis situated below the place altered. If the alterations are in the upper, the middle, or the lower parts of the pons, on one side, as the decussation must take place below the seat of the injury, we are led to the conclusion that it must be in the medulla oblongata or in the spinal cord. At last, in examining what occurs when the injury exists in the medulla oblongata, we find that the decussation must occur in the spinal cord.

As regards the spinal cord, we find also that, the injury existing in one lateral half, there is loss of sensibility in the opposite side. This, of course, is a direct and a better proof than the preceding that the conductors of sensitive impressions decussate in the spinal cord; but the cases of this kind are not numerous, so that, to give more power to our demonstration, I will relate the cases referring to the pons Varolii and the medulla oblongata. I will, therefore, divide into two series the cases I have to adduce in proof of the decussation of the conductors of sensitive impressions in the spinal cord. In the first series we place the cases of alterations of a lateral half of the spinal cord; and in the second series, those of alterations of a lateral half of the medulla oblongata, the pons Varolii, &c.

First Series of Cases proving that the Conductors of Sensitive Impressions make their Decussation in the Spinal Cord.

In the name of a committee of the Société de Biologie, we have published a report on a paper by Dr. Oré, of Bordeaux, in which there are two important cases observed by this physician, in the Hospital St. André in the wards of Professor Gintrac. Here is an abstract of these cases:—

Case 29.—A patient was admitted into the St. André Hospital. He had a paralysis of voluntary movements in the *right* side of the body, in which sensibility was preserved. In the *left* side, on the contrary, the voluntary movements existed, but there was a great diminution of sensibility.

Autopsy.—There was a fungoid growth (*végétation fungoïde*) pressing upon the *right* lateral half of the spinal cord. (*Mémoires de la Société de Biologie pour* 1854.)

CASE 30.—A patient had lost voluntary movements in the two limbs of the *left* side, in which sensibility was preserved. In the right side sensibility was much diminished (*très obtuse.*)

Autopsy.—A clot of blood was found in the *left* lateral half of the spinal cord in the cervical region. (*Mémoires de la Société de Biologie, pour* 1854.)

These two cases are certainly extremely valuable, and they agree perfectly with the results of my experiments on animals. It is so also with the following cases:—

CASE 31.—A man, after having felt a sudden pain in his back, became incompletely paralyzed of voluntary movements in the *right* lower limb. Sensibility was not altered in this limb, but in the *left* side, where voluntary movements were not impaired, sensibility was entirely lost from the breast to the foot.

Autopsy.—Brain and its membranes normal. In the spinal cord an hemorrhage had taken place, and blood was found in the *right* side of the gray matter, having destroyed also its horns, and a part of the right anterior column in the dorsal region. (Monod, in *Bulletin de la Société Anatomique*, No. XVIII., p. 349, Obs. 3, and in Ollivier, *loco cit.*, vol. ii. p. 177.)

This is a very remarkable case, teaching, not only that there is a decussation of the conductors of sensitive impressions in the spinal cord, but also that the gray matter is the principal channel for these impressions. The reporter of the case, M. Monod, I hardly need to say, is one of the best surgeons of Paris. I subjoin here three figures, representing sections of the spinal cord, to show the place where the blood was found.

If we had time, we could show, by some details of this case which we have not mentioned, that the hemorrhage was, at first, entirely confined to the gray matter of the right side of the spinal cord, high up in the dorsal region, and that afterwards the blood destroyed almost the whole of the gray matter and its horns, in a great extent, in that same side, and at last injured a little the central gray matter of the left side. Had the symptoms, as regards movement and sensibility, been noted after the first days, they would have been somewhat different from those above related. In another lecture we shall have to speak again of this most important case.

In the three preceding cases there is no mention of hyperæsthesia, although it must have existed on the side of the injury in the spinal cord; we shall find it mentioned in the following cases, and especially in the next one, which we give almost in full on account of its extreme importance:—

CASE 32.—On the 4th of February, 1850, a man, aged twenty-eight, was admitted into the St. Louis Hospital, in Professor Nélaton's ward, a short time after he had been wounded by a police officer. Besides a slight wound of the scalp, he had been wounded by a sword, in his back. The point of the sword was eight millimetres large; there was a transversal wound about one centimetre and a half (half an inch) between the ninth and tenth dorsal vertebræ, and three centimetres (an inch) from the line of the spinous processes. A physician, who had seen the patient at once, had introduced a stylet in the wound, and ascertained that its direction was oblique from the right to the left, and a little upwards. The patient complains of slight pains, only near the wound. The lower limbs are completely deprived of voluntary movements. The next morning a better examination is made; the patient has not slept; he has suffered violent pains, principally in the left lower limb; he feels a kind of burning and numbness, as if he were receiving electric shocks. The sensibility of the *left* lower limb is quite evidently increased. When a hand is simply applied upon this limb, the pains become very acute, and the very least pressure makes him shriek out. This morbid state of sensibility exists in the whole length of the limb, and also upon the left side of the sacrum and coccyx, and the upper and anterior part of the thigh. Higher up, sensibility is normal. Even cold air, when the sheet is drawn down, causes pain in the left lower limb. Voluntary movements are impossible in all this limb, except in the toes, which can slightly move.

The *right* lower limb has a diminution of sensibility; the patient knows when he is touched, but when pricked with a pin he does not feel pain, and he does not distinguish a pressure by the finger from the pricking of a pin. In both cases he has only a sensation of contact. This limb is not deprived of movement as it was the previous day. The flexion of the foot on the leg, and of the leg on the thigh, are executed; the movements are extensive, but the patient cannot altogether lift up his limb from the bed.

The temperature of the lower limbs is the same as that of the rest of the body, and there is no difference between those limbs. All the organic functions are in a normal condition, except that there is a retention of urine, and of the fecal matters. Voluntary movements and sensibility are not altered in the abdomen, and all the upper parts of the body. In the afternoon, the hyperæsthesia has extended a little higher on the left side in the upper parts of the abdomen, and the genital organs have also become very sensitive. When a cloth that has been dipped into water at 30° (probably centigrade, 86° Fahr.), is applied to the left limb, the patient has a feeling of burning, which makes him cry out. When the cloth has been dipped into water at the low temperature of the room, the patient has a very acute feeling of cold.

On the right limb the wet cloth does not give either a sensation of warmth or cold, or of dampness or dryness, although he feels he is touched. The tickling of the right foot is not felt as tickling, but only as a *contact.* On the left foot tickling is exceedingly painful.

Gradually this patient became more and more able to move the right limb, and partly also the left limb. The hyperæsthesia diminished, particularly in the upper parts of the left limb; but the right limb became, for a time, unable to feel the contact of a hand, and if pricked there was a sensation, but the patient did not know its place. On the 20th of February, a slough was found on the right side of the sacrum; the patient had not felt anything there. In April, voluntary movements had returned in the two limbs, but sensibility was still deficient in the right one. On the 15th of June, the patient could walk with the help of a cane, and he left the hospital, not having yet, however, recovered entirely the power of feeling, in his right limb.

Three years afterwards the patient was seen again, and he stated then that he was quite well, and that he could walk without difficulty or fatigue; but a year later, having walked a distance of many leagues, he found a large schar, produced, he said, by the friction of his pants on his right knee; he had felt no pain, and was surprised when he found this wound. Although sensibility was still deficient in this limb, all its movements were executed freely, and without fatigue. (Viguès, in *Moniteur des Hôpitaux*, Sept. 3, 1855, p. 838.)

This important case, so carefully reported by my friend, M. Viguès, has not the sanction of a *post-mortem* examination, but it is so much in accordance with the results of experiments in animals that we have thought there could be no objection to our giving it as a proof of the exactitude of our views. There are several points that are certain, or almost certain: in the first place, the sword entered the cord by its posterior surface; in the second place, its direction was oblique from behind forwards, and from the right to the left. These two facts being acknowledged, if we remember that the point was eight millimetres large, and that it penetrated *transversely—i. e.*, its edges being on a line perpendicular to the longitudinal axis of the cord—we are enabled to judge of the injury inflicted to the cord. Let us first admit the old theory, that the posterior column of the right side transmits the sensitive impressions of the right side of the body, and that the left anterior column transmits the orders of the will to the muscles of the left side of the body. Now let us suppose a section of the right posterior column and the left anterior column: there would have been then just what occurred in this case, loss of movement particularly in the left limb, and loss of sensibility in the right limb alone. But I will remark that such an injury was impossible with such a sword. Had the left anterior column been entirely, or almost entirely divided at the same time with the right posterior column, the left posterior column would also necessarily have been cut across, the sword having *at its point* almost the same diameter as the whole spinal cord; and had the left posterior column been divided, the left limb, according to the theory just exposed, would have lost its sensibility, and would not have been hyperæsthetic as it has been. We must therefore put aside the supposition which we have made. Now, if we take any of the theories that have been proposed concerning the transmission of the orders of the will to muscles, or of the sensitive impressions to the brain, through the spinal cord, we find that, except ours, they are all unable to explain the facts of this case. We think that the point of the sword entered the cord by only one of its edges (the right one), dividing entirely the left posterior column, and a part of the right one, and also almost the whole of the gray matter and of the lateral column on the left side, and a part of the anterior column of the same side, leaving the gray matter and the antero-lateral column of the right side uninjured, except by the pressure upon them by the blood which must have been effused on the withdrawal of the sword. In this way we can explain the rapid return of voluntary movements in the right limb, by the absorption of the blood; and we explain, 1st, the loss of sensibility and the persistence for years of a degree of anæsthesia in the right limb, by the section of almost the whole of the gray matter in the left side; 2d, the hyperæsthesia, by the peculiar influence we have found that a section (complete or incomplete) of a lateral half of the cord possesses on the sensitive nerves originating from the same side of the cord below the injured part; 3d, the more complete diminution of movements in the left than in the right limb, by the injury to the gray matter and anterior column of that side, and in a measure also to the left column of the same side.

There was no autopsy, also, in the two following cases.

CASE 33.—A man fell on his back, from a height of twenty feet. After having recovered his consciousness, he discovered that the whole left side of his body, from the shoulder down to the foot, was paralyzed of movement, but that there was not the slightest diminution of sensibility, and that the right side of the body, in which the movements were free, was completely deprived of sensibility.

Three months after this accident the patient was in the following state: When a needle or a lancet was introduced in the right limbs, the muscles of which obeyed the action of the will, there was no pain felt. The reverse existed in the left side, where sensibility was morbidly increased. The muscles of the right side were prominent, strong, and in good state of nutrition, and not paralyzed; while those on the left side were emaciated, and incapable of any voluntary movement. The temperature of the right side was one degree and a half lower (Reaumur's scale, nearly 4° Fahr.) than that of the left side, which was above the normal temperature. Although sensibility was entirely abolished in the right side, the patient was able to distinguish with the right hand the weight of external objects. The hand and the foot on the left side were œdematous. Above the fourth cervical vertebra sensibility and voluntary movements were in a normal condition. (Dundas, in the *Edin. Med. and Surg. Journ.*, April, 1825.)

When Dr. Dundas published this curious case (which I give here from a translation by Ollivier, *loco cit.*, vol. i. p. 509), the patient was living and improving, so that we do not know what was the alteration existing in the spinal cord, but the analogy between this case and other cases in which the autopsy was made, and with the results of my experiments on animals, renders it almost certain that the left lateral half of the cord had been altered. In the following case, the direction of the wound renders it almost certain that the same symptoms had followed a division of the lateral half of the spinal cord.

CASE 34.—A drummer of the National Guard of Paris received a wound in the back of the neck. A sword thrown at him had penetrated the superior part of the lateral half of the neck. An incomplete paralysis of movement took place in the right side of the body, and some time after it was *accidentally discovered* that sensibility was lost in many parts of the left side of the body. After twenty days the wound was cured, and the man went out of the hospital, but still paralyzed. (Boyer, in *Traité des Maladies Chirurgicales*, vol. vii. p. 9.)

The wound in the neck was in the right side; the paralysis of movement was limited to the right side of the body, so that the left side of the cord was not injured; and, from what is taught by experiments on animals, it seems certain that nearly all, if not all, the right lateral half of the cord had been divided transversely.

In the following case there was some complication, but, nevertheless, we think that such a case can be explained only by the theories we have proposed.

CASE 35.—A woman, aged twenty-three, after recovering from cholera, felt great weakness especially of the lower extremities. After two months, the motion of both legs was found greatly impaired, especially of the left, in which there was also diminished sensation, and a pain which extended from the origin of the sciatic nerve, quite to the extremity of the toes; and both limbs were affected with a sense of coldness and prickling. Soon after this she began to have pain in the lumbar region, and this was succeeded by acute pain in both limbs, with convulsive retraction of the toes. This pain was most acute in the *left* limb, and there was now increased sensibility of the *left foot, so that the slightest touch produced a sense of laceration*, and this morbid sensibility afterwards extended to the knee. *The right limb was continually numb*, but some degree of motion remained in both. She died, after gradual exhaustion, six or seven months from the commencement of the disease.

Autopsy.—At the lower extremity of the spinal cord was a firm, white tumor, the size of a filbert, inclosed in a cyst, and slightly softened in the centre. It lay between the two columns of the *left* side, and in some degree encroached upon those of the right; the left anterior column in particular was much distended and flattened by it. (Gendrin in *Pathological and Practical Researches on Diseases of the Brain*, &c., by J. Abercrombie, 4th edition, 1845, p. 369.)

It would be difficult to find a case presenting more interesting features than this one. Unfortunately, however, the precise place occupied by the tumor has not been mentioned, Mr. Gendrin merely stating that it was at the lower extremity of the cord. The tumor, as shown by this statement, as well as by the symptoms, was not above the place of decussation of the conductors of sensitive impressions from the lower limbs, and, besides, it was not entirely in one lateral half of the spinal cord. These two reasons explain that there was a diminution of sensibility in the upper part of the left leg, their conductors being injured while crossing the cord from the left to the right side. The left foot and also the left leg, up to the knee, had the most marked hyperæsthesia, their conductors having made their decussation below the tumor, and being able therefore to transmit sensitive impressions through the right side of the cord, which transmission they performed with the peculiar painful character which exists after an injury to either the anterior, the lateral, or the posterior columns. The right limb was continually numb, on account of the injury to many of its conductors of sensitive impressions in the gray matter and in the anterior columns of the left side of the cord.

This case is not only instructive in showing that there ought to be a decussation of the conductors of sensitive impressions in the spinal cord, but also in proving that the posterior columns are not the place through which these conductors go up to the brain, as we find here these columns uninjured, and sensibility diminished in many parts.

Some of the cases, already mentioned to establish the exactitude of my views concerning the decussation of the conductors of sensitive impressions in the spinal cord, are far from being *positive* proofs of these views, no autopsy having shown the real extent of the injury; but there are two reasons which have decided my relating them, as giving a strong additional evidence. The first of these reasons is, that the symptoms observed in these pathological facts (see Cases 32, 33, 34, and 35) are the same as those which I have shown to exist in animals after a section of a lateral half or some other injuries to the spinal cord, so that it seems quite certain that the same injuries existed in this organ in these cases. The second reason is, that there is no theory able to explain all that we know of these cases, except that the theory we are now trying to prove. I add to these reasons that in Cases 32 and 34 the direction of the sword and its shape and size were such that the injury must have been what we have already stated. It seems, therefore, that of the seven cases (from 29 to 35) which we have related to ground our theory, there are three (29, 30, 31) which are as direct and as positive proofs as possible of the exactitude of this theory, and there are four (32 to 35) which have an indirect but a great value for the establishment of this doctrine. We will now relate two more cases, which, although they do not give a positive proof, are very interesting by the symptoms which they have offered, and because they afford an additional testimony of inestimable value in support of the view that the conductors of sensitive impressions decussate in the spinal cord.

CASE 36.—A young man received a blow of a quadrangular and acute poniard, which entered the neck below the *left* ear, being directed towards the beginning of the spinal cord. Immediately all the parts below the head lost sensibility and motion. He was brought home and put in bed, and there, amongst other things that the impediment to his respiration allowed him to say, he complained of being cold, and without any feeling he was burnt on the thighs, the legs, and feet, in consequence of the application of a heated metallic vase to those parts. The *left* side of the body began for the first time to recover some feeling on the seventeenth day, and on the twentieth he began to move the toes and fingers of the same side, and these two faculties increased gradually until the thirtieth day in this side. Only on the thirty-second day there was a return of some feeling in the *right* side of the body; movement also, but later, returned slowly there. On the fortieth day there was sensibility and movement everywhere, but not enough to allow the patient to stand up, and still less to walk. The recovery was so slow, that four months after the accident he was hardly beginning to get out of bed, and to walk as a child learning to walk; even then there was less power of movement and feeling in the *right* than in the *left* side. (Morgagni, *De Sedibus et Causis Morborum*, &c. Nona ed., Lutetiæ, 1822, tomus sextus, pp. 515–517.)

In this interesting case, we find that, although the wound must have been more extensive in the *left* side of the spinal cord than in the right, the return of sensibility was quicker and greater in the *left* than in the *right* side of the body. It would not have been so if there was no decussation of the conductors of sensitive impressions in the spinal cord. In this respect, therefore, this case is a good one in support of my views; but how to explain that the power of voluntary motion returned quicker in the side most injured than in the other? It would be easy to understand all the phenomena observed in admitting that the medulla oblongata, just above the crossing of the pyramids, was the part injured; but death would have been an immediate, or almost immediate, result of such a wound, so that we must admit that the spinal cord is the organ that was injured. In trying experiments on animals to solve this difficulty, I have found that the introduction of an instrument in the spinal cord, obliquely from the left to the right, and a little from behind forwards and from below upwards, and dividing on the *left* side almost all the central gray matter, the posterior part of the lateral column, and a part of the posterior column, and, on the *right* side, a part of the central gray matter and the parts of the right lateral column just at the place where they approach the median line to make their crossing just below the medulla oblongata, I produced a more considerable loss of voluntary motion and sensibility in the right than in the left side. So that a greater injury to the gray matter on the left than on the right side, and a greater injury to the lateral column (particularly to its decussating part) on the right than on the left side, are probably the causes of a greater loss of voluntary movement and sensibility in the right than in the left side in the case recorded by Morgagni. We must add, that the complete loss of sensibility and motion in the beginning, in that case, depended upon the existence of some hemorrhage, with pressure upon the whole spinal cord, besides the section of certain parts of this organ.

The following case is less complicated than the preceding:—

CASE 37.—Mrs. W——, after a profuse hemorrhage, became paralytic. Upon one side of the body there was a loss of sensibility, without, however, any corresponding diminution of power in the muscles of volition. The breast, too, upon that side, partook of the insensibility, although the secretion of milk was as copious as in the other. Upon the opposite side of the body there was defective power of motion, without, however, any diminution of sensibility. The arm was incapable of supporting the child, the hand was powerless in its grasp, and the leg was moved with difficulty and with the ordinary rotatory movement of a paralytic patient; but the power of sensation was so far from being impaired that she constantly complained of an uncomfortable sense of heat, a painful tingling, and more than usual degree of tenderness from pressure, or other modes of slight mechanical violence.

Autopsy.—No positive disorganization of the brain could be detected; the ventricles, however, contained more serum than usual; and there were found thickening and increased vascularity of the membranes, with firm adhesion, in some parts; in others, an apparently gelatinous, transparent, and colorless deposit interposed between them. Unfortunately, the spinal cord was not examined. (H. Ley, in a letter to Sir C. Bell, in *The Nervous System of the Human Body*, 3d ed., 1844, p. 245.)

This case acquires importance from the fact that there was no alteration in the brain that could account for the symptoms, and from the similitude between the symptoms and those observed in animals after a section of a lateral half of the spinal cord.

Setting aside, in this lecture, what relates to temperature, we state that a transversal section of a lateral half of the spinal cord causes a loss of voluntary movement in the corresponding side of the body, and a loss of sensibility in the opposite side, and if, now, we look at the cases we have related to see how they agree with this general result, we find the following points:—

Cases.	Side of the injury.	Side of the paralysis.	Side of the anæsthesia.	Side of conservation of sensibility, or of hyperæsthesia.
29	*right*	*right*	*left*	*right*
30	*left*	*left*	*right*	*left*
31	*right*	*right*	*left*	*right*
32	*left* (probably)	*left*	*right*	*left*
34	*right* (ib.)	*right*	*left*	*right*
35	*left* (chiefly)	*left* (chiefly)	*right*	*left*

If we add to these cases those in which we have no other reason but the analogy of symptoms with those observed in animals, such as Cases 33 and 37, we have two more instances of this curious but simple morbid manifestation—*i. e.*, loss of movement in one side, loss of sensibility in the other. In animals, as I have often said and shown, the paralyzed parts are in a state of hyperæsthesia; in the cases I have related, hyperæsthesia has been noted in Cases 32, 33, 35, and 37. It was so great that the least touch produced pain in Cases 32 and 35. It would have been found in the other cases, had the physicians who attended the patients looked for it.

The cases of loss of movement in one side of the body with loss of sensibility in the opposite side, are not so rare as a great many of my hearers probably think. That very learned writer, Dr. Copland, says that the paralytic affection in epilepsy occasionally consists "of loss of sensation in one limb and of loss of movement in another, on the opposite side." (*Dict. of Pract. Medicine*, vol. i., 1844, p. 795.) There is a case of this kind in the *Ephemeridæ Naturæ Curios*, Cent. ii., obs. 196; and Dr. J. Cooke (*History and Method of Cure of Palsy*, 1821, p. 19) says that Ramazzini speaks of a person in whom one leg had lost its feeling, but not its power of motion, and the other its motion, but not its feeling. He also mentions Sénac as having related a case in which the most acute sensation (hyperæsthesia) was experienced in one arm, which had lost the power of motion; whilst in the other arm sensation was lost, though motion remained perfect. Burserius, he adds, quotes a similar case from Heister. (I have vainly looked for this case in Heister's works.) In a recently published work (*Des Paralysies des Membres Inférieurs*, 2de partie, 1857, p. 116, par R. Leroy d'Etiolles) there is a case of hysteric paralysis, with loss of movement in one side, and loss of sensibility in the other. Lastly, Dr. R. Bright has recorded a case of this kind, of which we will speak by and by.

I shall not stop now to show that these cases, or at least most of them, are cases of alteration limited to a lateral half of the spinal cord, as I shall have to treat of this subject again in a future lecture, in examining the symptoms of alterations of various parts of the cerebro-spinal axis. I set aside, also, for the present, cases which might be considered as in opposition to the theory I try to prove in this lecture, and I pass immediately to the second series of cases which I have to relate in favor of this theory.

Second Series of Cases proving that the Conductors of Sensitive Impressions make their Decussation in the Spinal Cord.

I begin this series by a most important case, indeed, from which many physiological and practical deductions may be drawn. It has been recorded by an able American physician, Dr. Samuel Annan.

CASE 38.—S. G——, aged twenty-eight, was, on the 14th of May, suddenly seized with an acute pain in the right side of the head, and fell down in a state of insensibility, remaining so for twenty-four hours. On recovering, she found she had lost the power of moving her *left* arm, and, in a great degree, that of moving the leg of the same side. The right side was unaffected, except the face, the muscles of which were paralyzed; those of the left side of the face retained their power. Sensibility of the *left* side of the body was destroyed, and likewise that of the right side of the face. She could not hear with the right ear. The right eye became inflamed several weeks before her death, and the cornea was slightly ulcerated; the upper eyelid was constantly raised. Her muttering was scarcely intelligible; paralysis of all the parts affected became complete; deglutition and mastication performed with great difficulty.

Autopsy, twelve hours after death.—A fibrous, semi-cartilaginous tumor was found on the *right* side of the tuber annulare and the medulla oblongata, seated in the substance of the dura mater and other membranes. It extended from the point where the fifth pair of nerves arises from the tuber annulare, covered the origin of this nerve and the whole of the right side of the tuber below this, and passed down along two-thirds of the medulla oblongata, and adhered to the right side of the basilar artery. The right vertebral artery was inclosed in the tumor, which was about two inches long. The surface of the root of the right crus cerebelli on which it pressed was softened, as was also that part of the tuber annulare on which it lay. It was incorporated with the substance of the right side of the medulla oblongata, and had produced softening as far as it reached. This softening extended through the posterior tract, but became less as it approached the posterior surface. The anterior tract was a pulpy mass. Neither the anterior nor the posterior tract of the left side was perceptibly affected. The tumor pressed upon the roots of the fifth, seventh, eighth, and ninth pairs of nerves. (S. Annan, in the *American Journal of the Medical Sciences*, vol, ii., July, 1841, p. 105.)

The author justly says: "The right side of the medulla oblongata was softened to the extent of complete disorganization; there was complete paralysis both of motion and sensation on the left side. The decussation of the fibres of the corpora pyramidalia explains the loss of motion in the opposite side, but as we have no facts proving a similar interlacement of the fibres of the posterior or sensory tract, it is not easy to discover how it happened that the right side was not deprived of sensation. Motion and sensation were unimpaired in the extremities of the side diseased; they were both destroyed in the same parts of the opposite or left side. Are we not justified from this in making the inference that there is a decussation of the fibres for sensation as well as those for motion?" Certainly this is a very proper inference; but this question remains: Where does the decussation of the "*fibres for sensation*" take place? Is it in the lower part of the medulla oblongata, where exists the decussation of the anterior pyramids, or in the spinal cord? Lately, Messrs. Vulpian and Philipeaux (*Comptus Rendus de la Société de Biologie*, Mars, 1858) have shown that there are in the anterior pyramids fibres originating from the posterior horns of gray matter, and decussating with the other decussating fibres of these pyramids; and they suggest that a crossing *for sensation* probably exists there. Admitting that they are right, these conductors of sensitive impressions would pass into the anterior pyramids, and they themselves state that it must be so. We will show, in the lecture on the medulla oblongata, that this view is in opposition to positive facts, and particularly to the celebrated case of alteration of the anterior pyramids, which has been recorded by our friend, Professor Lebert.

We think that the case of Dr. Annan, if we take into account the extent of the injury in the medulla oblongata, bears out clearly that most if not all of the conductors of sensitive impressions from the trunk and limbs make their decussation in the spinal cord. But the importance of this case is not limited to this demonstration: it shows at once the radical difference between the symptoms of an alteration of a lateral half of the medulla oblongata above the crossing of the pyramids, and an alteration of a lateral half of the spinal cord either in the cervical or in another region. In this last case, as we have shown a moment ago, there is loss of movement in one side and loss of sensibility in the opposite side; while in a case of alteration above the crossing of the pyramids, we find that the loss of movement and of sensibility are both in the opposite side. This case is also excellent to show that the functions attributed to the restiform body as a conductor of sensitive impressions, and to the cerebellum as either a centre of perception of these impressions, or as a regulator of our voluntary movements, or as a centre for the guiding sensation, whether by a reflex action or otherwise, are not performed by these parts, as the communication between the cerebellum and the right side of the body through the right side of the medulla oblongata was almost impossible, a small part only of the right restiform body remaining, and sensibility and voluntary movements being preserved in this side.

In the following case, which is related by Broussais, we find, with less detail, several of the features of the preceding one.

CASE 39.—An officer, recovered for some time, after having been attacked with stupor, vomiting, &c.; but, five months afterwards, hemiplegia gradually appeared in the *right* side; the leg could support him a little; the arm lost both movement and feeling. Soon after, the *left* eye lost its transparency and became atrophied; the left eyelids were paralyzed. A few weeks after, walking was still more difficult, and speech more impeded, and death occurred after coma.

Autopsy.—The left hemisphere was softened; cerebellum normal. At the upper part of the medulla oblongata, in the interior of the left pyramidal body, there was a cancerous tumor, the size of a chestnut, in continuity with the surrounding nervous tissue. (Broussais, in *Traité des Phlegmasies Chroniques*, troisième ed., 1822, p. 420.)

The state of sensibility of the right lower extremity is not mentioned, but we find that there was loss of feeling in the right upper limb, and a tumor in the left side of the medulla oblongata showing that the decussation of the conductors of sensitive impressions must have taken place below the point injured—*i. e.*, in the spinal cord or the lower part of the medulla oblongata. Now, as there is no proof that there is such a decussation in this part of this nervous centre; and as, on the contrary, there are facts in opposition to the view that there is such a crossing, we must admit that it exists in the spinal cord. The same thing may be concluded from a case of M. Carré (*Archives de Médecine*, p. 234, vol. v., 1834), in which a cancerous tumor in the *left* half of the pons Varolii, extending several lines in the medulla oblongata and the crus cerebri, had produced paralysis of movement and sensibility on the *right* side of the body, the left side remaining in the normal state. Nearly the same thing existed in a case of Friedreich, (*Beitraege zur Lehre von den Geschwülsten innerhalb der Schaedelhöhle*, 1853, p. 29.) The following case leads also to the same conclusions:—

CASE 40.—A young Pole, after a nervous fever, became paralyzed of sensibility and movement in the *left* side of the body, and in the right side of the face.

Autopsy.—The *right* side of the pons Varolii is twice its normal size; it extends forwards and backwards, where it passes under the right olive, compressing the neighboring parts. The enlargement was due to a very large clot of blood in the right half of the pons. (M. H. Romberg, in *Lehrbuch der Nervenkrankheiten*, 1851, vol. i., part 2, pp. 198, 202, and third edition, 1857, third part, p. 923.)

In many cases of alteration of a lateral half of the pons Varolii, the medulla oblongata not being injured, we find, also, the paralysis of movement and sensibility only in the opposite side (excepting, however, the face, which is paralyzed on the same side). Such cases are recorded by Gendrin,[1] Charcellay,[2] Greuzard[3] Friedreich (*loco cit.*, p. 15), Cruveilhier,[4] Dr. R. Bright,[5] Dr. J. W. Ogle,[6] &c. In many other cases, in which one-half of the pons was more altered than the other, there was paralysis and anæsthesia in the two sides of the body, but at a greater degree in the side opposite to the half of the pons most injured. Cases of this kind are recorded by Cruveilhier, Dr. R. Bright, Abercrombie (*loco cit.*, p. 235), Hermann Romberg[7]—whom we must not take for the great neuro-pathologist, Moritz Heinrich Romberg—Grenet,[8] Poisson,[9] Tacheron,[10] Dr. T. Inman,[11] etc.

These cases assuredly show that the decussation of the conductors of sensitive impressions does not take place in the pons Varolii, and that it has taken place before they reach this organ; and therefore that it occurs either in the spinal cord or the medulla oblongata, a question which is solved by the facts we have mentioned relating to these organs. But there is another consequence to be drawn from many of these cases: if the pons Varolii were a place of passage of only a part of the conductors of sensitive impressions, most of these conductors passing into the cerebellum from the posterior columns of the spinal cord and their continuation, the restiform bodies, we certainly should see but a diminution, and not a com-

[1] Hist. Anatom. des Inflammations, vol. ii. p. 155.

[2] In Ollivier, loco cit., vol. ii. p. 315.

[3] Archives de Médecine, 1834, vol. v. p. 458.

[4] Anatomie Pathologique, livre 21.

[5] Reports of Med. Cases, vol. ii. part 1.

[6] Edinburgh Monthly Journal of Medicine, March, 1855.

[7] Quædam de Ponte Varolii, 1838, p. 17.

[8] Gaz. Hebd. de Médec., No. 38, Sept. 1856.

[9] Bulletins de la Société Anatom., Mai et Juin, 1855.

[10] Rech. Anat. Pathol. sur la Médecine Pratique, 1823, vol. iii. p. 450.

[11] Edinburgh Medical and Surgical Journal, vol. 64, 1845, p. 294.

plete loss, of sensibility in those cases in which an alteration is limited to the central parts of the pons Varolii, and not interfering with the cerebellum and its peduncles. It is usually, however, a complete loss of sensibility which is observed, and not a diminution. The case of Greuzard, already mentioned, is particularly interesting in this respect; there was a softening, irregular in its shape, large, like an almond, and rose-colored, in the inferior and middle part of the right half of the pons Varolii, and the anæsthesia and paralysis of the left side of the body had been complete. In a case still more interesting, and which I shall have to relate by and by for another object, there was a tumor in the left half of the pons Varolii, with complete loss of sensibility in the right side of the body. (Stuart Cooper, in *Bulletins de la Soc. Anat.*, 1846, p. 68.)

In our Lecture on the Functions of the Medulla Oblongata and Pons Varolii, we shall have to treat at length of the place of decussation of the conductors of the orders of the will to muscles; but we must now point out the following characteristic features of alterations limited to one lateral half of those parts: 1st, the spinal cord; 2d, the medulla oblongata, at the place of the crossing of the pyramids; 3d, the encephalon, above this crossing.

In Fig. 21 may be seen what we think to be proved by pathological cases in this respect: 1st. In the spinal cord an alteration in a lateral half produces hyperæsthesia and paralysis of movement in the corresponding side, behind the place of the alteration, and the loss of sensibility, without loss of movement, in the opposite side. (See 3, Fig. 21.) 2d. In the lower part of the medulla oblongata, diminution of movement in the two sides of the body, hyperæsthesia on the side altered, anæsthesia in the opposite side. (See 2, Fig. 21.) 3d. Above the crossing of the pyramids, loss of movement and sensibility in the opposite side, and hyperæsthesia with conservation of movement in the side of the alteration. (See 1, Fig. 21.)

LECTURE VIII.

CONCLUSIONS FROM THE PATHOLOGICAL CASES RELATED IN THE PRECEDING LECTURES AND FROM SEVERAL OTHER CASES, AS REGARDS THE DIAGNOSIS OF ALTERATIONS OF THE VARIOUS PARTS OF THE SPINAL CORD.

Principal symptoms of the diseases of the spinal cord.—On a curious symptom which seems to belong especially to diseases of this organ.—Cases against the views of Bellingeri and Valentin, relative to the pretended motor functions of the posterior columns, and to certain symptoms of alterations of the anterior columns.—Differences in the degree of paralysis of voluntary movements, according to the extent of the alteration of the posterior columns.—Absence of paralysis, in cases in which these columns are entirely cut across, but not injured, in a great part of their length.—Causes and nature of the apparent paralysis observed when a great part of the length of the posterior columns is altered.—Alteration of the upper part of the anterior columns without paralysis.—Decussation of the lateral columns; their function and symptoms of their alteration.—Paralysis due to disease of the gray matter.—Alterations causing a loss of feeling a contact, a tickling, a muscular contraction, a painful impression, or a change of temperature.—Conclusions concerning anæsthesia.—When does anæsthesia exist without a notable paralysis.—Rarity of complete anæsthesia.—Referring of the various kinds of sensitive impressions to different parts of the body in cases of alteration of the spinal cord.—Absence of excitability of most of the conductors of the various kinds of sensitive impressions in the nerves and in the spinal cord.—Inflammation may render all these conductors excitable, and induce the production of all kinds of sensations, erroneously referred to the periphery.—Groups of symptoms which characterize alterations limited to certain parts of the various columns of the spinal cord and of its gray matter.

Mr. President and Gentlemen: Many conclusions having a practical bearing may be drawn from the facts concerning the spinal cord which I have mentioned in several of the preceding lectures. I will now point out those conclusions, and relate some new facts which bear them out as well as those I have already detailed. I will at first examine the signification of the various symptoms of disease of the spinal cord, and try to show how these symptoms may guide in the diagnosis of the place injured; then I will show how alterations in the principal parts of the spinal cord give different and characteristic symptoms.

The symptoms of injuries or alterations of the spinal cord consist in various degrees and forms of paralysis of voluntary movement; in a diminution or loss of the various kinds of sensibility, as regards contact, temperature, tickling, muscular sense, pain; in involuntary movements—spasmodic, choreic, epileptiform, &c.; in a morbid increase of the various kinds of sensibility; in a perversion of sensations; in errors as to the place of starting of a sensitive impression; in the referring of sensitive impressions to the extremities of the conductors of these impressions; in the absence, diminution, or increase of the reflex faculty, &c.

Paralysis of voluntary movement may occur in consequence of alterations existing almost anywhere in the spinal cord. This may seem to be very strange, particularly when we remember that a transversal section of the posterior columns of the spinal cord, in animals, is without influence upon voluntary movements. What are the deductions to be drawn from pathological cases observed in man as regards the share of the posterior columns of the spinal marrow in voluntary movements? Three questions must be examined in this respect: First, are there nerve-fibres going to muscles, and employed in voluntary movements, passing along the posterior columns, from the encephalon down to the spinal nerves? Are there volitional-motor nerve-fibres *passing, for a short distance*, through the posterior columns? Are there some peculiar causes of diminution of voluntary movements in cases of alterations of the posterior columns?

The first of these questions is very interesting, both in a physiological and in a practical point of view. To solve it, it may perhaps be sufficient to remind our hearers of three cases (see Lecture V., Cases 6, 7, and 8), which we have already related, and in which voluntary movements persisted, or returned after a time, although the posterior columns had been destroyed in a small part of their length, just as if they had been divided transversely. Of course, if there were a number of volitional nerve-fibres passing along these columns of the cord to go to the muscles of the limbs, there would have been a manifest diminution of voluntary movements in these cases; and, as this did not take place, we may conclude—first, that the posterior columns are not a channel between the will and muscles; and, secondly, that a paralysis of voluntary movements is not a symptom belonging to a section or a local destruction of the posterior columns by a tumor, or a piece of bone, &c.

According to the views of Bellingeri,[1] ably supported by the learned Prof. Valentin,[2] the posterior columns of the spinal cord contain the voluntary motor fibres going to the extensor muscles. I have already mentioned and shown experiments which are in opposition to this hypothesis. (See Lecture IV.) I will now show that clinical facts also disagree with it.

There is a very curious symptom which seems to belong exclusively to diseases of the spinal cord (at least we do not know of any case of disease of the encephalon in which this symptom has existed, the spinal cord being healthy). It consists in a spasm of the flexor muscles of the lower limbs, spasm which is so powerful that the anterior parts of the thighs come almost in contact with the abdomen, while the heels are drawn up so as to touch the back parts of the thighs.

Were it true, as admitted by Bellingeri and Valentin, that the anterior columns of the spinal cord are a bundle of nerve-fibres animating the flexor muscles, and that the posterior columns contain the nerve-fibres animating the extensor muscles; and were it true also, as admitted by almost all physiologists, that the nerve-fibres have the same excitability in the spinal cord as in the trunks and branches of nerves, we should see flexion produced in cases of tumors or diseases exciting the anterior columns, and extension in cases of excitation of the posterior columns. Now, in examining pathological cases in this respect, we find that there are a great many more in which neither of these symptoms have existed than cases in which they have been observed with the peculiar alteration which should be connected with them.

We can say more: there are cases in which an irritation, or at least an alteration, of the posterior columns has produced flexion. For instance, in a case we have already related (Case 10, Lecture V.), the knees were drawn up towards the abdomen, the legs were bent upon the thighs, so that the heels rested firmly upon the soft parts covering the tuber ischii, and the posterior columns in the cervical region were *semi-fluid*. In another case, that of a young patient whom I have observed at the Charité Hospital, in Paris (see Case 9, Lecture V.), there was also a flexion of the lower limbs,

[1] De Medulla Spinalis Nervisque ex ea Prodeuntibus, &c. Torino, 1823.
[2] De Functionibus Nervorum Cerebralium, &c., p. 135. 1839.

and the anterior columns were healthy, while the posterior columns were softened in the cervical region. In a case recorded by Mr. Colin,[1] the knees were drawn up towards the chest, and the heels were in contact with the back parts of the thighs, pressing against them; there was a tumor, two inches long, pressing against the posterior surface of the spinal cord at the level of the tenth dorsal vertebra. In another case of tumor pressing upon the posterior columns, in the cervical region, the same thing existed. (See Case 12, Lecture V.) Besides, there are several other cases in which the alteration was certainly not a simple irritation of the anterior columns, and in which the symptom we study (flexion of the lower limbs) has existed. So it was in a very interesting case recorded by Mr. Pilcher,[2] in which tubercles were found in the cerebral meninges and in the theca vertebralis, some attached to the roots of the spinal nerves. So it was, also, in two cases mentioned by Ollivier (*loco cit.*, vol. ii. p. 444 and p. 388), in one of which there was an atrophy of the lumbar swelling of the cord, while in the other there was a destruction of the gray matter in the cervical region of the cord. It is true, however, that there are several cases of alteration of the anterior columns, in which this symptom has existed. Valentin quotes cases of this kind observed by Marshall Hall, Cruveilhier, Herbert Mayo (*Outlines of Physiology*, p. 156), and Ollivier.

From these facts it results that the spasmodic flexion of the thighs and legs is a symptom which does not belong exclusively to alterations of either the anterior or the posterior columns of the spinal cord, and that it is impossible to find a proof of the exactitude of the views of Bellingeri and Valentin in establishing a connection between this sympton and certain parts of the cord. And we may be permitted to add that alterations of the posterior columns, when they cause paralysis without contraction, do not cause simply a paralysis of the extensor muscles, but at the same time a paralysis of the extensor and the flexor muscles: and that, on the other hand, when there is paralysis due to an alteration of the anterior columns, it exists also in the flexor and in the extensor muscles. Besides, in cases of tetanus, in which almost always the extensor muscles are those which are chiefly convulsed, the parts of the cord which are most frequently found altered are precisely the anterior columns.

[1] Revue Médicale, Avril, 1824.

[2] The Lancet, April 1, 1848, p. 368.

Several of the above mentioned facts seem to be decisive against the view that the posterior columns contain voluntary motor fibres descending through them to pass into motor nerves. But there are other facts which *seem to prove* what is disproved by the preceding. For instance, in several cases which we have related in another lecture (see Lecture V., Cases 10, 13, 14, 16), although sensibility persisted, there was almost a complete paralysis, with an alteration of the posterior columns. The details of these cases show that they differed from the others (Lecture V., Cases 6, 7, 8), which have been mentioned a moment ago, as to the extent of the injury. In all the last cases there was a considerable alteration occupying the whole length of the posterior columns, either in the cervical region alone (as in Case 10), or in both the cervical and dorso-lumbar regions.

In reviewing carefully all the cases that we know of alteration of the posterior columns of the spinal cord, we find that usually an alteration, limited to a small part of the length of these columns, does not affect the voluntary movements, while, on the contrary, there is no case in which an alteration extending a few inches in either the cervical or the dorso-lumbar regions, has not produced a diminution of voluntary movements in either the upper or the lower limbs. When the alteration exists along the cervico-brachial enlargement, the paralysis exists in the upper limbs and not in the lower ones. (See Case 17, Lecture V.) There are several cases, however, in which an alteration in the cervical region *co-existed* with a paralysis of the lower limbs, but the cause of this loss of power may be found in other circumstances than the alteration of the posterior columns, as we shall show in a moment.

Certainly one of the most embarrassing features of the diseases of the spinal cord consists in a complete paralysis in cases where the posterior columns alone are said to be affected. The celebrated case, reported by Mr. Edward Stanley, is one of this kind. (Case 14, Lecture V.) The following clinical fact is extremely interesting in this respect, and also as regards the conservation of sensibility.

CASE 41.—R. B——, aged seventeen, was admitted into the Pennsylvania Hospital, with complete paralysis of all the limbs, which had followed an attack of typhoid fever. From first to last his intellect was perfectly clear: he had no pain in his head; his senses were perfect; his countenance natural, and he had no spasms or convulsions. During a part of the time his bladder and rectum were involved in the paralysis. Although the loss of power was complete, or nearly so, the sensation in the limbs was preserved. Some time after his admission, the limbs, especially the upper ones, became the seat of permanent contractions, the forearm being flexed upon the arm, the hand upon the forearm, and the fingers upon the hand. For some time previous to his death, the power of the bladder and rectum was restored, and there was a slight return of motion in the limbs. The patient died of pulmonary consumption.

Autopsy fourteen hours after death.—Substance of the brain perfectly healthy. Vault and septum lucidum softened, as well as the surface of the thalami and of the corpora striata, forming the walls of the ventricles. Some effusion in the ventricles; some adhesions between the opposing surfaces of the arachnoid and between the pia mater and the cord. Upon dividing the posterior fissure, the substance of the spinal marrow was found perfectly pulpy, and of a milk-white color. This softening extended throughout the whole length of the column, but was most marked inferiorly, less so in the cervical, and least of all in the dorsal portion. It was limited to the posterior columns, which were softened throughout, its limits being distinctly marked by the posterior horns of the gray matter, which was rather paler and less distinct than natural. The anterior columns were of natural consistence and color. (*The Medical Examiner*, vol. i. p. 273. Philadelphia, 1838.)

This curious case is certainly a good additional proof against the view that the posterior columns of the cord are the only channels for sensitive impressions. Its signification concerning voluntary movements, we will discuss presently.

To make out the diagnostic value of paralysis, in cases of alteration of the posterior columns, it will prove useful to examine what degree and what kind of paralysis existed in connection with alterations in the spinal cord. We shall see that in most of the cases of alterations of, or injuries to, the posterior columns that we have related in the preceding lectures, there was some other part of the cerebro-spinal axis altered, and that in the few cases in which the posterior columns were alone altered, the paralysis of voluntary movements was not complete.

Cases.	Altered Parts.	Degree of Paralysis.
1.	Posterior columns, posterior roots, gray matter.	Probably complete.
2.	" " " " " "	Incomplete.
3.	" " " " " "	Incomplete.
4.	The whole cord (atrophy), median posterior columns (induration), and posterior roots (atrophy).	Probably complete.
5.	Posterior columns, and most probably the posterior roots.	Incomplete.
6.	Posterior columns (tumor, cervical region).	*No paralysis.*
7.	Posterior surface (bayonet wound below last dorsal vertebra).	*No paralysis.*
8.	Posterior columns (probably divided with some parts around).	At first paralysis, but afterwards entire return of voluntary movements.
9.	Posterior columns, also various other parts.	Complete.
10.	Back part (semi-fluid), the rest softened in cervical region.	Almost complete.
11.	One of the posterior columns (in medulla oblongata) and neighboring parts (pressure by a tumor).	Not very marked.
12.	Posterior columns (chiefly the left), rest of the cord reduced to two-thirds of its size (tumor, level of second dorsal vertebra).	Probably complete.
13.	Posterior columns, in all their length and thickness.	Incomplete.
14.	Posterior columns, from the pons to the other end.	Complete (*but only in lower limbs*).
15.	Posterior columns (about two inches, level of fifth dorsal vertebra).	Probably complete.
16.	Posterior columns, and also, though less, the rest of the cord (cervical region).	Complete.
17.	Posterior columns (cervico-brachial swelling), posterior roots also.	Complete in upper limbs(?)
18.	Posterior columns (lumbar swelling).	Incomplete.
19.	Posterior columns, and some parts of the brain.	Complete(?)
41.	Posterior columns (the whole length).	Almost complete.

We find the paralysis complete, or probably complete, in Cases 1, 4, 9, 12, 14, 15, 16, 17, and 19. But Case 1 cannot prove anything, because the gray matter was altered; Case 4, because the whole cord was atrophied; Case 9, because various alterations existed in the brain, and the state of the limbs, which were in a permanent spasmodic flexion probably due to an old spinal meningitis, prevented the action of the will; Case 12, because the rest of the cord was also altered, the organ being reduced to two-thirds of its volume; Case 14, because the alteration does not answer to the symptoms observed (*no paralysis at all* in the upper limbs and complete paralysis in the lower ones, with an alteration of the whole length of the posterior columns); Case 16, because the rest of the cord was also altered; Case 19, because some parts of the brain were altered.

Two cases, 15 and 17, are the only ones about which we may have doubts. However, in Case 15 there was a curvature of the spine, and most probably the curved part of the anterior half of the cord had some alteration which was not sufficiently evident to be detected with the naked eye. This is, at any rate, the only case that I know of an alteration said to be limited to the posterior columns, with a complete loss of voluntary movements; and this case, which would be quite insufficient to prove that these columns are the channels of the orders of the will to muscles, is entirely in opposition to many other cases (see Cases 6, 7, 8, 11, &c.), which establish the reverse.[1] As regards Case 17, there has certainly been some mistake made by the author who reported it, as he states that the posterior roots were in a state of putrilage and that sensibility was preserved.

In two of the cases of the above list there was almost a complete paralysis (Cases 10 and 41). In one of these there was softening in the whole thickness of the cord, though less than in the posterior columns (Case 10). The state of voluntary movements had partly its cause in this condition of the cord, but there was also another cause of paralysis—the spasmodic flexion of the limbs. As regards Case 41, although there was a softening of the walls of the lateral ventricles, we think the principal cause of the paralysis was in the spinal cord. If we remark that there was no hyperæsthesia (as we know that hyperæsthesia always exists in diseases of the posterior columns, unless there is a cause of diminution of sensibility, which reduces hyperæsthesia so much that the degree of sensibility seems to be normal), and if we remark also that the gray matter is said to have been paler and less distinct than natural, we have sufficient explanation of the paralysis, without admitting that the whole of it was due to the alteration of the posterior columns.

Now we must point out a capital distinction which relates to the extent (in length) of the alteration in the posterior columns. If the alteration is very little extended, it allows reflex actions to take

[1] For other remarks on this interesting case, I will refer to Lecture V.

place; but if, for instance, it extends to the whole of the lumbar swelling, it prevents these actions, and as walking, standing, &c., cannot be perfected without them, it follows that there is a degree of apparent paralysis of voluntary movements. If the alteration extends to the whole length of the posterior columns, the loss of reflex action in the muscles of the limbs renders their voluntary movements much less powerful. It is not so in cases in which the alteration of the posterior columns occupies only a small part of their length (as in Cases 6, 7, 8 and 11); reflex action persisting, voluntary movements are hardly diminished.

It might be supposed that there are some of the voluntary motor conductors that pass into the posterior columns for a short distance, so that an alteration existing in the whole length of these columns destroys all these conductors, while a local alteration destroys but very few of them. It may be so, but we do not see any proof of it, either in experiments or in pathological cases.

It remains now to examine what kind of alteration in voluntary movements there is in cases of alteration of the posterior columns. When the posterior roots are also altered, there is an absence of the power of guiding the movements which renders walking almost completely impossible (see Cases 2 and 3). When in bed, the patients, looking at their limbs, can make any movements; but they cannot walk, or stand on their feet, and when their eyes are shut they can hardly make the least movement.

From the facts we have just discussed, and from the reasonings we have exposed, it results—

1st. That a complete loss of voluntary movements is not a symptom depending upon an alteration limited to the posterior columns,

2d. That in cases of alterations limited to the posterior columns, but occupying all their length and thickness, or only the whole of the lumbar swelling, there is an impossibility of standing or walking, depending upon the loss of the reflex actions of the limbs; but that, in bed, the patients in such cases can move their lower limbs pretty freely.

3d. That there is no loss of the reflex actions of the limbs, and that the voluntary movements persist in cases of alteration of the posterior columns, limited to a small part of their length.

Physiologists and medical men agree in admitting that deep alterations of the anterior columns of the spinal cord always cause a more or less complete paralysis of voluntary movements. They may be right in this view as long as we consider only what relates to these columns in the dorsal and lumbar regions; but, as we have tried to prove, by experiments on animals (see Lecture IV.), this view is wrong as regards the anterior columns in the upper part of the cervical region. Anatomy, experiments upon animals, and pathological cases, contribute, each and all, to prove that the anterior columns in the neighborhood of the medulla oblongata are not the channels for the orders of the will to muscles.

In the first place, it is well known that the decussating part of the anterior pyramids of the medulla oblongata is almost entirely composed of fibres coming from the lateral columns of the spinal cord. Some anatomists have even gone so far as to say that none of the decussating fibres of the pyramids proceed into the anterior columns of the opposite side.[1] Now experiments have shown to me that the section of the anterior columns of the spinal cord, near the medulla oblongata, does not affect, in a very marked manner, the voluntary movements; while, on the contrary, a section of the lateral columns usually produces a complete paralysis of the voluntary movements.

Clinical observation teaches, as I have already shown (see Lecture VII.), that an alteration of a lateral half of the pons Varolii or of the medulla oblongata, above the decussation of the anterior pyramids, causes a paralysis of voluntary movements in the opposite side of the body, and not at all in the corresponding side. This fact, assuredly, proves that the decussation of the fibres employed in voluntary movements takes place entirely below the place altered, because if the decussation were not achieved below this place, there would be some degree of paralysis in the side of the body corresponding to the side altered in the basis of the encephalon—which is not the case—and the paralysis in the opposite side would not be complete, which also is not the case. From these facts we could, therefore, conclude already, that the anterior columns of the spinal cord near the medulla oblongata are not the channels for the orders of the will to muscles, as anatomy shows that these columns do not decussate in the lower part of the medulla oblongata. It might be said, however, that these columns, perhaps, make their decussation in the spinal cord itself; but this hypothesis is disproved by many pathological cases, showing that

[1] See the remarkable paper of Dr. J. Reid, on the Anatomy of the Medulla Oblongata, in his "Physiological, Anat., and Pathol. Researches," 1848, p. 307.

an alteration of a lateral half of the spinal cord causes a loss of voluntary movements only in the corresponding side.

In Fig. 22 may be seen what ought to be the results of an alteration of a lateral half of the medulla oblongata, if we admit one of the three following opinions: 1st. That the anterior columns of the spinal cord are the only channels for voluntary movements. 2d. That the lateral columns are the only channels for these movements. 3d. That these two parts of the spinal cord have almost an equal share in this function.

If we suppose an alteration occupying the whole lateral half of the medulla oblongata (as in Cases 38 and 39), the loss of voluntary movements would be only in the right side of the body, if the first of the three opinions just exposed were the true one; on the contrary, we find that the paralysis is in the left side of the body. Were the third opinion the true one, there would be paralysis in the right side of the body, on account of the alteration of the anterior column (A A, Fig. 22), and paralysis in the left side on account of the alteration of the anterior pyramid, which is the continuation of the left lateral column of the spinal cord. This is not what takes place, the paralysis being only in the left side. It results that we must admit the second opinion—which is, that the lateral columns of the spinal cord, near their decussation, are the channels for the orders of the will to muscles, adding, however, that most probably there are some conductors for this influence of the will in the gray matter. (See Lecture VII.)

This view concerning the anterior and the lateral columns, near the medulla oblongata, is also borne out by cases of disease of the spinal cord, as well as by cases of alterations in the medulla oblongata. I will relate, as a decisive proof, a very interesting case which has been observed and published by one of the most able physiologists of our age, the late Dr. John Reid.

CASE 42.—G. S——, aged thirty, was admitted into the Infirmary of Edinburgh, on the 29th of June, 1840. For many months he had felt pains in the lumbar region, in several joints, and in the back of the neck, and his head was turned towards the right shoulder. He had pains in both arms, from the shoulder to the elbow, and the forearm and hand felt numb and stiff. He complained much of cold sweats. Pulse, quick and small. On the 7th of July, pulse 46. On the 11th and 12th, skin warm. In August increased headache. The symptoms much the same until October, when he was attacked by typhus fever, and died. He was able *to rise up to stool* during this attack, which lasted six days.

Autopsy.—The spinal cord was compressed opposite the upper part of the second cervical vertebra by a conical exostosis, about one-third of an inch in length, growing from the posterior part of the root of the odontoid process. This exostosis had produced a marked depression in the centre of the spinal cord, *immediately below the decussation of the pyramidal bodies.* On cutting into the cord at this part, the whole of the central portion was found to consist of a soft, reddish-brown pulp. The only part of the cord which here appeared healthy, was a thin layer of the lateral portions, varying in thickness in different parts, but in some places not thicker than one line. (*Physiol., Anat., and Pathol. Researches,* by J. Reid, 1848, p. 418.)

Dr. Reid says: "In this case we find that though the whole of the central portion of the spinal cord was in a state of *ramollissement,* from the effects of external pressure, the portion of the cord thus altered could nevertheless transmit downwards the motive influence of volition and of the excito-motory respiratory movements, and convey upwards those impressions which excite sensations." Dr. Reid does not say *when* he ascertained that sensibility and voluntary movements were still existing. As regards volition, it is probable, from his saying that five days before death "the stools were *now* passed in bed," that it was before that time that the patient had been able to rise up to stool. The softening found was certainly an inflammatory one, and it is most probable that the inflammation began only a day or two before death. But there is one thing beyond question: it is that the anterior columns of the spinal cord, which were the first parts exposed to the pressure from the exostosis, must have been crushed for a long while. In this respect this case is a decisive one, and it positively proves that near the medulla oblongata the anterior columns contain hardly any fibre used in voluntary movements.

As a complement to this case, we might relate cases showing that an alteration of the anterior part of the medulla oblongata causes paralysis. The contrast, indeed, is striking between the case of Dr. Reid and cases of alteration of the anterior pyramids: at a distance of a few lines one from the other, an alteration of the anterior part of the spinal cord hardly causes paralysis, and an alteration of the anterior pyramids, on the contrary, causes a complete paralysis. So it was in many cases, and particularly in one recorded by Dr. R. Bright,[1] and in another by Professor Lebert.[2]

There are so many cases on record in which the anterior columns of the spinal cord (in the lumbar and dorsal regions and in the lower part of the cervical region), were alone altered, and in which the voluntary movements were lost, and many of these cases are so well known, that it is useless to relate any of them. We will merely say that the paralysis is not absolutely complete in all these cases.

Before we leave the subject of paralysis of the voluntary movements, we must say that this symptom exists also in cases of alteration of the gray matter. We will refer, as a proof of the correctness of this assertion, to the cases of alteration of the gray matter that we have related. (See Lecture VI., Case 27, and several others, which are mentioned after this one, and Lecture VII., Cases 28 and 31.)

In summing up now all that relates to paralysis of movement in connection with the alterations of the various parts of the spinal cord, we find—

1st. That it is not an essential symptom of an alteration of the posterior columns.

2d. That it is an essential symptom of an alteration of the anterior columns everywhere, except in the upper part of the spinal cord, near the medulla oblongata.

3d. That it is an essential symptom of an alteration of the lateral columns, near their decussation at the upper part of the spinal cord, and, perhaps, not in the other parts of this organ.

4th. That it is an essential symptom of an alteration of the whole central part of the gray matter.

These results lead to the conclusion that a paralysis of voluntary movements alone could not be of service in the diagnosis of the place altered in the spinal cord; but we will show hereafter that various modifications in the degree, in the extent and place, and in the kind of a paralysis of voluntary movements, and the co-existence of this symptom with others, &c., are able to guide more or less surely in the diagnosis of the seat, and, also, of the nature of an alteration in the spinal cord.

We pass now to conclusions relating to the different kinds of

[1] Reports of Medical Cases, vol. ii. p. 548–9.

[2] In Traité des Maladies de la Moelle, by Ollivier, vol. i. p. 455.

anæsthesia in cases of alteration of various parts of the spinal cord. We have shown that a loss of sensibility is not a symptom depending upon an alteration of the posterior columns of this organ in any part of their length, and that this symptom, on the contrary, chiefly belongs to alterations of the central gray matter. It remains to examine if there is some difference between the various kinds of sensitive impressions as regards their place of passage in the spinal cord.

There are many cases on record showing that the loss of each of the various kinds of sensibility of the skin may exist alone, the other kinds continuing to exist. For a long while several cases of this species of anæsthesia have been known, but it is only recently that their relation with alterations of the spinal cord has been observed.

We think, and for many years already we have tried to prove, that the nerve-fibres employed in the transmission of each of the following sensitive impressions are as distinct one from the other as they all are from the nerve-fibres employed in the transmission of the orders of the will to muscles. We have not time enough to give the reasons we have for adopting this view: we will merely state that of the three hypotheses that may be made to explain a loss of one or of a few only of the following sensations, there is but one which agrees with the facts at present known; and we repeat that this one is, that the conductors of the various sensitive impressions are distinct one from another. The kinds of sensitive impressions which have different conductors are those giving the sensations of *touch*, *tickling*, *pain*, *heat* and *cold*, and the peculiar sensation which accompanies muscular contraction.

The following analysis of many cases of alteration of the spinal cord shows that there is probably, in this organ, a special place of passage of some of these impressions, and that their principal channel is the gray matter.

1. Loss of tactile sensibility, loss of the faculty of feeling pinching, pricking, and the passage of a very powerful galvanic current (and, therefore, loss of muscular sensibility). Persistence of the power of feeling cold and tickling. (See for the autopsy, Case 24, Lecture VI.)

From this case, as also from a few others, we can draw the conclusions: 1st, that the conductors of the impressions of cold and tickling do not pass in the same parts of the spinal cord as those of the other sensitive impressions; 2d, that the conductors of cold and tickling impressions are not excitable by a galvanic current, as the passage of a powerful current in the skin did not produce the least sensation.

2. Loss of feeling, a tickling, or a contact. Persistence of feeling of pain. No mention of other sensations. (See for autopsy, Case 23, Lecture VI.)

Here also we have a proof that the various conductors of sensitive impressions do not pass in the same part of the spinal cord; but, unfortunately, this case, like the preceding, does not lead to any view as to what parts are employed for the different sensations. In both cases the cord was flattened and softened by tubercles pressing upon its posterior surface. In these cases, however, the posterior columns of the cord were more altered than any other part, as the tubercles pressed directly upon them. We are, therefore, entitled to draw the conclusion, that the persisting kinds of sensibility have not their conductors in these columns. In a case recorded by my friend, M. Laboulbène (see Case 22, Lecture VI.), not only were the posterior columns altered, but all the rest of the white parts of the spinal cord, and the various kinds of sensibility persisted. This fact shows that it is chiefly in the gray matter (which, in that case, was not altered), that the various sensitive impressions pass.

3. Loss of tactile sensibility in the fingers of the left hand; diminution of this sensibility in the two upper limbs, and particularly the left one. Increased sensibility to painful impressions. (See for autopsy, Case 13, Lecture V.)

It might be concluded from this case, that tactile impressions pass through the posterior columns which were altered; but the persistence of the tactile sensibility, in cases of alteration of these columns, is so frequent that certainly there was some peculiar alteration in that case producing that kind of anæsthesia.

4. In a very interesting case, recorded by Dr. W. Budd (*Medico-Chirurgical Transactions*, vol. xxii. p. 170), there was no sensation produced by heat, while contact was felt. The spinal cord had been injured in the cervical region; but the patient having recovered, we do not know what was the part altered.

5. Loss of feeling of pain or pinching; diminished sensibility to cold and heat, and touch. Fracture of the seventh cervical vertebra, and softening of the spinal cord. (Ollivier, *loc. cit.*, vol. i. p. 287.)

Most unfortunately, medical men usually neglect noticing the state of the various kinds of sensibility in cases of disease of the spinal cord. It is interesting, therefore, to collect the cases in which there is mention of some, if not all, the kinds of sensibility. We give here a list of some of such cases.

6. Return of general sensibility of the skin (probably to contact and pain), and of muscular sense. Local destruction of posterior columns. (See Case 8, Lecture V.)

7. All kinds of sensibility persisting. Alteration of the posterior columns. (Case 9, Lecture V.)

8. Scratching, pricking, and pinching the skin were felt. Alteration of the posterior columns. (Case 14, Lecture V.)

9. Touch and painful impressions acutely felt, as also any change of temperature. Alteration of the posterior columns, and slightly of the rest of the cord. (Case 16, Lecture V.)

10. All kinds of sensibility persisting. The whole of the white substance of the cord altered. (Case 22, Lecture VI.)

We might add to this list of facts, many cases of alteration of the anterior or of the lateral columns of the spinal cord, in which it has been noted that touch, heat and cold, and painful impressions have continued to be felt. But it is unnecessary to mention cases so frequent as those are.

Now, on the other hand, in some of the cases of alteration of the gray matter that we have related in the preceding lectures, it has been noted that there was a loss of the various kinds of sensibility.

From this review of facts, it results that what we have said of sensibility generally, may be applied to its various kinds. The gray matter is the principal channel of the various sensitive impressions, and the posterior columns are not the channels for any kind of these impressions. Therefore, as a means of diagnosis of the place where an alteration exists in the spinal cord, any kind of anæsthesia cannot be considered as a symptom of alteration of the posterior columns; while, on the contrary, the loss of one kind of sensibility, another kind remaining, may serve, as we will show hereafter, as a means of diagnosis of an alteration of the gray matter of the spinal cord.

Before proceeding farther, we must state that there are three series of facts to be added to those already mentioned, and leading to the same conclusions, concerning the place of passage of the various kinds of sensitive impressions in the spinal cord. The first of these series of facts includes the cases of alteration of a lateral half of the spinal cord, producing anæsthesia in the opposite side of the body. Of course, if the posterior columns, which have no decussation, were the conductors of any of the various kinds of sensitive impressions to the brain, we should find that in the side injured the peculiar kind of impressions supposed to be transmitted by the posterior columns is no more transmitted; while, on the contrary, transmission should continue to take place for impressions made upon the opposite side of the body. But it is not so.

In the first place, as regards the two kinds of sensitive impressions which are usually made—those which give a tactile sensation and a sensation of pain—we may be sure that the posterior columns are not their conductors, as these two kinds of sensibility existed in the side injured, and were lost or much diminished in the opposite side, in all the cases of alteration of a lateral half of the spinal cord that we know, in which the state of sensibility in the two sides of the body has been noted. (See Cases 29, 30, 31, 35, and several others, in Lecture VII.)

In the second place, we find that, of the other kinds of sensibility, which have been noticed in one case, the same thing has existed as for the two kinds just spoken of. Unfortunately, however, this is a case in which the injury to the spinal cord is not exactly known. Cold and heat and tickling in that case (see Lecture VII., Case 32), were not felt on the side opposite to that of the principal injury to the spinal cord, and were felt on the corresponding side. It seems, therefore, that the conductors of the various kinds of sensitive impressions decussate in the spinal cord, and consequently that none of them go up to the brain along the posterior columns which have no decussation, and are lying close beside each other, unable to have communication together except through the gray matter. It remains to be known, however, at what place the decussation exists for the conductors of the various kinds of sensitive impressions. This will be positively determined only by future cases; but we can already say that for all the kinds of conductors, except one, the place of decussation seems to be in the immediate neighborhood of the entrance of the posterior roots in the spinal cord. The conductors of the kind of sensitive impressions that originate in muscles when they contract—impressions which, on being felt, guide our movements—these conductors, perhaps, decussate very high in the spinal cord. This seems to be shown by the fact, that in most of the cases of alteration of a lateral half of the spinal cord that we have reported, the voluntary movements are said to have been free in the opposite side of the body, which would not have existed if the *guiding sensation* had not been felt. In one of the cases, however (Case 37), the patient had lost that peculiar muscular sensibility which guides voluntary movements, as she could not hold her child in her arm when she did not look at that arm.[1] But as we do not know what was the precise place of the alteration in this case, we cannot draw a positive conclusion from it.

We shall not insist on the second and third series of facts which militate against the view that there is at least some kind of sensitive impression going up to the brain along the posterior columns of the spinal cord. These columns go chiefly to the cerebellum, and a small part only of their fibres pass through the pons Varolii. Now, we find that, in a great many cases of alteration of the cerebellum, there is no loss of *any kind* of sensibility, while, on the contrary, in cases of alteration of the pons Varolii, there is a loss of *all kinds* of sensibility; and, still more, the loss is only in the side of the body opposite to the side of the alteration, if it occupies only a lateral half of the pons. These two series of facts concerning the cerebellum and the pons Varolii, united with the facts concerning the medulla oblongata (see Cases 38 and 39, Lecture VII.) and the spinal cord, constitute such a mass of proofs against the view that the posterior columns are not the channels to the brain of any of the various kinds of sensitive impressions, that we think it useless to insist any more on this point.[2]

From the above discussion, and also from facts that we have not time enough to relate, we draw the following conclusions:—

[1] It might be said that the sensibility of the skin being lost in this case, the impossibility of holding the child arose from this cutaneous anæsthesia. There is a decisive reply to this objection; it is, that muscular sensibility alone is sufficient for the direction of voluntary movements. I have seen a child completely deprived of cutaneous sensibility (unable to feel contact, pressure, pricking, pinching, tickling, cold, and heat), yet able to walk well without looking at his feet, and undoubtedly owing this power to the persistence of guiding sensations in the muscles. In this case, besides the peculiar sensibility which guides voluntary movements, the muscles had the power of giving pain. When they were excited to contract spasmodically, the patient had the feeling of pain which exists in cramps.

[2] We have insisted much on this subject, on account of the recent assertions made by an able experimentalist, M. Moritz Schiff, who, after having long maintained that the posterior columns transmit tactile and painful impressions, has given up one-half of this view, and now affirms that they transmit tactile impressions, while the gray matter transmits painful impressions. Pathological cases are quite in opposition to this view, and so are experiments upon animals, as we have already shown. (See Lecture IV.)

1st. Anæsthesia, in cases of disease of the spinal cord, is a symptom indicating that the gray matter is altered. This conclusion seems to hold good also with respect to the loss of each of the various kinds of sensibility.

2d. Alterations, limited to either of the white columns of the spinal cord, do not cause anæsthesia of any kind.

3d. Anæsthesia, limited to one-half of the body, in cases of disease of the spinal cord, is a symptom indicating that the gray matter in the opposite half of the cord is altered, except in cases of which we will now say a few words.

We have said already that anæsthesia alone—*i. e.*, without a paralysis of voluntary movements—is not a symptom of disease of the spinal cord, or at least of ordinary diseases of the organ, as we have acknowledged that there are two kinds of alterations that might produce a much more marked anæsthesia than a paralysis of voluntary motion, and even, perhaps, diminish voluntary movements almost only on account of the anæsthesia produced. One of these alterations would be an injury or a morbid transformation all along the posterior horns in which the posterior roots pass before going to the other parts of the spinal cord. In such a case there would be anæsthesia on the side where the alteration exists, if it is limited to one side of the cord, and the loss of sensibility would be localized to those parts which receive their sensitive nerve-fibres from the regions altered; so that, below and above, sensibility might exist. We do not know of a single case of this kind; some, however, may have been observed.

The other cause of anæsthesia, without paralysis of voluntary movements, consists in an injury to the decussating conductors of sensitive impressions in the spinal cord. Suppose, for instance, a sword introduced from below upwards, or in the opposite direction, in the spinal cord, and dividing this organ in its two lateral halves, and producing as little injury as possible to its anterior columns. The decussating fibres being then divided, sensibility would be lost in all the parts of the body from which these fibres come. It is hardly possible to conceive the production of such an injury, which is made with so much difficulty even in experimenting. But sometimes disease causes almost this kind of injury; for instance, a softening beginning in the very place where the decussation exists; or a slow increase of the amount of water in the central canal of the spinal cord may produce a greater diminution of sensibility than of voluntary movements. This is what occurs not rarely in the beginning of softening of the spinal cord, and in cases of spina bifida with hydrorachis. It would be very interesting to look for this symptom in cases of *diplomyelia.* Our learned friend Mr. Depaul has seen sensibility lost and voluntary movements partly preserved, in a case of division of the spinal cord (diplomyelia). This is a fact well worthy of attention, as it realizes in man what is shown in the most important of the experiments which I have shown in the preceding lectures.

We do not need to say that anæsthesia may be due to alterations of the posterior roots, and to the nerve-fibres of the various sensitive nerves in any part of their length. We do not need, also, to remind our hearers that anæsthesia may be due to diseases of the encephalon, to poisoning by lead, arsenic, belladonna, &c. But there is a kind of anæsthesia which is much less known, and about which we must say a few words. This peculiar anæsthesia depends upon a morbid reflex action; it may arise in diseases of all the viscera, and also from irritations upon any sensitive nerve, in any part of its course. If time allows, we will, in another lecture, give many illustrations of this kind of anæsthesia; at present, we will merely relate a curious case as an example of this affection.

CASE 43.—A man became paralyzed of sensibility in the whole left side of the body. Voluntary movements were only diminished. He stated that, fifteen years before, he had received a shot in the left side of the lumbar region. The ball had met with the last rib, followed it beneath the skin, and gone out at the level of the first lumbar vertebra, which, probably, had been fractured. The wounds quickly healed; but hardly had this taken place, when the patient perceived that a loss of sensibility began in the neighborhood of the cicatrix, and gradually extended from that to other parts. The wound in the lumbar region was opened, and sensibility reappeared, and from this time he was well: but at every time cicatrization was near being completed, he had threatening of a return of anæsthesia. At last the wound healed definitively, and then his condition was as above described. Four blisters in the neighborhood of the scar cured him. (Roche, in *Archives de Médec.*, Fév. 1823, vol. i. p. 262; and in Ollivier, *loco cit.*, vol. i. p. 360.)

This case assuredly is not an instance of anæsthesia due to an injury of the spinal cord, as the alteration, if there has been any in this organ, was in the lumbar region, and the loss of sensibility was in the whole left side of the body. Anæsthesia in this case was the result of a reflex influence on the nutrition of the sensitive nerves of the left side, due to an irritation of the sensitive nerve-fibres of the first lumbar nerve, as we shall prove in another lecture.

M. H. Romberg[1] lays great stress upon interesting facts recorded by Daniellsen and Bœck, to prove that alterations of the posterior columns of the spinal cord cause anæsthesia. It would be easy to show that no conclusion of this kind can be drawn from the facts observed by these physicians. In their important work upon Elephantiasis Græcorum,[2] they state that the posterior roots of the spinal nerves, and also the gray matter, are altered, and that sometimes the whole of the spinal cord is atrophied or hardened—alterations which sufficiently explain the anæsthesia observed in leprosy.

We now pass to another question, which is: How is it that sensibility is not lost in some parts of the body, in cases of considerable alteration of parts of the spinal cord; which we admit to be conductors of sensitive impressions? We have already given a solution to this question, by experiments which we have mentioned in one of the preceding lectures. (See Lecture IV.) Taking notice only of the conductors of painful impressions, we may imagine them scattered in the spinal cord, without any order whatever, or having there one of the two following dispositions: they may be so distributed, that those coming from the anterior surface of the body form a distinct layer in the cord, and so on for those from the posterior surface, or for any other longitudinal part of the body; or they may be arranged so that each layer of conductors, in the spinal cord, contains conducting elements from the anterior, the middle, and the posterior parts of the body. This last disposition is the one that seems to exist according to our experiments and to pathological cases. In this respect, pathology clearly shows that an alteration, of any limited part of the zone of the spinal cord, by which sensitive impressions are transmitted to the encephalon, does not produce anæsthesia, in any limited part of the body, below the place where the alteration lies. Pathology shows, on the other hand, that, when incomplete anæsthesia exists, it is in the same degree or very nearly so in all the parts which receive their sensitive nerves below the place altered, and whatever may be the part of the conducting zone that is altered. If any part of the skin, for

[1] Lehrbuch der Nervenkrankheiten, Bd. i. 3d ed., 1853, p. 317 et seq.

[2] Traité de la Spédalskhed, Paris, 1848, pp. 283–286.

instance, is connected with the sensorium by a hundred conductors of sensitive impressions, these conductors are not in a bundle in the spinal cord; they seem also not to be scattered without order in several parts of this organ. On the contrary, we may deduce from vivisections and pathological facts, that they are distributed in good order in all the parts of the conducting zone of the spinal cord.

In this way we can explain easily why sensibility is so rarely lost in cases of deep alteration of the spinal cord. But there is another cause to be added to this one, and explaining why anæsthesia may seem not to exist, where even one-third, one-half, or more of the conductors of sensitive impressions have been altered so much that they lose their function entirely. This is the hyperæsthesia, to which it is due that the sensitive impressions, transmitted by the remaining conductors, are felt with such an intensity that the cause of diminution of sensibility is more than compensated.

It seems extremely probable that, in a certain measure, what we have just said of painful impressions, is true also of the other kinds of sensitive impressions; but pathology shows that, besides a distribution of many of their conductors, in various parts of the conducting zone of the spinal cord, there is a place, and a special one, for each kind of these impressions, where there is an aggregation of many of their conductors. Much is to be discovered in this respect, and I hope that the opportunities of throwing light on this subject will not exist in vain in the future.

We may deduce, from the preceding discussion, that anæsthesia, existing in a limited part of the body, whether alone or with paralysis of voluntary movements, cannot be considered as a symptom of a local affection of the spinal cord, unless it be an alteration of the posterior gray horns destroying the posterior roots at their place of entrance, or an alteration of the gray matter in its centre destroying the conductors of sensitive impressions at the place where they decussate on the median line. (See Case 28, Lecture VII.)

There is a symptom of disease of the spinal cord, the study of which is full of interest, both in a physiological and a practical point of view: I mean the referring to the peripheral termination of conductors of sensitive impressions, the impressions made on them in any part of their length. As regards the trunks of nerves, it is well known that usually impressions on them are referred to the periphery. We have no time now to examine why it is usually so, and why, in so many cases, there are exceptions to this law. We will only examine what relates to the spinal cord concerning this phenomenon.

Taking as true for a moment the old view that the spinal cord contains nerve-fibres, which are the continuation of those of the posterior roots and of the nerves of the sensitive parts of the body, and possessing the same properties in this nervous centre as in these roots and nerves, what ought to be the result of pressure on this organ? According to the seat of the pressure, there ought to be pain felt as if it originated from a more or less considerable part of the body. We have read carefully the details of a great many cases of fracture or luxation of the spine, or of tumors pressing upon the spinal cord; we have also carefully questioned many patients, and we can state that the *referring to the periphery* is rare, and that it never exists unless the posterior roots are irritated or the spinal cord inflamed.

There is a remarkable fact concerning this *error loci*, in regard to the place irritated. The gray matter is not excitable in its normal condition, so that a pressure upon it cannot give origin to any sensation, and it is therefore very natural that a fractured or dislocated bone, pressing even much upon the whole spinal cord, and consequently upon its gray matter, should not cause sensations referred to all the parts of the body below the place compressed. But when inflammation has set in, it is not rare that this gray matter acquires the property of being excitable, and that then the pressure acts upon this matter, and causes that peculiar feeling called formication, and sometimes a pain, the character of which varies very much.

The referring of sensations to the periphery of the body, in diseases of the spinal cord, is a fact of great practical value. I hope, therefore, I shall be allowed to say a few words more on this subject.

If we inquire into the differences between the various conductors of the five kinds of sensitive impressions that may come from the different parts of the body, leaving aside the four higher senses and the peculiar sensation given by the genital organs, we find that, as regards their excitability, they differ extremely in different parts of their length, and also one from the other. We have shown, nearly six years ago,[1] that the degree of excitability of the conductors of painful impressions varies very much in the different parts of their length: they have no excitability in the central gray matter of the

[1] Experimental Researches applied to Physiology and Pathology. New York, 1853, p. 98.

cord, and they have the maximum of excitability in the part of the posterior roots attached to the cord, and the minimum in their passage through the ganglions. But it seems that some of them, ending in bones, in muscles, &c., have no excitability, except in their peripheric extremity; at least, when we press upon the trunk of a nerve in the arm or the leg, we find that there is but very little pain, if any, *referred* to muscles, bones, and some other parts. It seems probable, therefore, that a number of conductors of painful impressions have no excitability—at least, to a mechanical irritation—in some parts of their length, in nerves.

As regards the conductors of the other kinds of sensitive impressions, they seem to have no excitability at all, in the normal condition, in any part of their length, except at their termination in the skin or in muscles. E. H. Weber has shown,[1] that in a part that has lost its skin, there is a loss of feeling cold, heat, and touch. Perhaps, however, it would be right to make an exception for the conductors of impressions of tickling, in the trunks of nerves, as a certain degree of pressure upon them gives a feeling of tickling that we refer to the periphery. But whatever may be admitted in regard to this fact, there is something concerning, not only this kind of conductors, but also all the others, which seems quite certain. It is, that they all may acquire, particularly, if not exclusively, under the influence of inflammation, the power of being excitable, and of giving sensitive impressions which are referred to the periphery. This change may take place in all their length, from their terminal ramification in the different parts of the body, to their origin in different parts of the brain—*i. e.*, in the branches and trunks of nerves, in the gray matter of the spinal cord, in the medulla oblongata, the pons Varolii, and most of the other parts of the encephalon. This is true with respect to the conductors of the *guiding muscular sensations*, as also those of impressions of cold and heat, as well as the other kinds of conductors. If I had time, I could relate many cases in proof of this assertion. I will only mention two or three at present, and I will point out some others when I treat of the medulla oblongata and pons Varolii.

In an interesting case of tumor in the midst of the cauda equina, and pressing particularly on the posterior roots of the nerves of the left lower limb, there was a complete loss of sensibility in this limb; nevertheless, the patient complained strongly of a feeling of

[1] Wagner's Handwörterbuch der Physiol., vol. iii. Part ii. 1846, p. 498.

heat in the parts. (Dr. W. W. Fisher, in *Trans. of the Prov. Assoc.*, vol. x., and in *Philad. Med. Examiner*, 1842, p. 361.)

In a case recorded by Gall (*Sur les Fonctions du Cerveau*, vol. vi. 1825, p. 284), there was the feeling of a burning fire in the chest, the throat, and the tongue; the anterior parts of the spinal cord were very much inflamed, in the cervical and in the lumbar regions.

In a case of fracture of the twelfth dorsal vertebra, with considerable compression of the spinal cord, there was complete loss of sensibility, with a sense of burning in the legs. (Case recorded by Dr. Gay, in *A Descriptive Catalogue of the Boston Museum*, by J. B. S. Jackson, 1847, p. 30.)

It is of some importance, for the diagnosis of the locality of disease in the spinal cord, to bear in mind that sensations felt as if they came from the periphery, whatever be their kind, are not due to some irritation of the posterior columns, but to changes that take place in the gray matter, in consequence of an inflammation. This is the general conclusion to be drawn from all the facts I know concerning sensations referred to the periphery in cases of alteration of the spinal cord.

I should like to speak of the various other symptoms of disease of the spinal marrow; but, as I have but little time, and also as I shall have another opportunity of explaining some of these symptoms (such as hyperæsthesia, convulsions, cramps, and reflex actions), I will pass at once to the enunciation of the groups of symptoms existing in the cases of disease of the spinal cord, according to the place and extent of the alteration. I leave aside the symptoms concerning the movements of the heart, respiration, the state of the sphincters, animal heat, and nutrition.

1st. *Deep alteration of the posterior columns in all their length.*—Increased sensibility in the trunk and limbs for impressions of touch, or due to pricking, pinching, and galvanic excitations, and for changes of temperature (cold and heat). Loss, or a very great diminution, of reflex movements. All kinds of voluntary movements possible, and more or less easily executed when the patient is in bed. Walking and standing very difficult.[1]

[1] On account of the loss of reflex action, and of the morbid sensibility, and also on account of the alteration in the *guiding sensations* coming from muscles—alteration which is due to two causes, one of which is the loss of action of some of these conductors altered in the posterior columns through which they pass before reaching the gray matter, while the other is the morbid increase of sensibility of those conductors which go directly into gray matter.

2d. *Deep alteration of the posterior columns in the extent of the cervico-branchial swelling.*—Increased sensibility in the four limbs, and in the trunk, for all kinds of impressions. Diminution of reflex actions in the upper limbs, and increased reflex actions in the lower limbs. Some difficulty in the direction of the movements of the upper limbs, without the help of the sight. Standing and walking possible without any great difficulty.

3d. *Deep alteration of the posterior columns in the extent of the dorso-lumbar swelling.*—Increased sensibility in the lower limbs, and normal sensibility in the upper ones. Diminution or loss of reflex actions in the lower limbs. Movements of lower limbs possible, and even easy, when the patient is in bed; but walking and standing very difficult.

4th. *Deep alteration of a very limited part of the posterior columns.*—Increased sensibility, and increased reflex action, in all parts receiving their nerves from the spinal cord below the alteration. Voluntary movements possible, and even easy, everywhere. The place of the alteration may be detected by diminution of reflex actions in the zone round the body receiving nerves from the level of the part altered in the posterior columns.

5th. *Alteration of the posterior columns and posterior roots of the spinal nerves.*—Instead of hyperæsthesia, as in the preceding cases, diminution or loss of all kinds of sensibility, in places receiving the spinal nerves, which are the continuation of the altered roots. Voluntary movements still possible, in bed, and while the patient looks at his limbs, but walking and standing almost impossible. Reflex actions *completely* lost in all the anæsthetic parts. If the alterations are in the upper parts of the spinal cord, the other parts being healthy, then voluntary movements in the lower limbs, and even walking or standing, are possible, and may be easy, and these limbs have an increased sensibility and increased reflex actions.

6th. *Alteration of the posterior columns and of the gray matter in all their length.*—There is no difference between this case and the preceding, except that here there is a real paralysis of voluntary movements, which is complete if the alteration extends to the anterior gray cornua. Greater frequency of formication and of other sensations referred to the periphery.

7th. *Alteration of the posterior columns and gray matter in any limited part of the spinal cord.*—Very nearly complete loss of sensibility. Degrees of paralysis of voluntary movements varying with the place occupied by the alteration in the length of the spinal cord.

Reflex actions increased in parts receiving their nerves from the portions of the cord below the seat of the alteration.

8th. *Alteration limited to the gray matter.*—The same symptoms as in the preceding cases, except that at first there is a greater degree of anæsthesia than of paralysis, if the alteration begins in the very centre of the cord. Formication and other sensations referred to the periphery, in cases of inflammation.

9th. *Alteration of the anterior columns in the upper part of the cervical region.*—No paralysis, no anæsthesia, very slight hyperæsthesia, various sensations (particular pain) referred to several parts of the body.

10th. *Alteration of the lateral columns in the upper part of the cervical region.*—Paralysis of voluntary movements in the four limbs and the trunk. Increased sensibility and greatly increased reflex actions in the paralyzed parts.

11th. *Alteration of the anterior columns in any part of their length, except the neighborhood of the medulla oblongata.*—More or less complete paralysis of voluntary movements in all the parts receiving their nerves from or below the parts of the cord where the alteration exists. Slight hyperæsthesia. Reflex actions very much diminished in the parts which receive their nerves from the altered portion of the cord, and increased below these parts.

12th. *Alteration of the lateral columns in any part of their length, except the neighborhood of the medulla oblongata.*—Incomplete paralysis of movements. Hyperæsthesia. Diminution of reflex actions less than in the preceding case.

13th. *Alteration of the anterior half of the spinal cord, including the anterior columns, a good part of the gray matter, and a part of the lateral columns.*—Voluntary movements completely paralyzed. Sensibility very much diminished. For reflex actions, as in 11th.

14th. *Alteration of the various parts of the spinal cord, except the posterior columns.*—Loss of voluntary movements and of all kinds of sensibility. Reflex actions increased or diminished in certain parts of the body, according to the place of the alteration in the length of the spinal cord.

I know many cases in which one of the two last kinds of alteration has existed. In another lecture, I will relate three of them, which have been recorded by Mr. Cæsar Hawkins, by Dr. John W. Ogle, and by Dr. T. Inman.

LECTURE IX.

ON THE PHYSIOLOGICAL AND MORBID ACTIONS DUE TO THE GREAT SYMPATHETIC NERVE.

Effects of a section of the sympathetic nerve in the cervical region.—Effects of the excitation of the same nerve, in the same region, by a galvanic or an electro-magnetic current.—Almost all the effects due to the section or galvanization of this nerve are owing to the condition of bloodvessels after these operations.—The sympathetic nerve originates chiefly from the cerebro-spinal axis.—Similitude between the effects of a section of the sympathetic nerve, and those of a section of a lateral half of the spinal cord.—Persistence of a contraction of bloodvessels due to irritation of the cerebro-spinal axis in certain diseases.—Two kinds of normal or morbid influences of the nervous system upon nutrition, secretion, &c.; one upon bloodvessels, the other upon tissues.

I PASS now to quite a different subject. In the preceding lectures, I have chiefly examined what relates to voluntary movements and sensibility; I come now to the influence of the nervous system upon nutrition, animal heat, secretions, &c., and I begin by the peculiar influences of the sympathetic nerve on these functions in health and disease.

Before entering into the subject of the influence of the nervous system upon the functions of organic life, it is necessary to state what are the effects of the section and of the galvanization of the cervical sympathetic nerve. I hope I may be allowed to fix some dates of publication of the principal discoveries in this respect. Prof. Cl. Bernard published the results of his first researches on the effects of the section of the cervical sympathetic nerve in 1851, and in the beginning of 1852.[1] The only great fact announced in these publications was, that this section was constantly followed by a considerable afflux of blood in the parts of the head to which the sympathetic goes. Led by experiments that I had made several years before, with my friend Dr. Tholozan, on the influence of

[1] Comptes rendus de la Soc. de Biol., Dec. 1851, in Gaz. Méd., 1852, p. 74.—Comptes rendus de l'Acad. des Sciences; séance du 29 Mars, 1852.

nerves on bloodvessels, I understood at once that the fact discovered by Prof. Bernard was due to the paralysis of the bloodvessels after the section of the sympathetic; and I thought that, if this view were right, I should find galvanization of this nerve producing the reverse of the effects of the section. The experiment being made, I found, as I had foreseen, that the bloodvessels contracted, and that the quantity of blood and the temperature diminished. The date of my first publication is Aug. 1st, 1852.[1] Three or four months afterwards, Prof. Bernard not knowing what I had done, announced to the Société de Biologie (in October and November, 1852), that he had seen galvanization of the sympathetic nerve diminish the quantity of the blood and the temperature, &c.[2] In February, 1853, a very able English physiologist, Dr. Augustus Waller, being unaware of what I had published, and of the more recent paper of Prof. Bernard, announced to the Academy of Sciences of Paris,[3] that he had found the galvanization of the sympathetic nerve producing effects opposite to those of its section; and he gave the same theory that I had already proposed—a theory which has since been admitted by almost all the physiologists who have written on this subject.

As I consider that the knowledge of the effects of the paralysis, and the irritation of the sympathetic nerve, opens a new and most important field in physiology, in pathology, and in therapeutics, I will give at length two lists of the phenomena which have been observed after the section and after the galvanization of the cervical sympathetic nerve.

I. *Effects of the Section of the Cervical Sympathetic Nerve.*

Phenomena observed in the head, on the side of the operation.	Authors who have made the first observation.
1. Constriction of the pupil	Pourfour du Petit.
2. The eye seems to be smaller, or even truly shrinks .	Idem.
3. The eye is drawn backwards and a little inwards .	Idem.
4. The eyelids are partially closed . . .	Idem.

[1] Philadelphia Medical Examiner, August, 1852, p. 489. This paper has been reprinted in my work, "Exper. Researches applied to Physiol. and Pathol." p. 9. New York, 1853.

[2] Comptes rendus de la Soc. de Biol., in Gaz. Méd., 1852, p. 775; and 1853, p. 71.

[3] Comptes rendus de l'Acad. des Sciences, séance du 28 Février, 1853.—I will, by and by, point out what had already been done as regards the influence of nerves on bloodvessels, by Stilling, Henle, Mr. James Paget, and Mr. Wharton Jones, before the researches of Prof. Bernard.

Phenomena observed in the head, on the side of the operation.	Authors who have made the first observation.
5. The third eyelid, or nictitant membrane, advances upon the globe of the eye, and sometimes extends over a part of the cornea.	Pourfour du Petit.
6. The production of the palpebral mucus is increased	Idem.
7. The cornea becomes flatter and dimmer	Idem.
8. Almost all the muscles of the eye are contracted	Bernard.
9. The muscles of the angle of the mouth and of the nostril are contracted	Idem.
10. The ear is kept erect, partly on account of the contraction of some of its muscles	Brown-Séquard.
11. There is an evident increase in the quantity of blood	Dupuy and Bernard.
12. The temperature is notably increased	Idem.
13. Sensibility is increased	Bernard.
14. When the animal is killed, the reflex faculty lasts longer there than in the other side	Idem.
15. Voluntary movements seem also to last longer.	Brown-Séquard.
16. Sensibility also lasts longer	Idem.
17. The reflex movements of the iris last longer	Idem.
18. The sense of hearing *seems* to be more acute	Idem.
19. The sensibility of the retina *seems* to be increased	Idem.
20. Perspiration (particularly from the ears in horses), is increased	Dupuy.
21. The secretion of cerumen is increased	Schiff.
22. The secretion of tears is increased	(?)
23. Absorption is more rapid	Bernard.
24. Chloroform destroys sensibility there later than elsewhere	Idem.
25. The color of venous blood is changed	Martini and Bernard.
26. The quantity of fat diminishes (?)	Martini.
27. The first convulsions, after poisoning by strychnia, take place there	Brown-Séquard.
28. A galvanic current, too weak to act on the other side, may produce contractions there	Idem.
29. The so-called recurrent sensibility of the facial nerve is increased	Idem.
30. The pressure of blood on the walls of the arteries is increased	Bernard.
31. After death the motor nerves of the face *seem* to remain excitable longer than on the other side	Brown-Séquard.
32. The muscles, also, and the iris remain contractile longer	Idem.
33. The irritability of the arteries, and particularly of the principal auricular, is increased, at least for several weeks after the operation, and it lasts longer after death	Idem.
34. Cadaveric rigidity comes later, and lasts longer	Idem.
35. Putrefaction comes later	Idem.
36. The galvanic current of the muscles, detected with the galvanoscopic frog, is stronger than in those of the other side	Idem.

Phenomena observed in the head on the side of the operation.	Authors who have made the first observation.
37. Injections of red blood by the carotid and vertebral arteries, after death, are able to regenerate the vital properties of the nervous and of the contractile tissues, later there than on the other side . .	Brown-Séquard.
38. Various pathological alterations may take place, chiefly in the eye	Petit, Molinelli, Mayer, J. Reid, &c.

I pass now to the list of phenomena observed after the galvanization of the cervical sympathetic.

Phenomena observed.	Discoverers.
1. Dilatation of the pupil	Aug. Waller & Budge.
2. The eyelids are wide opened, and the globe of the eye protrudes	Bernard.
3. The bloodvessels contract, and the quantity of blood diminishes	Brown-Séquard.
4. The temperature diminishes	Idem.
5. Sensibility diminishes	Idem.
6. The conjunctiva and the cornea become dry . .	Idem.
7. Strychnia produces less convulsions there than on the other side	Idem.
8. After death, the vital properties of the motor and sensitive nerves disappear there sooner than on the other side	Idem.
9. The irritability of the iris and of the muscles disappears also sooner after death	Idem.
10. The contractility of the arteries lasts less time after death	Idem.
11. The galvanic current given by the muscles is very weak	Idem.
12. Cadaveric rigidity comes sooner, and lasts less time .	Idem.
13. Putrefaction comes sooner	Idem.
14. The faculty of regeneration of the vital properties in the muscles of the face after cadaveric rigidity has appeared, is lost sooner than on the other side .	Idem.

It is evident that all these phenomena are just the reverse of those which follow the section of the cervical sympathetic.

The phenomena observed after the section or the galvanization of this nerve, with the exception of a few, may be summed up under the three following heads:—

Section of the Nerve.	*Galvanization of the Nerve.*
1. Dilatation of Bloodvessels.	1. Contraction of Bloodvessels.
2. Afflux of Blood.	2. Diminution of Blood.
3. Increase of Vital Properties.	3. Decrease of Vital Properties.

The view, that the section of the cervical sympathetic is followed by a paralysis of the bloodvessels, in consequence of which more blood passes through these vessels in a given time, producing the increase of the vital properties of the contractile and nervous tissues—this view is now admitted by almost all physiologists. It is based on a great many various experiments made by Dr. Aug. Waller, Donders, and several of his pupils, Kussmaul, and Tenner, Moritz, Schiff, and myself, showing that all the circumstances, whatever they may be, which cause an increase in the quantity of blood passing in the bloodvessels of the head in a given time, produce there almost all, if not all, the phenomena following the section of the cervical sympathetic. The hanging down of an animal, by holding it by its hind-legs, in producing a congestion in the head, produces very nearly all the effects of this section.[1]

We regret very much not having time to relate the most decisive proofs of the view that we hold. Many of these facts not only prove the correctness of our view, but they show the untenability of a *vitalistic* theory, according to which the normal actions of the sympathetic nerve would be increased after it has been divided, and diminished when it is excited by galvanism, and according to which, also, nutrition and animal heat would be dependent upon the sympathetic nerve, which would produce an increase of these two functions after it has been divided (although it then ought to cease to act), and a diminution of these functions when it is galvanized (although it then ought to act more than normally).

However, we are ready to acknowledge that there are other causes of active circulation in the head, after the section of the cervical sympathetic, besides the paralysis of the bloodvessels. The very fact that there is more blood producing an increase in nutrition and secretion—a fact which depends chiefly, as we have said, upon the paralysis of bloodvessels, produces an increase in the normal *suction-power* of the capillaries. In other words, the greater afflux of arterial blood is itself, through the increased chemical changes of nutrition and secretion, a cause of attraction of arterial blood.[2] To this cause another one of the same kind ought to be

[1] See my paper, "Sur les Effets de la Section et de la Galvanization du Grand Sympathique. Paris, 1854.

[2] For the demonstration of the normal attraction of arterial blood by the living tissues, and of the participation of capillaries in the causes of the circulation of blood, I will refer to the learned treatises on Human and Comparative Physiology of Prof. Carpenter; to the original works of Professor Draper, of New York; and, especially to a most able and complete treatise on the subject—although modestly published as a review—by Mr. W. S. Savory. (*Brit. and For. Med.-Chir. Rev.*, April and July, 1855.)

added: it is, that as there is more blood, the temperature is increased, and as the temperature is augmented, the chemical changes, which are a cause of attraction of blood, are also augmented. From this statement it may be concluded that the primitive, and, I may say, by far the principal, cause of augmentation in the afflux of blood, is the absence of contraction of the bloodvessels, which allows this liquid to pass easier there than elsewhere.

We now come to the question, What is the origin of the cervical sympathetic nerve? That most ingenious physiologist, Dr. Augustus Waller, has made experiments, with Prof. J. Budge, which seem to prove that the nerve-fibres of the cervical sympathetic that go to the iris originate from the spinal cord, between the sixth cervical and the fourth dorsal vertebræ. We have ascertained that the origins of the fibres of the sympathetic going to the iris are more extended than they thought. A section of a lateral half of the spinal cord at the level of the fifth, the sixth, and even sometimes as low down as the ninth or tenth, dorsal vertebra, affect the iris like the section of the sympathetic, though in a less degree. On the other hand, we have seen, as Schiff also has, that some of the fibres animating the iris ascend the cervical part of the spinal cord, and most probably go up to the medulla oblongata.

As regards the other fibres of the sympathetic, those going to the bloodvessels of the various parts of the head, I found, as early as 1852,[1] that they come out chiefly from the spinal cord, by the roots of the last cervical, and first and second dorsal nerves. Their place of real origin I think to be, partly the spinal cord, partly the higher portions of the encephalon, but chiefly the medulla oblongata and the neighboring parts of the encephalon.

In the other parts of the body the nerves of bloodvessels seem to come chiefly from the cerebro-spinal centre, as well as the cervical sympathetic. If we divide transversely a lateral half of the spinal marrow in the dorsal region, we find in the lower limb on the same side most of the effects of a section of the sympathetic in the neck. Amongst these effects we may point out the following: 1st, dilatation of bloodvessels; 2d, greater afflux of blood; 3d, elevation of temperature; 4th, hyperæsthesia; 5th, increase of the vital properties of muscles, and of the motor nerves.[2]

The following list contains the most interesting features of this comparison:—

[1] Medical Examiner, Philadelphia, Aug. 1852, p. 489.

[2] See Proceedings of the Royal Society, vol. viii. No. 27, 1857, p. 594.

Section of the cervical sympathetic nerve; its effects on the corresponding side of the face.	*Section of a lateral half of the spinal cord in the dorsal region; its effects on the posterior limb on the corresponding side.*
1. Bloodvessels dilated (paralyzed).	1. The same effect.
2. As a consequence, more blood.	2. The same effect.
3. Elevation of temperature.	3. The same effect.
4. Sensibility slightly increased.	4. Very much increased.
5. Sensibility lasting longer there than on the other side, when the animal is chloroformized.	5. Lasting longer than anywhere else, during chloroformization.
6. Sensibility lasting longer there than on the other side, during agony.	6. Lasting longer than anywhere else during agony.
7. Many muscles contracted.	7. A state of slight contraction in many muscles.
8. Absorption more rapid.	8. The same effect.
9. Increase of sweat and other secretions.	9. Increase of sweat.
10. Reflex movements last longer there than elsewhere, after death.	10. The same effect.
11. After poisoning by strychnia, the first convulsions take place.	11. The same effect.
12. A galvanic current too weak to excite contraction elsewhere, may act there.	12. The same effect.
13. The motor nerves after death, remain longer excitable there than on the other side.	13. The motor nerves, after death, remain *notably longer* excitable there.
14. The muscles, after death, remain longer contractile there than on the other side.	14. The muscles after death remain *much longer* contractile there.
15. The contractility of bloodvessels is greater, and lasts longer there.	15. The same effect.
16. The galvanic muscular current (as ascertained with the rheoscopic frog), is stronger, and lasts longer there than on the other side.	16. The same effect (more marked).
17. Cadaveric rigidity appears later there than on the other side, and it lasts longer.	17. Cadaveric rigidity appears *notably later* there than elsewhere, and lasts longer.
18. It is easier to regenerate there than on the other side, the vital properties of nerves and muscles by injections of red blood, a short time after they have disappeared.	18. The same effect (more marked).
19. Putrefaction comes on later, and seems to progress more slowly there than on the other side.	19. The same effect (more marked).

The question concerning the real origin of the nerves of bloodvessels in the cerebro-spinal centres is not yet entirely solved, but many points are already established. I will postpone, however, all that I have still to say on this subject till I treat of the share these nerves take in certain pathological conditions.

We have already said what are the effects of the galvanization of the cervical sympathetic nerve. We will add only a few remarks to our previous statements. The motor nerve-fibres of the sympathetic which go to bloodvessels (the *vaso-motor* nerve-fibres), are able to act when directly excited; but there does not lie the principal feature of their physiological history; they are also able to produce the contraction of the bloodvessels by a reflex action. The first fact in science which established positively that such a phenomenon is possible, was observed by my friend Dr. Tholozan, and myself. We found that the bloodvessels of one hand contract very much when the other hand is dipped into water at a very low temperature (from 32° to 34° Fahr.). The more pain we felt from the influence of the cold water, the more and the sooner did the bloodvessels of the hand left out of the water contract.[1] Since the time we published these facts, several physiologists have found that the bloodvessels of the ear, which receive their motor nerve-fibres from the cervical sympathetic, contract when the cutaneous branches of some of the spinal nerves are excited. Various decisive experiments have proved that this contraction takes place by a reflex action. When we treat of epilepsy, we will show that one of the principal features of a fit depends upon a reflex contraction (through the sympathetic), of the bloodvessels of the brain proper.

The bloodvessels, like muscles of animal life, may have spasms, as well as they may be paralyzed. In certain injuries to the nervous centres there are spasms produced in the bloodvessels of many parts of one-half of the body, at the same time that there are paralysis and dilatation of those of the other half of the body. A section of a lateral half of the spinal cord near the medulla oblongata produces this curious effect; on the side injured, the bloodvessels of the extremities are paralyzed; while on the opposite side they are spasmodically contracted. Very often the spasm persists for days, and after temporary relaxations it alternately reappears and disappears again.

The spasm of bloodvessels may be so great that circulation is almost entirely suspended; the temperature of the limbs (especially

[1] See my Experimental Researches on Physiology and Pathology, 1853, p. 32, and Journal de la Physiologie de l'Homme, etc., Paris, Juillet, 1858, p. 497.

that of the toes) falls quicker than after death, and it is soon at nearly the same degree as that of the atmosphere. In one case, in a dog, we have seen the temperature of the toes on the left side, after the section of the right half of the cord in the cervical region, falling from 26° Centigrade (78.8° Fahr.) to 15½° (59.9° Fahr.), the atmosphere being at 15° (59° Fahr.). In the toes, on the right side, the temperature had increased extremely, and reached 36° Cent. (96.8° Fahr.).

If we have time, we will try to show, in another lecture, that this spasm of bloodvessels is the cause of the coldness of the feet and hands in epileptics and certain paralytics: it is a result of an irritation of the cerebro-spinal axis, and chiefly of the upper parts of the spinal cord and of the medulla oblongata. We will also try to show the share of this spasm in the cold stage in intermittent fever, in cholera, or after the introduction of a catheter in the urethra, &c.

In the posterior limb of a dog, in which the bloodvessels are in a state of spasm, the circulation is so much impeded, that the cutting of the skin hardly gives a drop of blood. As this state exists in cases of a section of a lateral half of the spinal cord, near the encephalon, and as the other posterior limb has then its bloodvessels paralyzed, and, therefore, dilated, it might be supposed that the diminution in the amount of blood in one limb depends on the increase of its amount in the other. Let us imagine, for instance, that the right lateral half of the spinal cord has been divided; the bloodvessels of the posterior limb, as, also, those of other parts on the same side, are paralyzed, and, therefore, they do not oppose any resistance to the causes of the circulation of the blood, while the left posterior limb continues to have its bloodvessels resisting to these causes. I suppose that the amount of blood passing in the aorta, where it divides into the two common iliac arteries, is, in a given time, twenty ounces, ten for each of the posterior limbs, and that, after the operation (the aorta continuing to give the same amount of blood), sixteen ounces, instead of ten, pass in the right common iliac, on account of the paralyzed state of its branches, and of their ramifications. The result of such a change ought to be, that only four ounces will pass in the left common iliac. Supposing this to be the case, the diminution of circulation in the left limb might be explained, without our admitting the existence of a spasm of bloodvessels. But it is not on the simple fact that circulation is diminished, that I ground the opinion that there is a spasm: it is on the result of direct experiments, the detail of which I have not time to describe, but of which some show—1st, that if a ligature be put round the right iliac artery in a dog operated upon as we have already stated, the temperature rises but little, and slowly, in the extremity of the left limb, although almost the whole of the blood coming from the aorta passes into the left iliac, and it is quite evident that the small arteries, at least near the toes, do not allow the blood to pass freely; 2d, that an injection of blood by the femoral artery is difficult to be made in the left limb, compared to limbs of healthy dogs.

In those cases of gangrene in which no obstruction has been found after death in the vessels of the dead parts, it is extremely probable that a long persistent spasm of the bloodvessels has existed, rather than simply a cessation of the attraction of blood, according to the explanation of Dr. Houston.[1]

Now, to sum up all that we have stated about the sympathetic nerve, we will say—first, that it is essentially (though not exclusively) a motor nerve of bloodvessels; secondly, that it originates chiefly from the cerebro-spinal axis; thirdly, that its paralysis is characterized by a dilatation of bloodvessels and an afflux of blood, with the results of this afflux; fourthly, that its excitation, direct or reflex, is characterized by a contraction of bloodvessels, and the results of this contraction.

The question now comes: Can we explain all the phenomena, normal and pathologic, showing the direct or the reflex influence of the nervous system on nutrition and secretion, by the above notions concerning the effects of paralysis or excitation of the sympathetic nerve on bloodvessels? For several years I have felt inclined to admit the possibility of an explanation of these phenomena founded only upon these notions, but I must say, that facts discovered by Ludwig, by Czermak, and, especially, by Professor Bernard, seem to have solved the question in the most positive manner, and that it seems absolutely certain that there is some agency of the nervous system which is not simply an influence on the constricting muscular fibres of the bloodvessels, in the normal or pathological phenomena of nutrition and secretion. I must add, also, that the views held, in this respect, by the most eminent British physiologists (Mr. J. Paget, Dr. Carpenter, Dr. Todd, and

[1] See his interesting remarks on a case of Mortification after Fever, in the Dublin Medical Journal, 1836, pp. 217–219.

others) have, by the discovery of the facts I allude to, received a sanction which, I confess, they needed. The principal amongst these facts is the following: Instead of contracting, the blood-vessels of the salivary glands become enlarged, when certain nerves are excited.[1] I think that this enlargement in the blood-vessels must be due to a greater attraction of the arterial blood by the tissue of the gland; and we explain this increased attraction by the production of the chemical interchanges between the secretory tissue and the blood, which are rendered manifest by the secretion of saliva, then taking place.

The researches of Czermak and of Professor Bernard tend to show that the increase in the salivary secretion does not depend on the sympathetic nerve, but on the lingual; and we have now, in this discovery, the explanation of the following apparent contradiction: how can it be that the glands of the eye, of the ear, &c., secrete more when their bloodvessels are paralyzed and enlarged after the section of the sympathetic nerve, and that an increase in the secretion of the salivary and other glands is due to a nervous excitation? How can it be that, in one case, secretion is increased when the bloodvessels are dilated, and that, in other cases, it would be increased while their vessels ought (according to what we thought) to be contracted? This contradiction disappears now that Bernard shows that, instead of being contracted, the bloodvessels are dilated in these last cases. Besides, the experiments of Czermak and Bernard show that the salivary secretion is arrested when the sympathetic nerve is excited; and we know that this nerve, when excited, has the same stopping influence on the lachrymal and on the mucous glands of the eye and ear, &c.

From this discussion we conclude that there are two kinds, at least, of immediate influences of the nervous system, either by a direct or by a reflex action, on nutrition and secretion, normal or pathologic. By one, which we see plainly when the cervical sympathetic nerve is excited, the bloodvessels contract, and there is a diminution of secretion and nutrition; by the other, the discovery of which is chiefly due to Prof. Bernard, the bloodvessels dilate in consequence of a greater attraction for arterial blood developed in the tissues.[2] Which of these two modes of action is the most fre-

[1] This had been found by Professor Bernard. See the Journal de la Physiol. de l'Homme, &c., April, 1858, p. 240, and especially October, 1858, pp. 646–665.

[2] Recently, Professor Bernard has considered this dilatation as an active phenomenon; and he has imagined that the *capillaries* have two properties, one of

quent? and which is the most powerful in producing the normal and the morbid phenomena of nutrition and secretion? These are questions very difficult to be solved. If we have time, however, we will, in our next lecture, mention facts throwing some light upon them.

contraction and the other of dilatation; and that the first of these properties is put in play by one set of nerves, and the other by another set. We have no doubt that he will soon abandon these hypothetic and untenable views. (See *Journal de Physiol.*, pp. 646–665.)

LECTURE X.

ON THE INFLUENCE OF THE NERVOUS SYSTEM UPON NUTRITION AND SECRETION; WITH REMARKS ON THE IMPORTANCE OF THE KNOWLEDGE OF THIS INFLUENCE FOR THE TREATMENT AND THE EXPLANATION OF THE PRODUCTION OF MANY DISEASES.

Distinction between the effects of the excitation of the nervous system and those of the absence of action of this system.—Three kinds of reflex actions: contraction, secretion, and modification of nutrition.—Normal and morbid reflex secretions.—Normal and morbid reflex changes in nutrition.—Reflex influence of injuries of the trigeminal nerve upon the eye.—Reflex influence of one eye upon the nutrition of the other.—Sudden arrest of the heart's movements by a reflex action.—Cause of the rapid death after injuries of the abdominal sympathetic nerve.—Stoppage of the heart's movements by the application of cold to the skin, by the influence of cold drinks, and in some cases of death by chloroform.—Reflex influence of burns on the principal viscera.—Inflammation of the eyes, of the testicles, of the nervous centres, &c., by a reflex action.—Muscular atrophy due to an irritation of sensitive nerves.—Paralysis and anæsthesia due to a reflex action.—Disturbance of the functions of the brain and of the senses produced by irritation of centripetal nerves.—Other instances of reflex changes of nutrition.—Mode of production of the secretory and nutritive reflex actions.—Importance of the knowledge of the reflex secretory and nutritive phenomena for the treatment of disease.—Influence of the irritation of the nervous centres and of the centrifugal nerves on nutrition and secretion.—Influence of the absence of nervous action on nutrition, repair and secretion.

MR. PRESIDENT AND GENTLEMEN: To understand fully the mode of influence of the nervous system, in health and disease, upon nutrition, secretion, and animal heat, it is necessary to distinguish clearly the effects due to this influence from those due to its absence. Although these two kinds of effects are very different one from the other, they have very often been confounded. For instance, it might be easily shown that many of the best writers on physiology and pathology, when trying to prove that an influence of the nervous system is necessary to nutrition and secretion, bring forward facts showing the effects of excitation of the nervous system, together with facts depending upon the absence of action of this system.

The influence of the nervous system on organic functions cannot be proved to be necessary by facts showing only that this system can act upon these functions. There is no question at all that the nervous centres and most of the nerves, directly, or by a reflex action, can produce the greatest and the most varied effects on nutrition and secretions; but this power of acting of the nervous system does not and cannot show that these organic functions require for their normal existence a peculiar influence of the nervous organs. The only facts that can prove positively that a nervous influence is necessary to the organic functions, are to be found in the effects of the absence of any influence of the nervous system. We will, by and by, examine this kind of effects; at present, we propose to study the effects of excitation of the nervous system upon those functions.

The influence of the nervous system on the organic functions as well as upon contractile tissues, may take place in consequence of irritations on centrifugal nerve-fibres, on nervous centres, or on centripetal or sensitive nerve-fibres. We will first study the effects of the irritation of the centripetal nerve-fibres. It is well known that three kinds of reflex phenomena may be due to such an irritation: 1st, a contraction of muscles or of any kind of contractile element; 2d, a secretion; 3d, a change in the nutrition of some part of the body.[1] These three kinds of reflex actions are represented in Fig. 23.

[1] A short time before his death, Dr. Marshall Hall (*The Lancet*, 1857, vol. i. pp. 4 and 108) announced, as a new discovery, the *supposed* existence of a system of *excito-secretory* and *secretory* nerves. Dr. H. F. Campbell, of Georgia (U. S.), has claimed the priority of this discovery, which Dr. Hall has, in a great measure, candidly conceded to him (*ibid.*, pp. 462–464). We will merely remark here, that Dr. Campbell seems really to have been the first to introduce in science the hypothesis that there exists a secretory and excito-secretory system of nerves, but that neither he nor Dr. Hall has adduced a *single* fact to prove the existence of this pretended independent or distinct *system of nerves*. Both these physiologists seem not to have been aware that reflex secretions and reflex changes in nutrition were perfectly known, and that the question was, not to prove that there are such reflex phenomena, but whether they are to be explained by a reflex influence on blood-vessels or otherwise. Any one desirous to know the state of science, in this respect, before the first publication of Dr. Campbell, will find, easily, that it was more advanced than in the last paper of this able physiologist, in Mueller's *Manual of Physiology* (2d German edition, 1837), in Stilling's *Treatise on Spinal Irritation* (1840), and in several works of Henle published in 1840 and 1841. Since that time there has been no treatise on Physiology or General Pathology, and no paper nor other work on Inflammation, that does not speak of reflex phenomena of nutrition or secretion as of something well known. However, we are pleased to be able

The first decisive experimental proofs that secretions may take place by a reflex action have been given by Ludwig,[1] Colin,[2] Czermak, and Prof. Bernard for the salivary secretion, and by this last physiologist for the secretion of sugar in the liver.

The laws of reflex secretions seem to be the same as those of reflex movements: 1st, the peripheric ramification of centripetal nerves has much more power than their trunks for the production of a reflex secretion; 2d, there are certain centripetal nerves which normally can produce certain secretions by a reflex action, while others cannot; but a morbid condition of a nerve or of the nervous centres is able to render almost any nerve capable of producing any secretion; 3d, certain kinds of irritation produce reflex secretions which other kinds cannot produce, except in morbid states.

These laws are proved by many facts, some of which I will relate as illustrations of reflex secretions. The *consensus* between the various digestive organs affords the most positive demonstrations of reflex secretions. For instance, we find saliva secreted when the mucous membrane of the stomach is irritated by food. Dr. Gairdner[3] speaks of a man, whose œsophagus being divided, had a secretion of from six to eight ounces of saliva during a meal of broth injected into the stomach. The reverse takes place also; the excitation of the nerves of taste produces an abundant reflex secretion of gastric juice, and also a flow of bile and pancreatic juice in the bowels. Several times I have seen injections of warm water in the rectum of a dog, having a gastric fistula, producing a secretion of gastric juice. There is some importance in the knowledge of these facts; for instance, guided by this knowledge, we can, if necessary, increase or decrease the quantity of gastric juice, in recommending the use of very sapid or of nearly insipid food, &c.

The morbid influences acting upon the digestive organs to produce secretions are very well known. I shall only point out that the curious effects of the ligature of the œsophagus (congestions and secretions in the stomach and bowels, efforts of vomiting, &c.),

to declare that, as if it were impossible for Dr. Marshall Hall to write, even on a well-known subject, without putting upon it the stamp of his inventive genius, he has suggested a very important explanation of the alterations in the mucous secretions of the lungs after a section of the par vagum, in his first paper on reflex secretions (*loco cit.*, p. 4).

[1] Zeitschrift fuer Rationelle Medicin, 1851, N. F., vol. i. 1851, p. 260.

[2] Comptes Rendus de l'Acad. des Sciences, 1852, vol. xxxv. p. 130.

[3] Edinburgh Med. and Surg. Journal, vol. xvi. p. 355.

which have been observed by Messrs. Bouley and Reynal,[1] are very simple phenomena, if we look upon them as reflex actions resulting from the irritation of the centripetal nerve-fibres of the œsophagus.

It is important to know that the gastric juice may be so altered by a reflex action due to an irritation on the nerves of the anus or of the rectum, that digestion becomes almost impossible. The late Dr. Chapman,[2] of Philadelphia, relates two cases of dyspepsia (in one of which the gastric juice is said to have been extremely corrosive) which were cured almost immediately after the extirpation of painful piles. I know a case in which vomiting of a great quantity of unduly-acid gastric juice took place under the irritating influence of worms in the rectum. R. Whytt says, that "the pain of hæmorrhoids is, sometimes, accompanied by a sickness of the stomach and faintness." (*Observations, etc.*, p. 26.)

The ptyalism due to neuralgia is a good example of morbid reflex secretion. Dr. Notta (*Archives de Médecine*, Sept., 1854, p. 298) states that ptyalism has been observed 14 times out of 128 cases of trifacial neuralgia.

Dr. Cain, of Charleston,[3] in a very interesting paper, in which he gives many instances of reflex disturbances of secretion and nutrition, relates cases which seem to show that croup may be produced by a reflex irritation starting from the stomach. Facts of this kind were already known; but here the theory of the *modus agendi* of the gastric irritation on the larynx is clearly exposed and based upon many facts and very sound reasonings.

The production of tears affords decided instances of reflex secretions. We find that any irritation of the eye, or of the mucous membrane of the nose, causes an increase in the production of tears. Two cases mentioned by Henle[4] as having been observed, one by Sir Charles Bell, the other by Vogt, prove that it is through a nervous excitation that the shedding of tears takes place when we touch the eye. In two patients, the eye having lost its sensibility, tears were no more shed when this organ was irritated. Mr. Castorani has recently confirmed, by decisive facts, the view that it

[1] See the Report of Prof. Trousseau to the Academy of Medicine of Paris, and my remarks on this Report in the Journal de Physiol., October, 1858.

[2] Lectures on the more important Diseases of the Thoracic and Abdominal Viscera, 1844, pp. 216–7.

[3] The Southern Journal of Medicine, &c., 1847, p. 377.

[4] Anatomie Générale, French translation, 1843, vol. ii. p. 255.

is not through the optic nerve that the secretion of tears is increased in cases of photophobia, when the eye is exposed to the irritation of light: it is through the exalted excitability of the trigeminal nerve. A curious fact observed by Deslandes[1] is in harmony with this view: a man totally blind, had an abundant secretion of tears at every time that he passed from a dark place to a lighted one. The shedding of tears under the influence of irritation of other parts than the eye and nose is less and less the farther the irritation is from the eye. I have experimented upon myself, and found that the pinching of the neck or of the back parts of the head hardly produce lachrymation, while that of the face produces it more and more the nearer to the eye the irritation is made. This increased secretion exists only on the side irritated, except when the pinching is made very near the median line. Mr. Notta[2] mentions that lachrymation has been noted as an effect of neuralgia of the fifth pair of nerves 61 times out of 128 cases. It is chiefly in cases of neuralgia of the supra-orbitary branch that lachrymation is produced. The fact that the irritation of the cornea by a foreign body causes lachrymation, and that the removal of this irritative agent is at once followed by a cessation of this abundant and abnormal secretion, is a good illustration of its mode of production.

If I had time, I would show that we must admit that it is by a reflex action that the following secretions take place in the circumstances that I will point out: 1. Secretion of milk by an irritation of the uterus, of the skin of the mammæ, or of the mucous membrane of the vagina (particularly by the steam of a decoction of the *jatropha curcas*, as done at the Cape de Verde Islands). 2. Menstruation in consequence of an irritation of the ovaries of the vagina or of the mammæ by warm poultices, &c. 3. Secretion of nasal mucus increased by application of cold water to the feet, and sometimes stopped at once by dipping of the feet in iced water,[3] and increased by a draught of cold air on the neck. 4. Secretion of semen increased by the irritation of the genital organs. 5. Perspiration due to neuralgia, as in a case by Dr. Galliet, or due to the excitation of the nerves of taste, by salt or sugar, etc., as in a case I have mentioned to the Society of Biology, in a communication on reflex secretions in 1849. (See *Comptes Rendus de la Soc. de Biol.*, vol. i. p. 104.)

[1] Dictionn. de Méd. et de Chir. Pratiques, vol. ii. p. 179.
[2] Archives Génér. de Médecine, etc., Juillet, 1854.
[3] Hyp. Cloquet, Thèse sur les Odeurs, p. 162.

Before treating of the reflex changes in nutrition, which are by far more frequent, and more important to be well investigated, than the reflex secretions, I must remark that the reflex character of facts more or less similar to those I have to mention has been known for a long while, and that the modern theory is not far in advance of that given, in this respect, by Robert Whytt[1] in the last century. In one of his important works he has shown that the normal and morbid sympathies, either for movements, nutrition, or secretion, are reflex phenomena. Still more, he has shown that the share of bloodvessels is very great in many of these phenomena.

Although Robert Whytt and several other writers, amongst whom I will name Tissot, Prochaska, Barthez, J. Mueller, Henle, and Prof. Martyn Paine, have published so many interesting facts concerning the sympathy between various parts of the body, physiologists and practitioners have not paid a sufficient attention to this most important subject. I regret that I cannot enter into great developments on the capital points concerning this subject; but I will, at least, endeavor to show their importance.

Reflex changes in nutrition ought to be known as being amongst the most frequent causes of many diseases. An irritation starts from an excitable part of a nerve, it reaches the nervous centres, and thence, being reflected to a more or less distant part of the body, it produces either a contraction of a bloodvessel, and, through this, effects a diminution of nutrition, or it acts directly upon the tissues, and produces an alteration of the interchanges between them and the blood. The eye, amongst all the other organs in the body, is the one that gives the most evident and the most frequent instances of this kind of affection. The most positive of these facts, as regards the production by a reflex action, are the following: 1st. When the supra-orbitalis nerve has been crushed or injured, in such a way that it remains irritated, an inflammation or some other affection of the corresponding eye supervenes, which is cured either by the means that diminish the irritation of the injured nerve, or by its section between the nervous centre and the injured part, so as to prevent reflex actions starting from this irritated part. 2d. When an eye is the seat of a violent inflammation, and particularly if it be of traumatic origin, it is not rare for the other eye to become affected, and the successful treatment for the affection of this last eye consists in preventing, by various means, the irritation

[1] Observations on the Nature, Causes, and Cure of Nervous Disorders, pp. 1–65.

from the first one reaching the nervous centre, by which a reflex action is operated upon the secondarily attacked eye.

These two facts are now proved by so many cases, that there can be no doubt as to the mode of production of the consecutive affection of the eye, in both kinds of facts. However, there have been men of great reputation who have doubted the correctness of the etiology of these affections of the eye. For instance, Walther[1] denies that there is a single fact proving that amaurosis may be due to an injury of the frontal nerve. J. Mueller[2] says that it is much more natural to attribute amaurosis, following a blow upon the forehead, to the commotion of the eye and of the optic nerve; and Mr. Sichel[3] expresses the same opinions. But most of the recent works on the diseases of the eyes contain many, and the most positive facts, showing that several kinds of affection of the eye may be the result of an injury to the frontal or of other branches of the trigeminal nerves. Besides some facts that I shall relate, I will mention the publications of Mr. Deval, as containing many facts of this kind.[4]

A paper of Mr. Notta, on Neuralgia,[5] shows that this kind of irritation very often causes congestion of the eye and photophobia. Out of 128 cases of neuralgia of the trigeminal nerve, the eye was congested *thirty-four* times; and in most of those cases the nerve attacked was the supra-orbitalis. Photophobia existed in *eighteen* cases; and a real ophthalmia has sometimes been observed. Mr. James,[6] a pupil of Magendie, has seen amaurosis caused by a neuralgia. Mr. Notta (*loc. cit.*, Juillet, pp. 12–21) mentions ten cases of amaurosis due to neuralgia. The short duration of this amaurosis, its relapsing character, and, moreover, its appearance during, or immediately after, an attack of neuralgia, and the fact that it was cured when the neuralgia was cured, prove that it resulted from the irritation of the trigeminal nerve. Alterations in the cornea have been observed in a very curious case of neuralgia of the face, by Mr. Mazade.[7] In a case of hyperæmia of the eye, which had resisted for a year many kinds of treatment, Dr. Emmerich,

1 Journal füer Chirurgie und Augenheilkunde, 1840, vol. xxix. p. 505.
2 Manuel de Physiologie, Trad. Française, 1851, p. 707.
3 Traité de l'Ophthalmie, 1837, p. 697.
4 See particularly his Traité de l'Amaurose, Paris, 1850, 8vo.
5 Archives de Médecine, Juillet, Septembre, et Novembre, 1854.
6 Gazette Médicale de Paris, 1840, p. 678.
7 Annales d'Oculistique, 1848, p. 128.

quoted by Schiff,[1] states that an immediate cure was obtained after the extraction of a tooth. Prof. Paul F. Eve, of Tennessee, U.S., suggested the idea of the extirpation of a carious tooth to Dr. H. F. Campbell,[2] in a case of ophthalmia, and, the operation having been performed, the patient was at once cured. In a case recorded by Vallez, quoted by Schiff (*loc. cit.*, p. 116), there was strong hyperæmia of one eye, with abundant mucous secretion, followed by an ulceration of the cornea, in a man who had received a deep wound in the face, dividing the supra-maxillary nerve. Dr. Alcock, in his important article on the Fifth Pair of Nerves,[3] relates experiments on animals, in which an injury to the infra-orbitalis nerve had produced inflammation and suppuration of the eye. It is worthy of remark that, in these experiments, when the wound healed the eye returned to its normal condition. Morgagni,[4] says that Valsalva has seen amaurosis instantly produced in a woman whose eyebrow had been struck by the beak of a cock.

The cases which prove the reflex influence of one eye upon the other are more numerous than those showing the influence of various branches of the trigeminal nerve of one side upon the corresponding eye. Schenk, Richter, Bidloo, and many other writers of the two preceding centuries, have mentioned facts proving that one eye may be affected by a disease or an injury of the other. In this century, particularly in England, facts of this kind have been very well studied, and the treatment, consisting in the extirpation of a wounded eye to save the other, has been applied many times.[5] The happy influence of such a treatment shows, if this were necessary, that it is on account of an irritation starting from the first injured eye, that the other is affected.

Even a cataract may be produced in a healthy eye by a nervous reflex influence, either from some part of the trigeminal nerve on the same side, or from the other eye. Mr. Notta mentions two cases, one of a wound of the frontal nerve, and another of neuralgia, both followed by cataract. (*Loc. cit.*, Juillet, 1854, p. 28.) Albers

[1] Untersuchungen zur Physiol. des Nervensystems, 1855, p. 115.

[2] The Secretory and Excito-Secretory System of Nerves, 1857, p. 98.

[3] The Cyclopædia of Anat. and Physiol., vol. ii. p. 312.

[4] De Sedibus et Causis Morborum, Epist. xiii., s. 5, vol. ii. p. 14.

[5] I will refer to an inaugural dissertation (Thèse pour le Doctorat, Paris, 24 Juillet, 1858, par M. de Brondeau), in which there is a relation of no less than twenty-four cases observed by the author, showing the influence of one eye upon the other, for the production of disease.

relates a case of a wound of the cornea and the iris on the *right* side, followed, in three days, by an opacity of the cornea of the *left* eye, and in eight days by a cataract in this last eye. (De Brondeau, *loc. cit.*, p. 16.) Aug. Bérard has insisted extremely[1] on the necessity of operating on one eye attacked with cataract to prevent the other from being attacked.

As a second series of examples of reflex changes in nutrition, I will mention what takes place in cases of sudden stopping of the movements of the heart, in consequence of an irritation of some peripheric parts of the nervous system. Whether the heart's movements depend, as I have tried to show long ago,[2] upon an excitation from some substance contained in the blood circulating through the tissue of this organ upon its muscular fibres, or whether they depend upon some peculiar rhythmical change in nutrition, as ingeniously suggested by Mr. James Paget,[3] their stoppage in the cases I shall mention is produced by a reflex action.

The sudden death which sometimes occurs when very cold water is drunk in a warm day, or in cases of a blow on the abdomen, of a sudden perforation of the stomach or intestine, of a wound of some abdominal viscus (without a notable hemorrhage), &c., seems to be due to a reflex stopping of the heart's action. I have made a great many experiments, which show positively that a sudden excitation of the abdominal sympathetic nerve sometimes kills, and often diminishes the movements of the heart, by a reflex action.[4] The excitation goes up to the spinal cord, chiefly along the great splanchnic nerve, and ascends the spinal cord until the place of origin of the par vagum, and through this pair of nerves it comes to the heart. This is proved by the fact that a section of either the par vagum, or the spinal cord, or the splanchnic nerves, allows any kind of irritation to be made on the abdominal sympathetic without a stopping taking place in the heart. In some animals, the influence of the irritation of the sympathetic in the abdomen is much more marked than in others; it is so, probably, in man. I have seen a gentleman suddenly drop down pulseless, in the most complete syncope, from a pain in the abdomen. The same gentleman is easily attacked by syncope from any kind of pain. One day, while

[1] Annales d'Oculistique, vol. xi. p. 183.

[2] Experimental Researches applied to Physiology and Pathology, 1853, pp. 77 and 114.

[3] Proceedings of the Royal Society, May 28, 1857.

[4] Recherches sur les Capsules surrénales. Paris, 1856.

I was trying to bleed him with the assistance of my learned friend Professor Natalis Guillot, he had, as soon as pricked by the lancet, a complete stopping of the heart's movements, and we thought, for two minutes, that he would die. I took him by his feet, which I put on my shoulders, and then rising, I held him, the head hanging down, and he gradually recovered.

It is by the reflex influence due to the *sudden* irritation of the branches of the par vagum in the lungs that chloroform has killed in the very rare cases in which the heart's action has been stopped before the respiration. In dogs, in which we can cause death in this way rather easier than in other animals, I have found that this mode of death never exists after the section of the par vagum. On the other hand, I have ascertained, in the same kind of animals, that the state of the heart is just the same as when death has been produced by the irritation (by galvanism) of the medulla oblongata and par vagum, or by the extirpation of the so-called *vital knot*.[1] Besides, another proof that it is in this way that chloroform kills in the cases which I try to elucidate is, that in some dogs, on which the heart's action has been suddenly stopped by the inhalation of a very large quantity of chloroform, I have been able to restore life by merely exciting the heart to contract by mechanical excitation (pressure on the chest).

I must point out, *apropos* of the stopping of the heart's action by a reflex mechanism, that one of the means employed to restore life in asphyxiated children—which consists in the alternative dipping of the body in warm and cold water—is a most dangerous one. No doubt that it is a powerful means of producing reflex actions, as long as any reflex power remains in the cerebro-spinal axis, but in this very thing lies the danger. I have seen puppies asphyxiated, and having no more respiration, while the heart was still beating fifteen or twenty times in a minute, killed at once on being dipped into cold water, the heart stopping by a reflex action. I do not intend to say that such a means ought not to be employed; I wish only to point out the chance of a sudden arrest of the heart's action, so that practitioners may be on the watch respecting this accident.

An extensive burn may also produce a stopping of the heart's movements, but it frequently produces other effects, which are much more interesting, and prove the great power of the nervous

[1] See Journal de la Physiol. de l'Homme, etc., No. 2, Avril, 1858, p. 217 et seq.

system on nutrition. In an important paper of Mr. Long, of Liverpool,[1] it is stated that death was caused, in many cases of extensive burns, by an inflammation of the various viscera. The three following conclusions have been arrived at by Mr. Long: 1st. That in almost every burn, indeed in every burn, lesions of one or more of the viscera contained in the three great cavities exist, being according to their frequency as follows: abdomen, chest, head. 2d. That the lesions of the different tissues contained in the abdomen are in the following order: mucous membranes, serous membranes, parenchymatous tissues; in the chest it is quite the reverse—namely, parenchymatous tissues, serous tissues, and lastly mucous; in the head—membranes, brain. 3d. That the seat of internal inflammation corresponds sufficiently often with the external position of the burn, but that in a precisely equal number of instances no such correspondence can be traced. Mr. Curling, in a paper on the Influence of Burns on the Bowels,[2] relates ten cases of ulceration of the duodenum as a consequence of this powerful irritation of the skin. Lastly, in a very remarkable paper, Mr. J. E. Erichsen[3] gives the following as the result of observations of many cases of burns:—

The cerebral organs	were	diseased	in 33 out of 37	cases.
The thoracic viscera	"	"	in 30 out of 40	"
The abdominal viscera	"	"	in 31 out of 42	"

I have given these numbers to show the frequency of this reflex influence of burns. When I come to the deductions to be drawn from the facts I have mentioned in this lecture, for the treatment of disease, I will show the importance of the knowledge of this influence of burns, and I will show, also, what should be done against this frequently deathly influence, according to the view that it acts by a reflection from the nervous centres upon themselves, or upon the thoracic or the abdominal viscera.[4]

When we come to the demonstration that the phenomena which we have mentioned in this lecture are really to be attributed to a reflex action, we will show what parts of the alterations in the various viscera, after extensive burns, belong to a reflex influence, and what parts are due to other causes. But we will, at once,

[1] Philadelphia Medical Examiner, 1840, p. 492; from the London Medical Gazette, Feb. 1840.

[2] Medico-Chirurgical Transactions, 2d Series, vol. vii.

[3] London Medical Gazette, Jan. 1843, pp. 544 and 588.

[4] That the nervous centres may act upon themselves, just as upon other organs, by a *reflex* action, will be shown hereafter.

relate cases which show that several of the inflammations of internal organs after burns may be due to a reflex action, in showing that inflammations in various parts of the body may be caused by an irritation of the nerves of the skin or of other sensitive nerves.

Inflammation by a reflex action.—In his admirable "Lectures on Inflammation," delivered in this College, Mr. James Paget said that whoever has worked much with microscopes may have observed, as he has upon himself, that the eye not employed becomes inflamed; and he adds that the fact cannot be explained except by the supposition that the excited state of the optic nerve of the working eye is transferred or communicated to the nerves of the conjunctiva of the other eye. He thinks that the communication must take place through the encephalon, and therefore by a reflex action.[1] I know of a most curious case of inflammation of the cornea and conjunctiva, followed by ulceration and opacity of the cornea, due to that very cause: overwork with the microscope. It has occurred in a distinguished friend of mine, Dr. F——, now Professor, at Lille. In this case, anæsthesia and a degree of atrophy of the face were produced at the same time as the ophthalmia, on the *left* side, the micrographer making use of the *right* eye. If I had time I would endeavor to prove that it is not by a reflex action from the optic nerve, but from the filaments of the trigeminal, in one eye, that this inflammation of the other eye has proceeded. The recent works on diseases of the eye contain many cases of inflammation of this organ by a reflex action, and I will refer for some cases of ophthalmia due to this influence to the cases of irritation of the dental nerves, observed by Emmerich and by Dr. Eve, and to the experiments of Dr. Alcock, which I have already mentioned.

It is not rare that an inflammation of the testicle takes place by a reflex action. Barras, quoted by Notta (*loc. cit.*, Nov., p. 547), and Marotte[2] relate cases of orchitis due to ileo-scrotal neuralgia. Sir B. Brodie[3] mentions a case of inflammation of one testicle due to the irritation of the ureter by a calculus, and a case of inflammatory swelling of the face due to a neuralgia. Mr. J. Paget (*loco cit.*, p. 54) says that it is through a nervous action that the urethra excites inflammation of the testicle; that the irritation of teething excites this morbid nutrition in any distant part, and that inflam-

[1] Lectures on Inflammation, 1850, p. 12.
[2] L'Union Médicale, 1851, p. 155.
[3] Lectures Illustrative of certain Local Affections. London, 1837, p. 16.

mation of the brain has been caused by the application of a ligature to the brachial plexus, as in a case observed by Lallemand.

Inflammation of the brain seems manifestly to have been generated by a reflex influence in a case recorded by M. P. Meynier.[1] The same thing may be said of a great many cases of inflammation of the spinal cord or medulla oblongata, in tetanus or trismus nascentium.[2] Other inflammations may be produced by a reflex action: I have seen purulent otorrhœa taking place at every attack of neuralgia of the auriculo-temporalis nerve in a young girl. I have seen a real inflammation of the stomach, in a dog, after the irritation of the filaments of the par vagum in the œsophagus, and Professor Trousseau has made a similar observation. My learned friend, Mr. P. Broca, has seen several cases of pleurisy due to an irritation of the nerves of the breast, by some operations.

Muscular atrophy by a reflex action.—My friend and pupil, M. Clément Bonnefin, is now collecting facts of this kind, and already he has found a great many. He has observed a very evident one in which the atrophy is due to a neuralgia. M. Notta says (*loco cit.*, Nov., p. 557) that in seven cases of neuralgia a more or less extensive atrophy has been observed. I have seen two cases: one of sciatica, having producéd an atrophy of some of the muscles of the leg; the other, in which pain starting from the cicatrix of a wound on the *left* forearm has caused atrophy of *both arms*. In the case of an injury to the supra-maxillary nerve which I have already mentioned,[3] there was atrophy of the face. In the case of my friend, Dr. F——, the ulceration of the eye, due to irritation of the other, is accompanied by an atrophy of some muscles of the face.

In several of the cases of muscular atrophy collected by Dr. W. Roberts,[4] there is sufficient evidence that this condition of the muscles has been caused by a reflex action (particularly in some cases of Sir Charles Bell, of H. Mayo, of Aran, of Romberg, of Frerichs, and of Diemer).

That the paralysis of atrophied muscles is not the only cause of

[1] Gazette Médicale de Paris. Décembre, 1856.

[2] It is probable that it is in the same way that inflammation of the spinal cord was produced in those very interesting cases recorded by Dr. W. W. Gull, and in which a disease of the viscera of the pelvis or diphtheria has preceded the symptoms of myelitis. (See the *Medico-Chirurgical Transactions* for 1856, and the *Lancet*, July, 1858, p. 4.)

[3] Vallez, quoted by Schiff (*loco cit.*, p. 115).

[4] An Essay on Wasting Palsy. London, 1858.

atrophy is shown by the fact that this state of the muscles has often existed without paralysis, or at least before paralysis, and sometimes although there were convulsions in the muscles. Notta mentions three cases in which constant or frequent convulsions occurred while atrophy was increasing.

Paralysis and anæsthesia by a reflex action.—The number of facts of this kind is immense, as shown in the voluminous papers and works of R. Leroy d'Etiolles,[1] of Landry,[2] and of Macario.[3] It would be most important to review these cases to show that they cannot have been produced otherwise than by a reflex action, producing an alteration of either the spinal cord or of some of its nerves; but we have not time enough for such a review, and we must therefore be content to mention a few amongst those facts which, more than the others, seem to prove that the cause of the paralysis or of the anæsthesia is truly in a reflex action.

It is well known that we owe to Mr. Edward Stanley[4] the proof that diseases of the genito-urinary organs can be the cause of paraplegia. Rayer,[5] Leroy d'Etiolles (*loco cit.*), Macario (*loco cit.*), and others, have related many facts which leave no doubt as to the possibility of existence of a more or less complete paraplegia without any visible alteration of the spinal cord or of its nerves, and due to a disease of either the bladder, the prostate, or the kidney. Other viscera of the abdominal and thoracic cavities may also be the starting point of a paralysis; Dr. R. Graves[6] is the first who has well established this etiology of certain kinds of paralysis. In children, the pretended essential paralysis, so well studied by Heine, Kennedy, Dr. West, Fliess, and Rilliet,[7] is evidently analogous in its mode of production with the reflex paralysis of adults. This paralysis of children is almost always due to the irritation of the dental nerves or of the bowels.

Marchal de Calvi[8] relates four cases of neuralgia of the fifth pair

[1] Des Paralysies des Membres Inférieurs ou Paraplégies, 1ère partie, 1855; 2de p., 1857.

[2] Recherches sur les Causes et les Indications Curatives des Maladies Nerveuses, 1855.

[3] Gazette Médicale de Paris, 1857, pp. 564 and 606.

[4] Medico-Chirurgical Transactions, vol. xviii. p. 260.

[5] Traité des Maladies des Reins, vol. iii. 1851, p. 168 *et seq.*

[6] Clinical Lectures on the Practice of Medicine. Ed. by Neligan.

[7] Traité des Maladies des Enfants, par Rilliet et Barthez, 2d edition, 1853, vol. ii. p. 547.

[8] Archives de Médecine, 1846, vol. xi. p. 261.

of nerves which had produced a paralysis of the third pair. Notta (*loco cit.*, Sept. 1854, p. 293) has seen two cases of paralysis of the elevator palpebræ, due to a neuralgia. Neucourt[1] and M. Gola[2] have each seen one case of facial paralysis cured at the same time that a neuralgia, which had caused it, was cured. Dr. Badin d'Hurtebise[3] has seen a neuralgia of the supra-orbitalis nerve producing a paralysis of the third and sixth pairs of nerves, which paralysis ceased quickly after the cure of the neuralgia. Sciatica, also, may produce a paralysis: Notta (p. 556) mentions a case in which the paralysis of the extensor muscles lasted two months after the cure of the sciatica. Irritation of the bowels in adults has often produced paralysis: besides cases recorded by Dr. Graves and by Leroy, there are two mentioned by Professor Trousseau,[4] several by Zabriskie[5] and by Camper.[6] Irritation of the lungs or the pleuræ may also produce paralysis: I have seen a case of this kind, in 1850, at the Charité Hospital in Paris; and Landry (*loco cit.*, Obs. 118 and 119) relates two cases. The same thing has occurred in diseases of the liver, without our being able, in some cases, to explain the paralysis by the presence of bile in the blood. I will point out especially a case of hepatic colic observed by Professor Fouquier (quoted by Landry, p. 99) and a case by Zabriskie.[7] A simple pressure on some sensitive nerve, or a wound, may cause an extensive paralysis: so it was in a case that I have observed with my friend M. Charcot, and in cases recorded or mentioned by Fabricius Hildanus (quoted by Whytt, *loco cit.*, p. 18), and by Barthez (*loco cit.*, vol. ii. pp. 41 and 42, *notes*, and p. 127).

The production of anæsthesia from irritation of centripetal nerves is as common as that of paralysis of movement. I have seen a case of anæsthesia of the two lower limbs due to sciatica. M. Notta (*loco cit.*, Nov., pp. 552–54) mentions five cases like this one—three observed by himself, one by Grisolle, and one by Martinet. A case of anæsthesia of the arm in consequence of a cervico-brachial neuralgia, is also related by Mr. Notta. Several cases of more or less extended anæsthesia, due to some kind of irritation of the skin,

[1] Arch., 1849, vol. xx. p. 172.
[2] Bulletin de Thérapeutique, 1846, vol. xxxi. p. 389.
[3] Annales d'Oculistique, 1849, vol. xxii. p. 12.
[4] Gazette des Hôpitaux, 1841, p. 192.
[5] Med. Examiner, 1841, vol. iv. p. 750; and Gaz. Méd. de Paris, 1842, p. 296.
[6] Quoted by Barthez, "Science de l'Homme," 2d ed., 1806, p. 11, *notes*.
[7] Gaz. Méd. de Paris, 1842, p. 296.

have been collected in an excellent thesis of Mr. O'Brien.[1] In one it followed a bite of the skin of the arm. I have seen a young woman who had a partial anæsthesia of the face, with swelling and infiltration of the cheek, and complete paralysis of the facial nerve, in consequence of neuralgia of the infra-orbitalis nerve. I must say that, in this case, as also in all the cases of paralysis and anæsthesia I have mentioned, the patients were not hysteric.

I will add that in those cases—1st, the supposed cause has always preceded the paralysis of movement or sensibility; 2d, the changes in the intensity of the cause have usually been accompanied by corresponding changes in the paralytic symptoms; 3d, the remedies against paralysis and anæsthesia have proved useless; 4th, these two affections, in many cases, have been speedily cured after the cessation of the irritating cause; 5th, there was no visible alteration of the nervous system in several cases in which an autopsy was made. All these facts assuredly tend to show that the paralytic symptoms were not due to a disease of the central nervous system, but to an irritation of some centripetal nerve; and we will show hereafter that it was in producing a peculiar reflex action that this irritation had acted.

Morbid changes in the nutrition of the brain, of the spinal cord, and of the senses produced by an irritation of some centripetal nerve.—I shall not insist upon the demonstration of the influence that an irritation of almost every centripetal nerve may have on the production of nervous affections, which show that a change in the nutrition of the nervous centres has taken place. In one of the lectures I have still to deliver, I will show, by an *immense* number of recorded cases, that insanity in its various forms, epilepsy, chorea, catalepsy, extasis, hydrophobia, hysteria, and all the varieties of nervous complaints, may be the result of a simple, and often slightly felt, irritation of some centripetal nerve. I will also then prove, or, at least, endeavor to prove, that it is by a reflex action of the cerebro-spinal axis upon itself, through the nerves going to its bloodvessels, that this irritation acts to alter the nutrition of this nervous centre.

As regards the influence of the irritation of centripetal nerves on the nutrition of the senses, I will refer to what I have already said of amaurosis, adding only that the influence by which worms acting on the bowels cause the paralysis of the retina is just the same as

[1] Recherches sur l'Anesthésie. Paris, 1834, pp. 14, 19, 21, and 24.

that by which a neuralgia acts in causing the same effect.[1] Deafness has also been caused by an irritation of the nerves of the bowels, as it has been in two cases of facial neuralgia. (Notta, *loco cit.*, p. 297.)

Neuralgia due to a reflex action.—Dr. Rowland mentions a girl, who had paroxysms of darting pain in the *left* temple and side of the head. Upon inquiry, it was found that several years previously she had received a severe cut over the *right* parietal bone, which cut was long in healing, and this spot had been tender ever since. A large uneven cicatrix was discovered, and a blister over this part relieved the pain for several weeks. (Parsons, Prize Essay on Neuralgia.[2]) Sir Benjamin Brodie mentions a case of stricture of the urethra inducing lameness and pain in the foot, which were relieved by the introduction of a bougie in the urethra. The irritation caused by a carious tooth has produced neuralgia in the arm in two cases. (Parsons, *loco cit.*, pp. 423 and 424.) Neuralgic hemicrania is very frequently due to gastralgia. Romberg[3] mentions several cases observed by Wardrop, Abernethy, Denmark, and others, in which a neuralgia in many nerves has been caused by the injury of one.

Various morbid influences due to an irritation of centripetal nerves.— I will only point out some of the most interesting facts. In the first place, I will mention the herpes zoster, which is now almost universally admitted as being often due to a neuralgia. Rayer, G. Simon, Notta, Dr. Parsons, Delioux, Romberg and Parrot,[4] have related many cases, which leave no doubt on this point. Hasse[5] mentions, besides the zona, the following skin affections as having been caused by neuralgia: erythema, pemphigus, and urticaria. In the second place, I will say that hypertrophy of a bone, in cases of neuralgia, is frequent enough to explain how Sir Henry Halford has been led to imagine that tic douloureux depends upon this affection of bones. There is no doubt that a disease of bones can produce neuralgia—and such is the case for the reflex neuralgia of

[1] As some persons deny that worms may have this influence, I will refer to a paper of Mondière, in which several unquestionable cases are recorded. (*Gazette des Hôpitaux*, 1840, p. 139 and p. 248.) In some cases an *immediate* cure has followed the expulsion of worms. (*L'Expérience*, 1840, p. 47, and *Gaz. Méd. de Paris*, 1845, p. 655.)

[2] American Journal of Medical Science, Oct. 1854, p. 421.

[3] Lehrbuch der Nervenkrankheiten des Menschen, 3d ed., 1856, pp. 23-35.

[4] Considérations sur le Zona, par J. Parrot. Paris, 1857.

[5] Krankheiten des Nervenapparates, in Virchow's Handb. d. sp. Pathol., vol. iv., 1855, p. 48.

most of the branches of the trigeminal nerve in cases of caries of a part of the cranium—but it seems certain also that hypertrophy of bone may be due to neuralgia, as is shown by cases of Romberg, Bouillaud, Neucourt, and Bellingeri. (Notta, *loco cit.*, Sept. 1854, pp. 311, 312.)

I will only add to the list of effects of irritation of centripetal nerves, that œdema, a change in the color and thickness of the hair, and several other morbid alterations, have been observed, in cases in which they were evidently due to that cause.

Many interesting facts might be added to those which I have mentioned as illustrations of the power of an excitation of centripetal nerves to act on glands, so as to produce an increase of all the secretions, or to change their nature, or to stop them, and to act also, at a great or small distance, on the various tissues, so as to increase, diminish, or alter their nutrition.[1] I come now to the explanation of the mode of action of the excitation of a centripetal nerve in those various cases.

The phenomena of sympathy between distant parts of the body have, at first, been explained by direct communications, which were supposed to exist between the nerves of the parts which have some sympathetic influence one upon the other. A second opinion was that the communications take place, partly through the nervous centres, partly through anastomoses of nerves. At last, after Claude Perrault and others, Robert Whytt held the view that all nerves producing sympathetic actions communicate only in the brain or spinal cord.[2] Since the times of Whytt and Haller, who agreed as regards this opinion, it had been admitted by most physiologists until 1835, when Tiedemann[3] tried again to show that it is through anastomoses of nerves that sympathies take place. But after the microscope had proved definitively that nerve-fibres remain usually quite distinct one from the other (a few only uniting together), and also, after the experiments of Kronenberg, of Van Deen, and others, had proved that the excitation of nerve-fibres passing through anastomoses remains isolated in them, the old theory, renewed by Tiedemann, has been totally ruined, and now

[1] For several facts worthy of interest, I will refer to the learned work of Henle, "Handbuch der Rationelle Pathologie," vol. i. 3d ed., 1855, pp. 237–41.

[2] See his two important works, "An Essay on the Vital and other Involuntary Motions of Animals," 2d ed., 1763, and "Observations on the Nature, Causes, and Cure of Nervous Disorders," &c., 2d ed., 1765, pp. 9–84.

[3] Zeitschrift fuer Physiologie, vol. i., 1835.

it is universally acknowledged that real sympathies require the intervention of the nervous centres. But, although admitted as the right one, this view seems not to be sufficiently understood, and the efforts made by Mueller, by Stilling,[1] by Henle,[2] by Dr. Martyn Paine,[3] and others, have not convinced every one that changes in secretion and in nutrition, due to a sympathetic influence, are produced, in a great measure, by the same mechanism as that of the reflex movements.

Let us take inflammation as an illustration. An operation is made on the cervix uteri,[4] and, one or two days after, a peritonitis supervenes, and the patient dies. How has this inflammation been produced? Few persons will be ready to explain this affection by a reflex action from the uterus to the peritoneum, and many would laugh at the idea of such an explanation. It is evident, assuredly, that the inflammation may have begun in the uterus, and been propagated to the peritoneum by bloodvessels; but let us suppose that no inflammation is found in the uterus or in the vagina, how then can an inflammation have been produced in the peritoneum, in consequence of an operation upon the cervix uteri? If you do not admit that the excitation of the nerves of this part of the womb has been propagated to the spinal cord, and thence reflected by other nerves upon the peritoneum, you will not be able to explain the phenomena observed. If we take separately almost any one of the facts I have mentioned as instances of reflex secretory or nutritive actions, many persons will decline admitting with

[1] Physiol., Pathol., und Med. Pract. Untersuchungen ueber die Spinal Irritation. Leipzig, 1840, and Geschichte einer Exstirpation eines Krankhaft vergr. Ovarium's, *u. s. w.* Hanover, 1841.

[2] Handbuch der Rationellen Pathologie. Dritte auflage. Vol. i., 1855, and his Pathologische Untersuchungen, 1840, and Algemeine Anatomie, 1841.

[3] The Institutes of Medicine. New York, 1847. The learned author of this work is a solidist and a vitalist, who has carried the theory of sympathies of Whytt and others far beyond the limits within which it ought to be restricted.

[4] My learned friend, Mr. P. Broca, has recently communicated to the Société de Chirurgie of Paris the case of a woman on whom an application of the actual cautery to the cervix uteri, after the extirpation of a polypus, was followed by an intense peritonitis and rapid death. The state of the uterus showed that this was not a case of propagation of inflammation from this organ to the peritoneum. See, for a summary of the case, the *Lancet*, Nov. 20, 1858, p. 530, and, for the details, the *Gazette des Hôpitaux* and the *Moniteur des Hôpitaux*, Nov. 1858. While I was writing this Lecture another case, similar to this one, has occurred. A woman, whose uterus has been cauterized by Mr. Jobert, has died of peritonitis, shortly afterward.

us that it is perhaps really a reflex action. It is, therefore, necessary to say at least a few words, to show that the sympathetic phenomena we have mentioned, and many others of the same kind, daily observed by practitioners, are reflex phenomena.

Suppose a foreign body in the cornea of one eye; in a short time after the cornea has been submitted to this cause of irritation, we find that the conjunctiva is congested, photophobia begins, and tears are shed. There is no bloodvessel in the cornea; and, therefore, we cannot admit that it is through this kind of tissue that the irritation has been propagated. Shall we admit that it is through the corneal tissue itself, and by its continuity or contiguity with the other parts of the eye, that the propagation has taken place? If any one were tempted to imagine such an explanation, I would say that in cases of disease or section of the trigeminal nerve, in man and in animals, the irritation of the cornea is not followed by the least appearance of congestion of the conjunctiva. This congestion, therefore, in cases where the trigeminal nerve is uninjured, appears after an irritation of the cornea, in consequence of the transmission of the irritation to the encephalon by the corneal filaments of the trigeminal. Now, how can the congestion be produced after the irritation has reached the encephalon, unless it be by nerve-fibres going from this nervous centre to the eye? We may have doubts as regards the question, by what nerves the encephalon *reacts* upon the eye in such a case; but we cannot doubt that it *does react*, and that the congestion is due to this *reaction*, or, in other words, to a reflex action of the encephalon. Still more, in cases of irritation of one eye producing alterations in the other eye, it is clear that it is through the encephalon that the irritation is propagated.

Let us take another example: suppose we have placed a tube in one of the ureters of a dog, so as to know what is the quantity of urine flowing out in a given time, after the dog has recovered from the shock of the operation. We then pinch the internal surface of the abdominal wall, in a part receiving its nerves from one of the first lumbar pairs, and, almost at once, we find that the secretion of urine is either stopped or very much diminished. It is not in consequence of a change in the circulation, due to the pain caused by the pinching, that the secretion is so much diminished, as we find the same thing taking place whether the spinal cord in the dorsal region has been divided transversely, or left in communication with the encephalon. And if the part of the cord which gives origin to the lumbar pairs of nerves has been destroyed—in which case the urinary secretion, after a short stoppage, becomes normal (as regards its quantity, at least), and is rather more than less abundant than before—we find that the irritation of the abdominal wall remains without effect upon the kidney. We must conclude, therefore, that when the spinal cord exists, the irritation passes through it, or, in other words, that the stoppage of the urinary secretion is due to a reflex action of the spinal cord. I have ascertained, also, that it is through the spinal cord, and by a reflex action, that the irritation of one kidney acts upon the other, sometimes to diminish, sometimes to increase, its secretion.

Of course it is not by a reflex action only that some of the phenomena mentioned in this lecture are produced. In a case of extensive burns, for instance, there are several circumstances which contribute to the production of the visceral alterations so well described by Dupuytren, Mr. Long, and Prof. Erichsen. In the first place, a certain amount of blood is submitted to such a temperature that several of its parts (the globules especially) must be altered; in the second place, there is a more or less considerable diminution of the cutaneous secretions and exhalations, and, as shown by the experiments of Fourcault, Gluge, Gerlach, Ducros, Magendie, Becquerel, Breschet, Bouley, and my friend, Mr. Balbiani,[1] this is a cause of congestion of the various viscera. But as regards this last circumstance, there are many cases of burns in which visceral inflammations and rapid death have taken place when only a part of the skin, not larger than that of one limb, has been destroyed, so that it is impossible to admit that the cause of these inflammations and of death is only, or even chiefly, in the loss of the function of the skin, the greater part of which remains in a normal condition. As regards the other cause, the influence of heated blood on the viscera, I have made some experiments, the details of which I cannot relate now, which show that in animals in which the spinal cord has been divided at the level of the third or fourth lumbar vertebra, so that the posterior limbs cannot give any pain, and that, also, no irritation can be propagated from them to the viscera of the head, the chest, and most of those of the abdomen, I have not seen—when I killed them two or three days after I had burnt one of the legs with boiling water—any marked alterations similar to those which are so often observed in man and

[1] See his important thesis, "Essai sur les Fonctions de la Peau," &c. Paris, 1854, pp. 94–132.

animals accidentally burnt, except in the bladder and rectum, and neighboring organs. On the contrary, when the section of the spinal cord was made as high as the third dorsal vertebra, I have seen all the abdominal viscera in a state of congestion, very much resembling inflammation in many parts, with serous infiltrations and ecchymoses, two days after one of the legs had been burnt by boiling water.

It seems, therefore, that we are entitled to conclude that it is not only, and even not chiefly, to the cessation of function in a part of the skin, nor to the alterations of the blood, in cases of burns having destroyed all the skin, and most of the tissues of a limb, that we ought to attribute the inflammations, or the other alterations that the viscera present after burns. In two cases, on animals on which the trunks of the sciatic and crural nerves in one limb had been divided as high as possible, I have not found a state of marked congestion in any viscus, three days after I had carbonized this limb from the toes up to the middle of the thigh. From these experiments and the preceding, it results that it is, in a great measure, by a reflex action of the spinal cord that burns produce their deadly influence on the viscera.

In the cases of paralysis or of disease of the nervous centres, which appears after, and as a consequence of, an affection of a gland, as a kidney, or the liver, I do not need to say there may be a cause entirely different from that spoken of in this lecture, producing the paralysis or the disease of the nervous centres: I mean the presence of a poison in the blood on account of the diminution or alteration of an important secretion. There may be also other causes: for instance, Dr. R. B. Todd[1] relates a curious case, showing that a complete paralysis of motion and sensation of the lower limbs, apparently due to a disease of the kidney (which he supposed depended upon suppressed gout), was cured, simultaneously with the renal disease, shortly after gout had been attracted to the feet.

We have now to examine how a reflex action may produce or stop a secretion, how it may produce an atrophy or an hypertrophy, an inflammation, or some other of the various changes in nutrition which we have mentioned. In the preceding lecture (see Lecture IX.) we have said that there are two modes of action of the nervous system upon the production of the phenomena of nutrition and

[1] Cyclopædia of Anat. and Physiol., vol. iv. p. 721.

secretion. By one of these actions the nervous system determines an increase in the attraction of blood by the living tissues, and in this case the phenomena are accompanied by a dilatation of the bloodvessels; while the reverse exists when the nervous system, instead of acting upon the *parenchyma* of the tissues, acts upon the walls of the bloodvessels and produces a contraction. In the first case, the quantity of blood, passing through the part on which the nervous system has acted is increased; while in the second case it is diminished: in the first case the secretions are increased; in the second, diminished: in the first case nutrition is more active, and there is a tendency to hypertrophy and an augmentation of the vital properties of nerves and muscles; in the second case nutrition is not active, and there is a tendency to atrophy and a diminution of the vital properties of nerves and muscles: lastly, in the first case there is an augmentation of the temperature; while in the second, there is diminution. There is, therefore, the most complete difference between these two nervous influences.

Let us now employ the knowledge of these two modes of action of the nervous system to explain what occurs in some cases of secretory or nutritive reflex phenomena. Suppose, for instance, a calculus in one of the ureters: it irritates the centripetal nerve-fibres of this canal, the irritation is transmitted to the spinal cord, which reflects it upon the muscular coat of the bloodvessels of the two kidneys, and produces a contraction, in consequence of which there is much less blood passing through these organs, so that the urinary secretion is stopped or much diminished. Suppose a worm in the bowels, irritating their centripetal nerve-fibres: the irritation is propagated to the spinal cord, which *reflects* it upon the roots of the cervical sympathetic nerve, by which it reaches the bloodvessels of the retina, produces their contraction, and, as a consequence of this cause of diminution in the amount of blood, an amaurosis. If instead of the reflex action on the bloodvessels there is an action on the tissues, as in the case of the experiments of Czermak and Prof. Bernard (see Lecture IX.), the bloodvessels dilate, and more blood passes through them. The cornea, for instance, is irritated; its centripetal nerve-fibres transmit the irritation to the pons Varolii, which reflects it upon the retina, the lachrymal gland, the conjunctiva, &c.; more blood is attracted by all these parts, their bloodvessels dilate, and the consequences of a greater amount of blood become manifest (increase of tears, photophobia, &c.).

The two kinds of effects produced by the nervous system on nutrition and secretion, may coexist or follow each other; and we have instances of such a combination or alternation in cases of neuralgia, of worms, &c.

The simple fact of an increase or a diminution in the quantity of blood passing through a part, in a given time, is assuredly enough to explain the physiological and some of the morbid changes in secretion and nutrition which are usually observed; but some other morbid changes seem to require more than a simple change in the amount of blood for their production. For instance, an inflammation cannot be explained by such a change only, as we see that after the section of the cervical sympathetic nerve a very considerable increase in the quantity of blood exists in the eye, the ear, &c., and lasts for many weeks or months without an inflammation. It is true that this morbid process supervenes much easier by far in those parts than in others; but, we repeat, that it does not appear spontaneously, and simply on account of the quantity of blood. We must, therefore, admit, that when a nervous influence acts upon certain tissues to produce inflammation, the principal cause of this morbid process is not in the augmentation of the quantity of blood, but in the change in the tissues which produces a greater attraction of arterial blood.[1]

The history of the treatment of disease by means of the powerful influence of an excitation of centripetal nerves on remote organs, could afford us as many interesting facts as the history of the reflex production of inflammation and other morbid changes. But as I have not time enough to dwell on this subject, I will content myself by indicating some rules of treatment founded upon the knowledge of reflex actions.

1st. When we wish to produce a modification in the condition of any organ, we must apply the means of irritation that we prefer to the part of the skin or of the mucous membranes which have the

[1] We regret very much not to be able to examine fully here this great question of the production of inflammation, either by a reflex action or by other causes. We regret also not to be able to show how much the recent advances of science agree with most of the observations made by Dr. Hughes Bennett, Dr. C. J. B. Williams, Mr. Wharton Jones, and Mr. James Paget. We do not agree entirely with Mr. Joseph Lister, whose very important researches we know only by a summary of his paper (*Proceedings of the Royal Society*, vol. viii., No. 27, 1857, p. 581), but we can say that his view, that a change occurring in the tissues around the bloodvessels is the primary act in inflammation, might be supported by many facts entirely different from those so interesting which he has discovered.

most evident nervous relations with it. In most cases the parts acting with the greatest power upon another are those which receive their nerves from the same segment of the cerebro-spinal axis. If we wish, for instance, to act upon the kidney, the skin of the abdomen in its upper part is the best for the application of any kind of irritation. Do we wish to act on the eye, in cases of amaurosis due to insufficiency in the amount of blood, the irritation ought to be applied chiefly to the supra or infra-orbitalis nerves. If the amaurosis co-exists with hyperæmia, the irritation of those nerves must be avoided, and the means of revulsion ought to be applied on the back of the neck, so as to act on the spinal cord, and, through it, by the sympathetic nerve, which has on the eye an influence entirely different from that of the trigeminal nerve. In cases of diarrhœa, an influence upon the nerves of the bowels originating from nearly the middle of the dorsal region might be obtained by the irritation of the skin of the middle of the chest. The ovaries and the uterus being able to influence the nutrition of the mammæ, and these glands being able to act upon the genital organs, irritation will be applied to one group of these organs when we wish to act upon the other. In amenorrhœa, for instance, various means of irritation to the breast have produced menstruation.

2d. The kinds of irritation which produce the most powerful effects are a great and sudden change of temperature, heat or cold, or the application of a very strong galvanic current. Frequent irritations, with periods of interruption between them, are better than permanent irritations.

3d. The suppression of the cause of irritation, when a disease is produced by a reflex action, is of course the principal mode of treatment. In cases of paralysis, of anæsthesia, or of a convulsive affection, &c., we must try to find out if there is an irritation on any centripetal nerve, and employ the most energetic means for its removal. But I must say that it is entirely useless to amputate a limb, or a part of it, as has been done sometimes in cases of convulsive affections produced by an external irritation. The section of a nerve will do as well, and this is already proved by many cases, and perhaps, as I will show in my last lecture, a simpler means might be employed.

4th. Time pressing me to go on, I will only add here that in cases of reflex congestions or inflammations due to burns or to congelation, or, in fact, in any case in which we have to avoid a reflex influence, we must diminish the reflex faculty of the spinal cord and encephalon, and we know no medicine having so much power in this respect as belladonna.

Direct influence of the nervous centres and of the centrifugal nerves upon nutrition and secretion.—I will only say here, that the same phenomena, which we have described as taking place by reflex actions, can be produced also in consequence of a direct irritation upon the nervous centres and the centrifugal nerves. The phenomena due to this *direct* irritation have very often been mistaken for consequences of absence of action of the nervous centres. I will merely point out here the rapid sloughs that are observed after a fracture or a luxation of the vertebral column, and the rapid change in the urinary secretion in similar cases. As regards the effects of direct irritation of centrifugal nerves, the following case, in which, however, there was probably some indirect influence of the nervous centres, has been observed by Mr. Hilton, and published by Mr. Paget: "A man was at Guy's Hospital, who, in consequence of a fracture at the lower end of the radius, repaired by an excessive quantity of new bone, suffered compression of the median nerve. He had ulceration of the thumb and fore and middle fingers, which resisted various treatment, and was cured only by so binding the wrist that, the parts on the palmar aspect being relaxed, the pressure on the nerve was removed. So long as this was done, the ulcers became and remained well; but as soon as the man was allowed to use his hand, the pressure on the nerves was renewed, and the ulceration of the parts supplied by them returned."[1] Mr. Paget also relates a case of Mr. Swan, which has great analogy with the preceding. These two patients might have been cured at once by the section of the irritated nerves.

I will only add, as regards the influence of the pressure on the spinal cord producing sloughs on the nates and other morbid changes, that it is chiefly in exciting a persistent contraction in the bloodvessels of the parts where nutrition or secretion is morbidly altered, that the pressure on the cord acts. As it often happens that death, after a fracture or a luxation of the spine, is due to the slough formed on the nates, I think I must remark that a very good means of *dilating* bloodvessels consists in exhausting their irritability by applications of powerful galvanic currents.

Influence of the absence of the nervous system upon nutrition and secretion.—If I had time, I would show that most of the morbid

[1] Lectures on Surgical Pathology, vol. i. pp. 42–43.

changes which have been attributed to paralysis do not belong to it, but are the results of irritation upon either the nervous centres or the nerves; and that the effects which are truly the consequences of a paralysis are due, only in an indirect way, to the absence of nervous action. For instance, atrophy of muscles is chiefly due to the state of rest; changes in secretion are chiefly due to the paralytic dilatation of bloodvessels; ulcerations of the toes, in animals in which the nerves of the limbs have been divided, only show an effect of the rubbing of the same parts on a hard floor; ulceration and inflammation of the eye after the section of the trigeminal nerve, are chiefly due to physical causes (the drying of the cornea and the conjunctiva, the prolonged action of light, &c.). All these effects of paralysis may be, and have sometimes been, avoided.

On the other hand, if we try to find out what is the power of cicatrization and repair, in cases of paralysis not complicated by irritation of nerves, we ascertain, as has long ago been done by Sir Benjamin Brodie,[1] and as we have done since, and in varying more the mode of experimenting,[2] that wounds, burns, and fractures may be cured as quickly in paralyzed parts as in others. Many facts might be advanced to prove (as in the preceding) that if the influence of the nervous system is indirectly necessary to nutrition and secretion, it is nevertheless true that all the phenomena of nutrition and secretion may remain normal when the action of the nervous system on the various tissues is missing.

Influence of the nervous system on animal heat.—We do not propose, in these lectures, to treat *ex professo* of this influence; we only wish to show what is the cause of the local diminution or augmentation of temperature in paralyzed parts. As it is chiefly in cases of disease of the pons Varolii and medulla oblongata that these local changes of temperature are interesting in a practical point of view, we will postpone, till our lecture on these organs, the development of our views on this subject. We will say here, however, that the temperature of a superficial part of the body, or of a whole limb, depends greatly upon the state of the central nervous system; and that we may judge pretty well of this state by the degree of temperature of the feet, of the hands, &c.

[1] See the "Treatise on Nervous Diseases," by J. Cooke, vol. i., 1820, pp. 130–133.

[2] Experimental Researches applied to Physiology and Pathology, New York, 1853, pp. 6–17.

LECTURE XI.

ON THE ETIOLOGY, NATURE, AND TREATMENT OF EPILEPSY, WITH A FEW REMARKS ON SEVERAL OTHER AFFECTIONS OF THE NERVOUS CENTRES.

Artificial production of an epileptiform affection in animals.—Influence of certain injuries to the spinal cord as a cause of real epilepsy.—Existence of an unfelt aura epileptica in many cases.—Means of detecting the existence of an unfelt aura and its point of starting.—Seat and nature of epilepsy.—Principles of treatment of this affection.—Analogy between epilepsy and many other nervous affections, as regards their mode of production and their treatment.—Curious case of convulsions and insanity, in illustration of some views advanced in this letter.

Mr. President and Gentlemen: It is impossible in the narrow compass of a lecture, to treat fully of the great variety of interesting points concerning several grave affections of the cerebro-spinal centre. I must, therefore, though I much regret it, limit myself to a short sketch of some new views, which, perhaps, deserve the attention of both practitioners and men of science. Although I will only mention here a few of the principal facts which have led me to these views, I hope it will be understood that, if I do not try to give a complete demonstration of them, it is because such a thing is impossible in a single lecture.

I have found that a convulsive affection, very much resembling epilepsy, may be produced in animals. A few weeks after certain injuries to the spinal cord, in the dorsal or the lumbar region, especially in guinea-pigs, fits appear spontaneously several times a day, or, at least, once every two or three days. But the most interesting point is, that it is possible to produce a fit when we choose, by simply pinching a certain part of the skin. These fits consist in clonic convulsions of almost all the muscles of the head, the trunk, and the limbs, except those muscles which are paralyzed. The animal seems to have lost its consciousness, or, at least, its sensibility. There is an evident laryngismus in the beginning of the fit, and, after it, when it has lasted long, a state of drowsiness or unwillingness to move.[1] I have ascertained that one part only of the skin has the power of producing the fit, and this part is that which covers the angle of the lower jaw, and extends from thence to the eye, the ear, and nearly to the shoulder. It is only the skin that has the power of generating the fit, as even the three nerves that send filaments to this part of the skin can be irritated without the occurrence of convulsions.

When the spinal cord has been injured only on the right side, it is only on that side that the skin of a part of the face and neck has the power of inducing fits, *et vice versâ* when the injury exists on the left side. If the two sides of the cord are injured, the two sides of the face can produce fits. It is not the pain due to the irritation of the skin which causes convulsions, as I have ascertained that the degree of sensibility of that part of the face and neck is not greater than that of the neighboring skin, and is less (by far) than that of some parts of the skin in one of the abdominal limbs. It is evidently a peculiar kind of irritation, starting from the cutaneous ramifications of some centripetal nerves, which alone possesses the power of producing the epileptiform convulsions which are observed in animals in which the spinal cord has been submitted to certain injuries.

It results from the facts which have led me to the above assertions:[2]—

1st. That the spinal cord in animals may be the *cause* (I do not say the *seat*) of an epileptic affection.

2d. That there is a mysterious relation between certain parts of the spinal cord and remote parts of the skin of the face and neck.

3d. That epileptiform convulsions may be the constant consequence of slight irritations upon certain nerves.

4th. That the trunk of a nerve may not have the power of producing convulsions, whilst its cutaneous ramifications possess this power.

5th. That even when an epileptiform affection has its primitive *cause* in the nervous centres, some cutaneous filaments of nerves,

[1] For more details on this point, and on others concerning epilepsy in this lecture, see my "Researches on Epilepsy," &c., Boston, 1857, and the *Journal de la Physiologie de l'Homme et des Animaux*, 1858, pp. 241 and 472.

[2] To those readers of these lectures who have not been amongst my hearers, I must say that I have shown the principal experiments relative to this subject, as well as to most of the principal subjects of my lectures, so that my *assertions* were, very often, accompanied by an actual and direct demonstration.

not directly connected with the injured parts of these centres, have a power of producing convulsions, which other nerves, even directly connected with them, have not.

In man, epilepsy very frequently presents most of these peculiarities. As regards the first of them, it cannot be doubted that a disease of the spinal cord or of its membranes, as well as an affection of any centripetal nerve in the human body, may be the primitive origin of a real epilepsy, quite similar to the erroneously-called idiopathic epilepsy. I will refer to cases recorded by Bonet, Lieutaud, Morgagni, Musel, Portal, Esquirol, and a great many other excellent observers. The careful study of these cases shows clearly that in a number of them epilepsy has truly been generated by the disease of the spinal cord.

I do not know yet of any case in which, in man, just the same thing has been observed as in my epileptic animals. But there are only very few cases on record in which the very injury which in them has caused epilepsy, has been observed in man; and in those cases in which probably this injury has existed, we either do not know what have become of the patients, or they have died before the time after which epilepsy appears in animals after the injury to the spinal cord. But there are many cases on record in which an irritation of some point of the skin, or of some centripetal nerve, and sometimes even an *unfelt irritation*, has produced fits, just as, in my animals, the excitation of a part of the skin produces them.

I have collected such a number of facts in this respect, that the analogy between epilepsy in man and in my animals seems to be as great as possible; and I may add that, in most cases of genuine and complete epilepsy, as well as in cases of simple vertigo, there is an irritation starting from some point of a centripetal nerve, especially from its peripheric parts in the skin, or in the various mucous membranes. There is no medical man who has been in practice for a few years, who has not seen some cases of this kind; but almost all the recent writers on epilepsy having considered those cases as quite special, I must insist on saying, that even in the so-called idiopathic epilepsy there may be found an irritation starting from some centripetal nerve, and generating the convulsions; and I must add, also, that there is no radical difference between the symptoms of the sympathetic epilepsy, and those of the pretended idiopathic.

I will leave aside here all the cases in which an evident irritation on a centripetal nerve has caused epilepsy, such as cases of worms in the bowels, in the biliary ducts, or in the frontal sinus; of calculi in the ureter, in the biliary ducts, &c.; of foreign bodies in the ear or beneath the skin; of tumors pressing on nerves; of decayed teeth; of necrosed bones, &c. But I must say that in several cases the peripheric origin of fits has been quite evident, as it was sufficient to press upon a certain part of the skin to produce the epileptic seizure.[1] In other cases, a draught of cold air, the application of a galvanic current to certain parts of the skin, a sound, a smell, or the sight of a certain color, were always followed by a fit.

In cases of aura epileptica there is the greatest variety in the sensations felt, and the degree and the painfulness of the sensations are not such that we could explain by them the production of convulsions. It results from a thorough examination of a great many cases of aura, that we must admit that an unfelt irritation starts, at the same time as the aura, from some centripetal nerve, and is the real cause of the epileptic seizure. We will call this irritation an unfelt aura; and it would be well, indeed, if we could employ the name of "aura epileptica" for this unfelt irritation alone, so as to distinguish it completely from the vague and variable sensations which accompany it in many cases. There are facts proving that an unfelt aura may exist without any kind of sensation, either because the first effect of the irritation has been to destroy consciousness, or because the irritation does not start from sensitive nerve-fibres, but from centripetal nerve-fibres endowed only with the excito-motory power.[2]

It is very important, on account of the treatment, to find out if there is an unfelt aura, and what is its starting point. In consequence of this view, the condition of all the organs of the body ought to be carefully inquired into.

If the unfelt aura starts from some parts of the skin, or from some organ not deep-seated, as the testicle, or some part of mucous membranes, near the skin, either the first contractions in a fit, or the most violent or the most prolonged, are found in the neighbor-

[1] See my "Researches on Epilepsy," pp. 31, 32, 38, and 48. I might add several other cases observed by myself or others.

[2] See the curious cases of Pontier, of Joseph Frank, and of Henricus ab Heer, in my "Researches on Epilepsy," p. 32. In cases of worms producing epileptic fits, there is, sometimes, no sensation at all accompanying the unfelt irritation which causes the convulsions.

hood of the point of starting of the aura. If no indication of this kind can be furnished by the persons who have seen the fits, it will be well to try the application of a very powerful galvanic current, with dry conductors, on the various parts of the skin, when the patient expects to have a fit. I have, in this way, twice ascertained the point of starting of an unfelt aura: a fit has been produced by the galvanization of certain parts of the skin. Of course there are many cases where such a means of diagnosis ought not to be employed: every one will understand what are those cases.

Another and the best means (so far as the limbs alone are concerned), to detect the existence of an unfelt aura, consists in applications of ligatures on each limb alternately. Suppose a case of epilepsy in which the fits are frequent, and come at nearly fixed times, or after warnings of any kind, so that it may be known that it is to take place in a given time, or nearly so: a very tight ligature is put on one limb; and if the fit does not come, it is extremely probable that it depends on the irritation of an unfelt aura; if it comes, the ligature is applied on the other limbs at other times. I am sorry not to be able to give more details in this respect; but I think it will be easy to understand how, by such a means, it may be ascertained if an aura comes from the upper part of a limb, or from a toe or a finger, and from which one.

Even in cases of epilepsy due to a disease of the encephalon, the cause of the fits may originate from some points of the skin, and the prevention of the passage of the aura, in such cases, can prevent the fits. There are four cases of this kind that I know, in three of which the disease consisted in a tumor in the brain. In my animals the same thing exists; although the alteration of the spinal cord—which is the cause of epilepsy—persists, the aura being interrupted by the section of the nerves which go to the skin of the neck and face, epilepsy, so far as I have been able to ascertain, ceases. The aura may originate from any part of any centripetal nerve, and there is no doubt that its place varies according to the location of disease in the nervous centres, when it is due to such a disease.

A great many cases in which, by various means, the aura epileptica has been prevented from going up to the encephalon, show that the fit is very often due to a simple outside irritation. Applications of ligatures, sections of nerves, amputations, &c., act in this way. We might say the same thing of the elongation of muscles (the first ones that are convulsed), and, in a certain measure, of various means of revulsion (such as burning, blistering, &c.), although the principal mode of action then consists in producing, by a reflex action, a change in the nutrition of the nervous centres, and of the nerves which are the channels of the aura.

Epilepsy seems to consist essentially in an increased reflex excitability of certain parts of the cerebro-spinal axis, and in a loss of the control that, in normal conditions, the will possesses over the reflex faculty. The base of the encephalon, and especially the medulla oblongata, is the most frequent seat of the increase in the reflex excitability, so that this part of the nervous centre is the ordinary seat of epilepsy. The disturbance in the functions of the cerebral lobes, during and immediately after a fit, and in the interparoxysmal periods, is chiefly due to the alterations taking place in the brain during the fits. This hitherto mysterious coincidence of loss of consciousness, or, in other words, loss of the function of the cerebral lobes, with an increased action of the base of the encephalon, in a complete epileptic seizure, may now be easily explained. I have tried to show that the same cause that produces the first convulsions in some muscles of the neck, the eye, the larynx, and the face, produces also a contraction of the bloodvessels of the brain proper, which contraction is necessarily followed by the loss of consciousness. I am happy to state that two very able German experimenters—Messrs. Kussmaul and Tenner,[1] led by researches in several respects different from mine, have arrived at the same explanation.

In reviewing the principal phenomena of a complete seizure of epilepsy, we find that they form a series of causes and effects, as shown in the following table:—

Causes.	Effects.
1. Excitation of certain parts of the excito-motory side of the nervous centre.	1. Contraction of bloodvessels of the brain proper and of the face, spasm of some muscles of the eye and face.
2. Contraction of the bloodvessels of the brain proper.	2. Loss of consciousness, and accumulation of blood in the base of the encephalon.
3. Extension of the first excitation, *partly* due to the accumulation of blood in the base of the encephalon.	3. Tonic contraction of the laryngeal, the cervical, and the thoracic expiratory muscles. (*Laryngismus* and *trachelismus*.)

[1] Untersuchungen zur Naturlehre, &c., von Moleschott, vol. iii., Part I., 1857. I must say that I had published the above explanation before these German physiologists; but they have arrived at it quite independently, and almost at the same time as myself.

Causes.	Effects.
4. Contraction of laryngeal and of thoracic expiratory muscles.	4. Crying, and stoppage of respiration.
5. Farther extension of the first excitation of the nervous centre.	5. Tonic contraction, extending to most of the muscles of the trunk and limbs.
6. Loss of consciousness, and tonic contraction in the trunk and limbs.	6. Falling.
7. Laryngismus, trachelismus, and the fixed state of the chest.	7. Asphyxia, with obstacles to the return of venous blood from the head and the spinal cavity.
8. Asphyxia, and the accumulation of black blood in the encephalon, and in the spinal cord.	8. *Clonic convulsions* everywhere; contractions of the bowels, the bladder, the uterus; erection; increase of many secretions; efforts at inspiration.
9. Exhaustion of nervous power generally, and of the reflex faculty especially, except for respiration, which gradually becomes normal.	9. Cessation of the convulsions; coma or heavy sleep, after which extreme fatigue and headache.

Of course this table shows only the most frequent filiation of phenomena, and it is useless to say that there are great varieties as regards the first phenomena. The admirable researches of Dr. Marshall Hall have shown how important are the laryngismus and trachelismus, in the causation of the epileptiform convulsions. I will only add that the asphyxia, to which so great a share is due in the phenomena of epilepsy and in its most grave consequences, depends not only upon the state of the larynx, but on that of the chest; and that, not only the blood cannot return easily from the head, on account of the trachelismus, but also it cannot enter the chest from either the spinal canal or the head, on account of the fixed state of expiration. Besides, the bronchiæ themselves are often contracted; and all these causes coexist with an increased production of carbonic acid, and with a change in the circulation of the encephalon, during which the blood accumulates in the base of this organ, and also in the spinal cord.

As regards the treatment of epilepsy, we will only say that the principal rule is to find out if the disease has an external cause—*i. e.*, if from any part of the centripetal nerves there is an irritation acting upon the nervous centres. To prevent this irritation reaching these centres, or to destroy the cause of this irritation, if it is known to exist, are the two things to be done. I must repeat that this will be found much more often than is generally supposed. Against the increased excitability of some part of the nervous centres, the best means, assuredly, are the powerful modificators of nutrition, which, I am sorry to say, are so little employed by regular practitioners—the cauterization of the back of the neck by moxas, or by the red-hot iron.

Other affections very often have the same characteristic features as epilepsy, as regards their production. If I had time, I could relate a very large number of facts to prove that, much more frequently than might be imagined by most of my hearers, the various forms of insanity, of vertigo, of hallucinations, and of illusions, and also extasis, catalepsy, hysteria, chorea, hydrophobia, tetanus, local cramps, and even the general paralysis connected with insanity, may be due to irritations starting from a centripetal nerve, and frequently slightly felt, or even unfelt; and that the suppression of these irritations may promptly cure the patient, just as in cases of epilepsy. Instead of a description of this kind of affection, I will give here a case which is full of interest, and which I owe to the kindness of Mr. Campbell de Morgan, who had received it from the late Mr. Standert, of Taunton, who, according to Mr. de Morgan, was one of the most original thinkers and best surgeons of his day:—

CASE 44.—On rising in the morning, a lad, fourteen years old, was heard by his father making a great disturbance in his bed-room, who, rushing in to know the cause, found his son in his shirt, violently agitated, speaking incoherently, and breaking to pieces the furniture. Mr. —— caught the lad in his arms, and threw him back on the bed, when he at once became composed, but did not seem conscious of the mischief he had done. He said that on getting out of bed he had *felt something odd*, but that he was very well, and thought that he might have had a frightful dream, although he could not recollect it. I was immediately sent for, and the lad ordered to remain in bed until I had seen him. About five hours after, I found the lad lying in bed, reading some amusing book; his tongue clean, pulse regular, countenance calm and cheerful. He said he was quite well, and wished to get up, but that his father had ordered him to remain in bed until I had seen him. I was informed, before I went up to his bed-room, that the lad had never before been heard to complain of disturbed dreams, or walked in his sleep, or exhibited any epileptic symptoms, and that his general health had been good, and all his functions regular. Finding the patient free from any apparent disease, and that he had eaten with good appetite, and no disturbance, his usual breakfast, I desired him to get up. When, sitting up in his bed, he drew on his stockings; but *on putting his feet on the floor and standing up, his countenance instantly changed, the jaw became violently convulsed*, and he was about to rush forward, when I seized and pushed him back on the bed. He was at once calm, but looked surprised, and asked what was the matter with him. He assured me that he had felt no pain, had slept well, but that he "*felt odd*" when he stood up. I found that he had been fishing on the preceding day, and, having entangled his line, had taken off his shoes and stockings, and waded into the river to disengage it; but he said he had not cut or scratched his feet or met with any other accident. To ascertain this point, I made him draw off his stockings, and examined his legs minutely. Not the slightest scratch or injury could be seen; but *on holding up the right great toe with my finger and thumb to examine the sole of that foot, the leg was drawn up, and the muscles of the jaws were suddenly convulsed, and on releasing the toe these effects instantly ceased.* I then closely inspected the toe. The nail was perfect; there was not the least swelling or redness in the surrounding parts, nor any tenderness or uneasiness felt when I compressed the toe laterally, or moved it, held thus, in any direction; but on the bulb of the toe, nearly at the point where the circumgyrations of the cuticle centre, there was a very small elevation, as if a bit of gravel, less than the head of a small pin, had been there pressed in beneath the cuticle. There was not the least redness on this spot, nor any sensation or effect produced by passing my finger over its surface; but *on compressing it with my finger and thumb against the nail very cautiously, a slight convulsion instantly ensued.* I asked the patient if anything pricked him? He said "No, but *something made him feel very odd.*" On examining the part well with a pocket lens, no scratch or puncture of the cuticle could be discerned. I then with a pair of scissors included and snipped away the slightly elevated part, but not so deeply as to denude the cutis beneath. In the bit of cuticle thus removed I expected to find some point of a thorn or particle of sand, but could not detect anything of the kind. I then pressed the toe in every direction; *the strange sensation was gone, and never returned.*

I do not know that any member of the patient's family had ever been under treatment for insanity, but two of his uncles and I believe an aunt were suicides, and the patient himself, many years afterwards, was "found drowned" by the cautious verdict of an inquest.

LECTURE XII.

ON THE MEDULLA OBLONGATA, THE PONS VAROLII, AND SOME PARTS OF THE SPINAL CORD, IN THEIR RELATIONS WITH RESPIRATORY MOVEMENTS; WITH VERTIGINOUS OR ROTATORY CONVULSIONS; WITH THE TRANSMISSION OF SENSITIVE IMPRESSIONS AND OF THE ORDERS OF THE WILL TO MUSCLES, AND WITH THE VASO-MOTOR NERVES AND ANIMAL HEAT.—GENERAL CONCLUSIONS OF THE COURSE.

Medulla oblongata erroneously considered as the source or focus of life.—Causes of death in cases of sudden injury to this organ.—Respiration depending upon other parts of the cerebro-spinal axis, besides the medulla oblongata.—Causes of the cessation of respiration in cases of a complete section of the medulla oblongata.—How are the respiratory movements produced?—Parts of the encephalon and spinal cord that may produce rotatory convulsions.—Causes of the vertiginous or rotatory convulsions.—The auditory nerve and its power of producing partial or general convulsions.—The olivary and restiform columns of the medulla oblongata and their relations with various nervous disturbances.—Reasons against the view that the fibres which decussate all along the median line of the base of the encephalon are voluntary motor fibres.—Reasons for admitting that the anterior pyramids contain nearly all the voluntary motor fibres of the body.—Three kinds of paralysis due to lesions in three different parts of the cerebro-spinal axis.—Anæsthesia and hyperæsthesia in their relations with the state of bloodvessels and the degree of animal heat.—Condition of voluntary movements, sensibility, and animal heat, in different cases of alteration of the central nervous system.—General conclusions.

Mr. President and Gentlemen: Since the time of Galen[1] most of the physiologists, and particularly Lorry, Cruikshank, Lorenz, Bartels, and Legallois, have ascertained that a sudden and deep injury to the lower part of the medulla oblongata, in animals, causes immediate death, and many cases observed in man have shown the same thing. It has been almost universally admitted that death is then due to the fact that respiration ceases because the lower part of the medulla oblongata is the centre for respiratory movements. But if we study carefully what takes place in most of the

[1] Galen clearly states that a section of the medullary axis, beneath the first or the second cervical vertebra in an animal, kills it at once. See *De Anat. Administr.*, lib. 8, cap. 9, pp. 696, 697. Kuhn's ed., Leipzig, 1821.

cases of immediate death caused by a sudden and deep injury to the lower part of the medulla oblongata, we find that it is impossible to explain this curious mode of death by admitting that it is only due to a sudden arrest of respiration.

If we take two living animals of the same species, and decapitate them by a section passing, in one of them, on the nib of the *calamus scriptorius*, and in the other, on the fourth or fifth cervical vertebra, and cutting also, in both, the principal nerves of the neck, and avoiding the section of the carotids, we often find that the first one has no convulsions, or, in other words, no agony; while the second almost always has very violent convulsions in the four limbs and in the trunk. In both cases the medulla oblongata is taken away and respiration is stopped; we cannot, therefore, attribute to the cessation of respiration the absence of convulsions in only one of the cases. We will see in a moment what is the cause of this absence of convulsions. Before we come to this explanation, we must say that a physiologist who has attained a very high situation in France, M. Flourens, one of the perpetual secretaries of the Academy of Sciences, to explain the sudden death after the destruction of a small part of the medulla oblongata, has proposed a theory of which we ought to take notice, on account of the standing of its author. M. Flourens imagines that life depends on a force springing from a very small part of the medulla oblongata, which small part he calls the *vital point* or the *vital knot*.[1]

If this hypothesis were true, certainly it would be very easy to understand why there are no convulsions, and hardly any sign of life in the heart and in other organs after the extirpation or destruction of the pretended vital knot. Unfortunately for this theory, the part which is supposed to be the *focus* or the *source of life* may be taken away, and life persist, without any marked trouble. My experiments not only show that life may last long after the extirpation of a much larger part of the medulla oblongata

[1] The paper of M. Flourens, containing his principal assertions in this respect is in the *Comptes Rendus de l'Acad. des Sciences*, vol. xxxiii., 1851, p. 437. He declares that the vital knot is not larger than the *head of a pin*, and that its place is at the *point* of the small V of gray matter, at the nib of the *calamus scriptorius*. Forgetting all that he had said as regards the size of this small point, M. Flourens has just read a paper to the Academy of Sciences (*Comptes Rendus*, 1858, vol. xlvii. p. 803), in which he acknowledges that the extirpation of that small point does not destroy life, and he now places the vital knot in the midst of the medulla oblongata, between the V of gray matter and the crossing of the anterior pyramids.

than this small amount of gray matter erroneously considered as the source of life, but that neither any part nor the whole of the oblong medulla can be considered as the source of a pretended vital force. In the first place, a sudden irritation of the spinal cord, as well as that of the medulla oblongata, may cause a sudden death, without agony or convulsions, although in both cases, and especially in the first one, the pretended *focus of life* remains almost or entirely uninjured. In the second place, the extirpation of this pretended only source of life, when made carefully by slow and partial sections, at a certain distance from it on the spinal cord and the pons Varolii, is followed by the most violent convulsions and by energetic movements of the heart, the bowels, the bladder, &c. In the third place, if the par vagum has been divided in a living animal, any kind of operation may be performed upon the medulla oblongata without destroying quickly or suddenly the movement of the heart; and, in this case, the convulsions of agony take place with energy.

From the above-mentioned facts and from several others, I have drawn the conclusions[1] that the irritation of the oblong medulla and of some parts of the spinal cord (a great portion of the cervical region) is able to produce a sudden stoppage or diminution of the movements of the heart, and that it is, in a great measure, to this influence on the heart that is due the absence of agony in most of the cases of sudden destruction of the oblong medulla.

More than ten years ago, I found that certain animals may live for many weeks, and, in more recent researches, for eight months, after the extirpation of the whole medulla oblongata.[2] In these animals all the functions of organic life, except pulmonary respiration, continue without any apparent alteration, showing that these functions do not depend upon the medulla oblongata, as some physiologists have thought. The persistence of life in these animals was possible on account of the cutaneous respiration; but in animals in which the skin absorbs but a small amount of oxygen, such as birds and mammals, death is said to be always rapid after the extirpation of the medulla oblongata, even when care is taken to avoid the influence of the operation upon the heart. It seems,

[1] See my paper, Recherches sur les Causes de Mort après l'Ablation du Point Vital, in *Journal de la Physiol. de l'Homme*, &c., Avril, 1858, pp. 217–233.

[2] Comptes Rendus de l'Acad. des Sciences, 1847, vol. xxiv. p. 363, and my Exper. Researches applied to Physiol. and Pathol., 1853, p. 40.

therefore, that the medulla oblongata is an organ absolutely necessary to respiratory movements. Against this view I will remark, 1st, that Dr. Bennet Dowler, of New Orleans, has seen thoracic respiratory movements continuing in decapitated alligators; 2d, that Dr. B. W. Richardson has observed the same fact in young mammals; 3d, that I have seen it also in birds, and in kittens and puppies.

It seems, therefore, quite certain that the respiratory movements do not depend only upon the medulla oblongata. I have already tried to show, in 1851, that many parts of the encephalon are employed in respiration, and, since then, I have collected a great many pathological facts, proving, I think, the correctness of this view. It is known that the only two appearances of proof that the medulla oblongata is the only centre of respiratory movements, or, in other words, the only source (direct or reflex) of these movements in the cerebro-spinal axis, are—1st, that a transversal section of the lower part of the medulla oblongata causes a sudden cessation of respiration; 2d, that when transversal sections are made on the encephalon, from its front to its back, taking away layer after layer, it is said that it is only after the greatest part of the medulla oblongata has been taken away, that respiration is destroyed. As regards the first of these two assertions, we have already shown the objections against it—objections which are also very good against the second assertion. But we must say a few words more of this second assertion. When, after a series of transversal sections of the encephalon, we have reached the medulla oblongata, just above the upper roots of the par vagum, we find that respiration continues almost normal. If now we cut away the part of the medulla giving origin to this pair of nerves, we find, in most cases, that respiration is suddenly stopped. This certainly *seems* to prove that the small part to which the par vagum is attached is the nervous centre for respiration. But is it truly so? I will try to prove that it is not.

1st. In weak animals, after many parts of the encephalon have been taken away, the whole of the medulla oblongata and of the pons Varolii remaining, respiration sometimes continues normal, but it suddenly stops after a small part of the pons is removed. It would be wrong to draw from this experiment the conclusion, that this small part is the central organ of respiration. To draw such a conclusion, however, would be to employ the same reasoning which has been adopted concerning the part of the medulla oblongata giving origin to the par vagum. The stronger an animal is, the more parts of its encephalon can be taken away before we destroy respiration. It is in animals in which the spinal cord is rich in gray matter, and possesses a powerful reflex faculty, that we find respiration persisting after the whole of the encephalon, including the oblong medulla, has been extirpated; such is the case in alligators, in birds, in young dogs and cats.

2d. In the strongest animals, death occurs in a few hours, and from insufficiency of respiration, after the ablation of the encephalon except the whole of the medulla oblongata; and so it often is with anencephalic monsters. These facts show clearly that, although respiration may be carried on, for a time, almost as well as in the normal condition of the central nervous system, when only the medulla oblongata and the spinal cord exist, these organs are insufficient for a long persistence of this function. A series of experiments on pigeons has given me the following results: with the spinal cord alone, respiration continues a few minutes; with the spinal cord and the part of the oblong medulla giving origin to the principal excitors of respiration—the vagi—this function continues many hours (the longest duration we have seen is thirteen hours); if there is also a great part of the base of the encephalon left, respiration continues longer, but I have never seen it last more than a day and a half; if the cerebrum alone is taken away, respiration remains undisturbed; and if death occurs, it is not on account of an insufficiency of the parts left of the cerebro-spinal axis to carry on respiration.

3d. In man, hemorrhage in the various parts of the base of the encephalon, near the median line or upon it, produces a trouble in respiration, which is more and more marked the greater the amount of effused blood, and the nearer it is to the medulla oblongata. Certainly, in many cases, the trouble of respiration may be partly attributed to pressure on the medulla oblongata, but it is not always so; and, at any rate, in several cases of softening of the pons Varolii, in which it cannot be said that there was a pressure on the oblong medulla, there has been a trouble in respiration. From the examination of a great many cases,[1] I have been led to the conclusion that the whole base of the encephalon is employed in respiration.

[1] Most of these cases have been published in the thesis of my pupil, Dr. J. B. Coste, *Recherches sur le Rôle de l'Encéphale dans la Respiration*, Paris, 1851.

4th. Many cases have been observed in which the medulla oblongata has been so much altered that almost all its actions as a nervous centre ought to have been destroyed, and, nevertheless, respiration has continued to take place; in those cases there was still, however, a more or less free communication between the pons Varolii and the spinal cord, and probably several of the filaments of the par vagum continued to act as excitors of respiratory movements.

All the facts just mentioned, and many others of which I have no time to speak, have led me, first, to abandon the view so generally admitted, that the medulla oblongata is the essential source of the respiratory movements in the nervous centres; and secondly, to propose the view that these movements depend upon all the *incito-motory* parts of the cerebro-spinal axis, and on the gray matter which connects those parts with the motor nerves going to the respiratory muscles. I must add that, according to the theory I have arrived at, the principal cause of respiration is in the lungs, as Dr. Marshall Hall has tried to prove; but that excitations coming from all parts of the body, as shown by Volkmann and Vierordt, and also direct irritations of the base of the encephalon and of the spinal cord, almost constantly taking place, contribute to the production of respiratory movements.

I pass now to another and a quite different subject, although it is connected with the physiology and pathology of the parts of the nervous centres which have the principal share in respiration. I wish to say at least a few words about rotatory or vertiginous movements. It seems, indeed, wonderful to see animals, sometimes after a slight puncture of some part of the encephalon with the point of a needle, *turn round*, just like a horse in a circus, or *roll over and over* for hours, and sometimes for days, with but short interruptions. The same phenomena having often been observed in man, I think it may prove interesting, if not useful, to point out the parts of the encephalon which may produce vertiginous or rotatory convulsions. The convulsions differ a great deal, according to the place injured and the depth and size of the injury. If we suppose that the right side of the encephalon, in the places I will name, has been injured, we find that the animal *turns* or *rolls*, and that in the first case the side on which it turns is either the left or the right; while, if it rolls, the rolling begins either by the left or the right side.

Parts producing turning or rolling after an injury on the right side.

Turning or rolling by the right side.	*Turning or rolling by the left side.*
1. Anterior part of the optic thalamus. (Schiff.)	1. Posterior part of the optic thalamus. (Schiff.)
2. The hind parts of the crus cerebri. (Schiff.)	2. Some parts of the crus cerebri, near the optic thalamus. (Brown-Séquard.)
3. The tubercula quadrigemina. (Flourens.)	3. Anterior and superior parts of the pons Varolii.
4. Posterior part of the processus cerebelli ad pontem. (Magendie.)	4. Anterior part of the processus cerebelli ad pontem. (Lafargue.)
5. Place of insertion of the auditory and of the facial nerves. (Brown-Séquard and Martin-Magron.)	5. Place of insertion of the glosso-pharyngeal nerve. (Brown-Séquard.)
6. Neighborhood of the insertion of the lower roots of the par vagum. (Brown-Séquard.)	6. Spinal cord, near the oblong medulla. (Brown-Séquard.)

While rotation takes place, it is easy to ascertain, 1st, that it is not its production by contractions resembling those of voluntary movements which causes the rolling or the turning; 2d, that some muscles are in a state of tonic contraction; 3d, that the trunk and neck of the animal are bent by a spasmodic action on the side of turning if it has a circus movement, and that it is bent like a cork-screw, as much as the bones allow, in cases of *rolling;* 4th, that sensibility and volition may remain, and that there are frequent efforts to resist the tendency to turn or roll. It seems clear from these observations and several others, that these rotatory movements depend chiefly upon the fact that certain muscles are in a state of spasm.

I shall not try to show that the theories of Magendie, of Flourens, and of Longet, are in opposition with many of the particularities of the experiments.[1] Any one knowing these theories may find out from the above statement of facts, that these hypotheses are not acceptable. The theory of Henle, who admits that convulsions are produced in the eyes, and that as a consequence a kind of vertigo is generated, which causes the rotatory movements, is not more acceptable, as there are some cases in man, and many in animals, in which the eyes had no convulsions at all, although rotation existed. My friend, Dr. Lebret, has seen a case of this kind in man. That a state of vertigo may sometimes be the prin-

[1] See my Experimental Researches on Physiology and Pathology, 1853, p. 18.

cipal cause of turning or rolling, is, I think, beyond question;[1] and that this state may be induced either by the irritation of some vaso-motor nerve in the encephalon, or by the too great attraction of blood by some parts of this organ, is, I think, also very probable; but I believe that in most cases the principal cause is in the irritation of a peculiar set of nerve-fibres not usually employed by the will—nerve-fibres, the division of which is not followed by paralysis, although they are able to act on muscles to produce contractions, and even more powerful than those caused by nerve-fibres employed by the will in voluntary movements. It is a fact worthy of attention, that a puncture with a needle through the anterior pyramids which contain, as I will soon prove, very nearly all, if not all, the nerve-fibres employed in voluntary movements, will hardly produce a momentary contraction in some muscles; while certain punctures through the olivary column of the medulla oblongata at once produce a spasm of many muscles, although this column does not contain more than very few (if any at all) voluntary motor-fibres! And, now, to add to the strangeness of the fact, in this last case, the muscles remain contracted sometimes for hours, sometimes for days and weeks! We have all been taught, and several probably in this room, where there are so many professors and lecturers, have taught that, after the removal of a cause of excitation in the nervous centres, as well as in the nerves, the effects of the excitation disappear until inflammation supervenes and produces a permanent excitation; while here, however, we see a puncture with a needle or a section with a knife, before any inflammation can have begun, followed by a persistent effect. There is, therefore, in some parts of the nervous centres, a property of acting in a persistent manner to produce muscular spasms, during and after a mechanical excitation.

The persistent spasmodic contractions, due to a mechanical injury to certain parts of the nervous centres, are always curious, but never so much so as when they result from some irritation of a part like the auditory nerve, which we were accustomed to consider simply as a nerve of sense. M. Flourens[2] has found that the section of the semicircular canals, in certain animals, is followed by a strange disorder of movements, and sometimes by a rotation

[1] See the very able and learned paper of Dr. Russell Reynolds, entitled Vertigo. London, 1854.

[2] Rech. sur les Propr. et les Fonctions du Syst. Nerveux. 2de ed., 1842, p. 454 *et seq.*

(circus movement). I have ascertained that the phenomena observed in these experiments do not depend on the section of these canals, as this operation may not cause these phenomena, but that they are the results of an irritation of the auditory nerve, from the drawing upon it by the membranous semicircular canals at the time we divide them. In frogs and in mammals, the direct irritation of the auditory nerve is followed by the most interesting phenomena. It is well known that in frogs the peripheric extremity of this nerve is inclosed in a bag containing carbonate of lime; as soon as this bag is laid bare and slightly touched, and still more if it be punctured with a needle or a bistoury, the anterior limb, *on the opposite side*, is thrown into a state of slight convulsion, and kept almost constantly in a spasmodic pronation; and almost at every attempt to move forwards the animal turns round on the side injured. As long as it lives (many days, or even many months), these phenomena may be observed, although not quite so marked as immediately after the injury, or after the first twenty-four hours. In mammals, the least puncture of the auditory nerve causes *rolling*, just as after the irritation of the processus cerebelli ad pontem; violent convulsions then occur in the eyes, the face, and many muscles of the neck and chest. The doctrine that the nerves of the higher senses are not endowed with general sensibility (*i. e.*, are not able to cause pain) seems not to be true with regard to the acoustic nerve; at least, the signs of pain given after an irritation of this pretended nerve are often as great as those observed after an irritation of the trunk of the trigeminal nerve.

In man, also, the auditory nerve seems to be able to act as it does after an injury in animals.

1st. Any one who has received an injection of cold water in the ear may know that it produces a kind of *vertigo*, and that it is difficult to walk straight for some time after this irritation.

2d. A sudden noise makes the whole body jump, particularly in old people, or in persons attacked with anæmia, chlorosis, epilepsy, chorea, hysteria, hydrophobia, and in certain cases of poisoning; in a word, in all circumstances in which the control of the will over reflex actions is lost or diminished.

3d. Vertigo and various convulsive movements, in cases of irritation of the acoustic nerve,[1] have been observed in adults and

[1] Walter and Lincke, quoted by Harless in art. "Horen," in Wagner's Handwörterbuch der Physiol., vol. iv., 1853, pp. 420, 423.

children. Rotatory movements have taken place in cases of suppurative inflammation of the ear, and twice immediately after an injection of a solution of nitrate of silver.[1] Quite recently Mr. Hinton has read a paper to one of the London medical societies, in which he relates several cases of convulsions in children, without any other visible alteration after death, except in the ear.

I could point out several other facts to prove that irritation of the auditory nerve may cause vertigo, rotatory movements, and various other kinds of convulsions; but I think I have said enough to call the attention of practitioners to this subject, and this was my principal object. I will only add a few words more to say that the causes of rotatory movements are numerous, and that, besides the one which is the principal in most cases (and that is the spasm produced in some muscles, as I have already said), there is a cause similar to that of simple vertigo, depending upon anæmia, or generated by an irritation upon some centripetal nerve (as, for instance, in cases of gastralgia), and producing a contraction of some blood-vessels of the brain, by a reflex action, and this cause is the insufficiency of blood, and the consequent alteration in the nutrition of certain parts of the brain.

The parts of the base of the encephalon, which are capable of producing persistent spasms, seem to be quite different from those employed in the transmission of sensitive impressions or of the orders of the will to muscles, at least in the medulla oblongata and the pons Varolii. They constitute a very large portion of these two organs, and perhaps the three-fourths of the first one; they are placed chiefly in the lateral and posterior columns of these organs; many of their fibres do not decussate, and produce spasms on the corresponding side of the body; they seem to contain most of the vaso-motor nerves, by which, directly or through a reflex action, they may act on other parts of the nervous system, as I will show hereafter; they have much to do with the phenomena of several, if not most, of the convulsive diseases; and, lastly, I will say that the history of their properties and actions throws a great deal of light on the effects of extirpation or diseases of the cerebellum.

The above assertions, which I advance with the greatest reluctance, as I have not time enough to show that they are based on

[1] See the case of Prof. Burggrœve, recorded by himself (*Gaz. Méd. de Paris*, 1842, p. 25). A most eminent military man, I am told, has twice been seized with rotatory convulsions after injections in the ear.

positive and numerous facts, are not the only ones to which I wish to call attention. Connected with them there is a theory of which I have already spoken (see Lecture VII.), and which I must now try to demonstrate. This theory is, that almost all, if not all, the voluntary motor fibres of the trunk and limbs that come from the brain pass by the anterior pyramids, or in the layer of gray matter in contact with them. This view, which is pretty nearly the one held already by Mistichelli, Pourfour du Petit, and others, has been universally abandoned, in this century, after the publication of the important researches of Foville[1] and of Valentin,[2] showing that there seems to be a complementary decussation of nerve-fibres, all along the median line of the base of the encephalon.

The small number of fibres in the anterior pyramids, on the one hand, has appeared to be insufficient for the conveyance of the orders of the will to all the muscles of the trunk and limbs; and the existence of paralysis on the side injured in the encephalon, on the other hand, has contributed to lead to the actually admitted opinion that the voluntary motor fibres make a part of their decussation in the medulla oblongata, and the other part in the pons Varolii, and also higher up between the two sets of tubercula quadrigemina and the two cerebral peduncles. Long ago Cruveilhier[3] had said that "the small fascicles, called anterior pyramids, cannot be sufficient for the extensive phenomena indicating a crossing of action in the brain." A man of great authority in physiology as well as in pathology, Dr. R. B. Todd,[4] says that "anatomy suggests that a lesion limited to either anterior pyramid would affect the *opposite* side of the trunk, for it is known that such an effect follows disease of the continuation of it in the meso-cephale or crus cerebri; and that lesion limited to the posterior half of the medulla oblongata, on either side, would affect the *same* side of the body, no decussation existing between the fibres of opposite restiform or posterior pyramidal bodies." Longet,[5] with Foville and Valentin, expresses the idea that there are two sets of voluntary motor columns in the medulla oblongata: one, the anterior pyramids, and the other the olivary or innominated columns; and that

[1] Traité Complet de l'Anatomie du Syst. Cérébro-Spinal, 1844, pp. 298–326.

[2] Traité de Névrologie, Trad. Franç., pp. 236, 237, 246.

[3] Article "Apoplexie," in "Dict. de Méd. et de Chir. Prat.," vol. iii. p. 226.

[4] Art. "Nervous System," in the Cyclop. of Anat. and Physiol.," vol. iii. p. 722. T.

[5] Anat. et Physiol. du Syst. Nerveux, 1843, vol. i. p. 383.

this last set has a decussation of fibres all along the pons Varolii and before it. (See Fig. 24, B, B.) Against this theory, the following decisive arguments may be advanced:—

1st. Suppose an alteration in one of the crura cerebri. (Fig. 25, *p*, *o*.) According to the theory, as a part of the decussation of the voluntary motor nerve-fibres takes place there, we should find that voluntary movements are diminished on both sides of the body—more, of course, in the side *opposite* to the alteration, but partly also in the *same* side of the body. This is not what exists. One side only of the body is paralyzed; and it is the *opposite* side. A number of cases prove that this is the rule. The hemiplegia may be complete or incomplete, according to many circumstances, and particularly the extent and the nature of the alteration, and the rapidity of its formation; but there is something constant coexisting with any one of these numerous varieties: it is that the seat of the paralysis is in the side of the body opposite to that of the disease. It is evident, in consequence, that the decussation of the voluntary motor nerve-fibres has entirely taken place before they reach the crura cerebri.

2d. The same thing may safely be said of the corpora quadrigemina. (Fig. 18, *n*, *t*, and Fig. 24, MN.) Although the cases relative to these organs are much less numerous than the cases relative to the crura cerebri, there are enough of them on record to prove that the crossing of the voluntary motor nerve-fibres must have taken place entirely before they reach the base of the corpora quadrigemina. Besides some other cases, there are two very interesting ones which have been published, one by Mohr, and the other by Burnet—both of which I have already quoted.

3d. As to the pons Varolii (Fig. 18, *p*, and Fig. 25, V), the question is much more interesting, because this is the place where the decussation of voluntary motor fibres, according to Foville, Valentin, and Longet, more particularly takes place. Here, according to the theory of these distinguished anatomists, we ought to find different symptoms in these three different cases: 1st, alteration limited to the superior part of the organ; 2d, alteration limited to the inferior parts (the nearest to the medulla oblongata); 3d, alteration occupying the whole of a lateral half of the organ. In the first case we should see an incomplete paralysis in both sides, but greater on the side of the body opposite to the side of the disease; and, in the second case, we should see also an incomplete paralysis in both sides, and almost to the same degree in both. Many cases are on record proving that it is not so, and that whatever is the part of the pons altered (the superior, the inferior, or the middle), the same effect is produced on voluntary movements. When paralysis is produced by the lesion, it exists, exclusively, in the *opposite* side of the body; and when the alteration is not limited to one side of the pons, and extends to the other, then the side most paralyzed in the body is the one *opposite* to the most altered side of the pons.

If the theory of Valentin, Longet, and others were true, we should find in cases where the whole of one-half of the pons is diseased, the two sides of the body partly paralyzed, and the side opposite to the alteration less than the other. On the contrary, we find that paralysis exists only in one side, and that is the one which, according to the theory, should be *less paralyzed.* I might prove that I am right by relating here many pathological facts; but as I have already mentioned some (see Lecture VII.), and as I shall have in a moment to mention several others, I will merely now affirm again that there are many.

4th. Still more, if the theory we disapprove were true, we should see in cases of alteration of a lateral half of the medulla oblongata, above the decussation of the anterior pyramids (Fig. 25, *p*, *o*), a paralysis nearly as marked in the same half of the body as in the opposite half. But this is not what is observed, and we find paralysis only in the opposite side. (See particularly Cases 38 and 39, Lecture VII.)

It seems absolutely certain, from the above facts and reasonings, that there is no decussation of the voluntary motor fibres of the trunk and limbs above the crossing of the pyramids. On the other hand, we have already shown, in a previous lecture, that there seems to be no decussation of these fibres in the spinal cord—*i. e.*, below the crossing of the pyramids; so that we are led to admit that most of, if not all, the conductors of the orders of the will to muscles decussate at the lower part of the medulla oblongata, and that these conductors chiefly form the anterior pyramids, after their decussation. An interesting fact, in addition to those already mentioned, concerning these pyramids, is, that when a lesion exists at the place of decussation, it produces a paralysis in the two sides of the body, because it destroys fibres belonging to them both. This is a feature quite peculiar to this part of the cerebro-spinal axis. (See Fig. 21—1, 2 and 3.)

From the preceding remarks, and from the facts and reasonings contained in our lectures (the third and seventh) on the decussation of the conductors of sensitive impressions, it results that, as regards anæsthesia and paralysis, three different groups of symptoms may be observed, according to the place of the alteration in a lateral half of the cerebro-spinal axis: 1st, above the decussation of the pyramids, a lesion on either the medulla oblongata, the pons Varolii, the crura cerebri, the optic thalami, the corpora striata, or the brain proper, if it produces anæsthesia and paralysis, produces them both in the opposite side of the body; 2d, below the decussation in the pyramids, a lesion in the spinal cord produces paralysis in the same side, and anæsthesia in the opposite side; 3d, at the level of the decussation of the pyramids, and upon the decussating fibres, and also behind them, a lesion produces paralysis in both sides of the body, and anæsthesia only in the opposite side. So that *wherever the lesion, in a lateral half of the cerebro-spinal axis, may be—below, above, or at the level of the crossing of the pyramids—if it produces anæsthesia, it is in the opposite side;*[1] *while paralysis, in these three cases, is either in the same or the opposite side, or in both sides.* (See Figs. 18 and 21.)

A striking proof of the exactitude of the view that the anterior pyramids are almost the only channels for the orders of the will to muscles in the medulla oblongata, and that the olivary or intermediate columns have no share in this function, is given by those very interesting cases of atrophy of one-half of the brain and of the corresponding anterior pyramid, with paralysis and atrophy of the two limbs of the opposite side, and also atrophy of the opposite half of the spinal cord, while the olivary and restiform columns are unaltered. There are now several cases of this kind on record; I have seen two, and Mr. Turner has given a complete description of three or four.[2]

Many persons have thought that the cases of paralysis depending upon an alteration in a lateral half of the encephalon, and existing in the same side of the body, could not be accounted for except by admitting that there are voluntary motor nerve-fibres that do not decussate in the medulla oblongata. I have not time

[1] Of course, a lesion in one-half of the cerebro-spinal axis, anywhere at the level of the entrance of a sensitive nerve, besides producing anæsthesia everywhere below the seat of the injury on the opposite side, causes it also in the same side, but only in parts receiving the nerve or nerves the roots of which pass through the altered part of the nervous centre.

[2] De l'Atrophie unilatérale du Cerveau, du Cervelet, &c. Thèse. Paris, 1855.

enough to examine fully the various explanations that may be proposed about paralysis in the same side as the encephalic lesion, but I will try to show—1st, that there is a part of the encephalon which almost always produces this kind of paralysis; 2d, that this paralysis ought to be regarded as similar to the reflex paralysis due to an irritation of centripetal nerve-fibres, in any viscus, any membrane, or the trunk of a nerve. (See my *Journal de Physiol.*, Juillet, 1857, p. 534.)

When a tumor exists, pressing upon the anterior surface of one of the crura cerebelli and upon the insertion of the trigeminal nerve (see Fig. 25, *c c*), if it causes paralysis, it is in the same side of the body. I have collected fourteen cases of this kind, all having the same features, which are *incomplete* paralysis in the side of the lesion, no anæsthesia (except in one case), and frequent fits of vertigo. Now, as to the explanation of this kind of paralysis, we will say, that it is either the result of the destruction of some conductors employed in voluntary movements (to regulate them or to act otherwise), or of the irritation of certain nervous fibres in the peduncle itself, or near it. Were the first hypothesis the true one, we should find that a destruction of the whole peduncle causes paralysis in the corresponding side only, or in it and in the other one, and not in this other alone; but there are several cases in which there has been, with such an alteration, a paralysis in the opposite side only.[1] We should find, also, that alterations of the parts by which the crus cerebelli communicates with the muscles produce a paralysis in the same side of the body, together with a paralysis in the opposite side. But this is not what is observed. I have collected more than thirty cases of alteration in a lateral half of the pons Varolii and medulla oblongata, in many of which the lesion extended to the crus cerebelli, and in all the paralysis was in the opposite side only.[2] For instance, in a case of Dr. Annan, which I have related (see Case 38, Lecture VII.), the whole connection of the *right* crus cerebelli with the *right* half of the medulla and of the pons was destroyed, and the paralysis existed only in the *left* limbs. (See Fig. 25, *c c*.)

As to the other hypothesis, we will say that it is the only one

[1] See especially a case carefully recorded by Serres (Traité d'Anatomie comparée du Cerveau, vol. ii. pp. 623-6).

[2] There are a few cases, however, in which a tumor has pushed backwards and upwards the crus cerebelli and the corresponding half of the pons, producing only a slight degree of paralysis in the same side of the body.

we can find able to explain the production of the paralysis in the side injured, in cases of irritation of the crus cerebelli; and we will add that, perhaps, the same explanation would be the right one for all the cases of the so-called *direct* paralysis. But whether it is the irritation of the fibres of the crus, or of those of the trigeminal nerve, which causes the paralysis, we cannot tell, and we have no time to discuss the question. The same reason prevents our examining why the anterior surface of the crus cerebelli, or the trigeminal nerve at its point of insertion, have more power than in their other parts, or than the rest of the encephalon, to cause a paralysis, in consequence of an irritation. I will only say that we find that the peripheric parts of the same nerve in the gums and the bulbs of the teeth, as also certain parts of the sympathetic nerve, have more power to produce a paralysis than other nervous ramifications in many parts of the body; and that, therefore, there is no ground for an objection to our hypothesis from the fact that such a paralysis is not caused by the irritation of other parts of the encephalon than the crus cerebelli. I may add, that when an irritation on a nerve causes a paralysis, it is usually in the corresponding side of the body that it appears, just as is the case when a tumor exists between the petrous bone and the crus cerebelli.

To complete, as much as time will allow, the exposition of my views on the physiology and pathology of the central nervous system, I have now to speak of the condition of animal heat in cases of alteration of the spinal cord and the encephalon. The following conclusions may be drawn from a great many facts bearing on this subject:—

1st. That usually anæsthesia is accompanied by a diminution of temperature.

2d. That hyperæsthesia almost always co-exists with an increased temperature.

3d. That in paralysis, without either a notable hyperæsthesia or anæsthesia, the temperature is nearly normal.

I must remark that the state of heat of a part is due to the amount of blood, the degree of heat of this fluid, the exposure of the part to the influence of the temperature of the surrounding medium, and the temperature of this medium. Now, in anæsthetic parts the bloodvessels are usually contracted, and, therefore, there is less blood in them, and also a lower temperature. In hyperæsthetic parts the reverse exists.

Pathological cases show that when there is an alteration in one-half of the spinal cord, the bloodvessels in that side are paralyzed, as are also the muscles. There is more blood in these paralyzed, parts, and the temperature is higher than it is normally. In the opposite side the reverse obtains. It seems from these facts, and from many experiments, that it is from paralysis of the vaso-motor nerves, and from their irritation in the cerebro-spinal axis, that arises the difference of temperature between the two sides of the body, in cases of alteration of a part of one-half of this axis. In combining what is taught by pathological cases, as regards temperature, with the symptoms concerning sensibility and voluntary movements, we are led to give the following indications of the usual phenomena to be observed in cases of disease in one part of a lateral half of the cerebro-spinal axis.

Table of symptoms in the trunk and limbs, according to the seat of a lesion in one lateral half of the cerebro-spinal axis.

1. Lesion in the brain proper, the optic thalamus, or the corpus striatum.

	On the opposite side.	On the same side.
Sensibility	Diminished or lost	Normal
Voluntary movements	Ditto, ditto	Ditto
Temperature (even without fever)	Increased	Ditto

2. Lesion of the pons Varolii or the medulla oblongata above the decussation of the anterior pyramids.

	On the opposite side.	On the same side.
Sensibility	Diminished or lost	Increased
Voluntary movements	Ditto, ditto	Normal
Temperature	Diminished	Increased

3. Lesion of the medulla oblongata at the level of the decussation of the anterior pyramids.

	On the opposite side.	On the same side.
Sensibility	Diminished or lost	Increased
Voluntary movements	Ditto, ditto	Diminished or lost
Temperature	Diminished	Increased

4. Lesion of the spinal cord.

	On the opposite side.	On the same side.
Sensibility	Diminished or lost	Notably increased
Voluntary movements	Ditto, ditto	Nearly normal
Temperature	Diminished	Increased

It is unnecessary to say that nothing is more variable than the degree of temperature of paralyzed or anæsthetic parts, and that, therefore, what is stated in the above table ought to be considered as the *most frequent* condition, and not as a *constant* one. Paralyzed bloodvessels may contract under the influence of cold, and the temperature and the hyperæsthesia of a part may, in this way, diminish for a time. On the other hand, contracted bloodvessels will necessarily relax after a long period of contraction, because they lose their power of contraction by a persistent and somewhat spasmodic action, and, in this way, anæsthetic and cold parts may temporarily become warm.[1]

GENERAL CONCLUSIONS OF THE COURSE.

Our principal object in these lectures has been, to prove, chiefly by experiments upon animals and by pathological cases observed in man, many new views concerning the physiology and pathology of the central nervous system. A number of these views have been proposed by myself; whilst the others, although advanced by several physiologists, have not yet been sufficiently proved.

At the same time that we have tried to build new doctrines, we have shown the insufficiency and, sometimes, the complete untenableness of certain theories which had been more or less generally admitted. In the following conclusions, which are only a very small part of those that might be drawn from the facts and reasonings which have been mentioned in our lectures, we will point out the most important views that we have tried to establish:—

1st. Excitations of the anterior roots of the spinal nerves may be a cause of pain, because these roots, being motor, produce a *cramp*. The pain due to this cramp is what has been erroneously called *recurring sensibility*. Cramps, and several other kinds of painful spasms (of the uterus during parturition, of the sphincter ani in certain cases, &c.), are painful on account of a galvanic irritation of sensitive nerves accompanying muscular contractions. (Lecture I.)

2d. Our movements seem to be guided by the peculiar sensations we derive from the galvanic irritation of certain sensitive nerves of muscles, while they contract. (Lecture I.)

3d. The power of transmitting sensitive impressions exists in many parts which are not able to give pain or any other sensation when they are excited by our usual means of irritation; so it is with the gray matter of the spinal cord, and with many parts of

[1] See for other parts concerning this subject my Experim. Researches applied to Physiol. and Pathol., 1853, pp. 73–78.

nerves, which, however, are conductors of sensitive impressions. (Lecture II.)

4th. Hyperæsthesia is a constant result of certain injuries upon, or alterations of, the posterior parts of the cerebro-spinal axis, from the tubercula quadrigemina down to the lower end of the spinal cord. (Lectures II., IV., and V.)

5th. The transmission of sensitive impressions, in the spinal cord, takes place chiefly through the gray matter, and partly through the anterior columns; but, before reaching the gray matter, the impressions, in a certain measure, pass through the posterior columns. (Lectures II., IV., and V.)

6th. The conductors of sensitive impressions from the trunk and limbs decussate in the spinal cord, and not in the encephalon, as was universally admitted. (Lectures III. and VII.)

7th. Although the spinal cord is greatly altered or injured, sensibility, more or less diminished, may persist everywhere, on account of a peculiar arrangement of the conductors of sensitive impressions. (Lectures IV. and VI.)

8th. The various kinds of sensitive impressions seem to be transmitted by quite distinct conductors, in the nerves and in the nervous centres, and the place of passage of some of these conductors, in the spinal cord, seems not to be the same as that of the others, but none of them go up to the sensorium *along* the posterior columns. (Lecture VII.)

9th. In the upper part of the cervical region of the spinal cord, near the medulla oblongata, most of the conductors of the orders of the will to muscles are in the lateral columns, and in the gray matter between these and the anterior columns. (Lectures IV. and VIII.)

10th. The voluntary motor conductors decussate at the lower part of the oblong medulla, and not all along the median line of the base of the encephalon. (Lectures VII. and XII.)

11th. The posterior columns of the spinal cord have a great share in reflex movements, and this is the principal cause of the peculiar kind of paralysis so often observed in cases of alteration of these columns. (Lecture VIII.)

12th. The effects of excitation of the vaso-motor nerves consist essentially in a contraction of bloodvessels, which is followed by a diminution of the quantity of blood, in the temperature, and in the activity of nutrition. The effects of interruption of continuity of the vaso-motor nerves (*i. e.*, their paralysis) consist essentially in a paralytic dilatation of bloodvessels, which is followed by a greater afflux of blood, an increase of temperature, and a greater activity of nutrition. (Lecture IX.)

13th. As a great many vaso-motor nerve-fibres go up to the brain and to the cerebellum along the spinal cord, the medulla oblongata and the pons Varolii, the diseases or injuries of the various parts of the cerebro-spinal axis, besides symptoms concerning sensibility and movement, present symptoms depending upon irritation or paralysis of vaso-motor nerves: contraction or relaxation of bloodvessels, diminution or augmentation in the quantity of blood, increase or diminution of temperature, alterations of nutrition, of secretions, &c. (Lectures IX. and XII.)

14th. Besides the kind of influence of the nervous system upon nutrition, absorption, and secretion, through the vaso-motor nerves, there is another kind, which seems to consist in changes in the elements of the tissues—changes producing various modifications in the quantity of blood attracted, and in the interchange of materials between the blood and the tissues. (Lectures IX. and X.)

15th. The absence of the influence of the nervous system on any part of the body is hardly a cause of other alterations of nutrition than atrophy, while the irritation of the nervous system is a most powerful direct or reflex cause of a great many morbid changes in nutrition, secretion, &c. (Lecture X.)

16th. The sympathetic, normal, and morbid changes of nutrition, secretion, &c., are reflex phenomena, the study of which shows how many diseases are produced by a reflex action, and how a rational mode of treatment might be arrived at. (Lectures X. and XI.)

17th. The loss of consciousness in simple vertigo or in complete attacks of epilepsy does not depend upon a disease of the brain, but upon a contraction of the bloodvessels of the cerebral lobes—contraction due to some irritation of the vaso-motor nerves of these vessels, either by some direct cause irritating them in the base of the encephalon or the spinal cord, or by a reflex influence.

18th. Much more frequently than has been imagined, all the following affections may be produced by a peculiar kind of irritation starting from almost any centripetal part of the nervous system; epilepsy, the various forms of insanity, chorea, catalepsy, hysteria, tetanus, hydrophobia, &c. (Lectures X. and XI.)

19th. The medulla oblongata is neither the only nor an essential nervous centre for the respiratory movements. (Lecture XII.)

20th. There are a great many nerve-fibres and nerve-cells in the medulla oblongata, the pons Varolii, and the other parts of the base of the encephalon, which are not employed in the transmission of sensitive impressions or of the orders of the will to muscles, and are endowed with the singular property of producing, after even a slight irritation, a *persistent* spasm in certain muscles, and especially in the neck. Rotatory convulsions very often depend chiefly upon the production of such spasms, and of changes in the bloodvessels of certain parts of the encephalon. (Lecture XII.)

21st. The irritation of the auditory nerve may cause rotatory or simple clonic convulsions. (Lecture XII.)

22d. The conductors of the orders of the will to muscles, of the sensitive impressions and of the nervous influences to bloodvessels, decussating at different places in the cerebro-spinal axis, various symptoms are to be observed, depending upon either the irritation or the paralysis of these three kinds of conductors, according to the part of a lateral half of the cerebro-spinal axis where an alteration exists. (Lecture XII.)

APPENDIX.

APPENDIX.

We propose to make here many additions, which, we hope, will increase the value our lectures may have, both in a scientific and in a practical point of view. There are objections to the opinions we have advanced, which we have not been willing to discuss in our lectures, for, had we stopped for such a discussion, this interruption might have proved injurious to the clearness of the demonstrations. It is one of the objects of this appendix to examine these objections. On the other hand, there are deductions for the treatment of many diseases, which are to be drawn from the principles that we have tried to establish in our lectures; it is also one of the objects of this appendix to give the most important of these deductions.

PART I. EXAMINATION OF OBJECTIONS THAT MIGHT BE MADE AGAINST MANY OF THE VIEWS WHICH ARE HELD IN THE PRECEDINC LECTURES.

We think that it is quite wrong to say—as many physiologists and practitioners do—that a fact is not true, simply because it is in opposition with generally admitted views. Many discoveries might be made by scientific inquirers, who, without prejudice, would collect facts, which, though they seem to have been well observed, *appear* to be contrary to admitted doctrines, and would try to find out an explanation of these facts. We will only say that there is no great discovery in science which has not been in opposition with previously admitted doctrines. The preceding assertion will serve as an apology for the discussion of certain facts, the existence or the exactitude of which has been generally doubted, although it seems to have been positive.

1. *Alleged existence of voluntary movements and of sensibility in children apparently deprived of the cerebro-spinal axis.*

I think that it is now impossible to deny that there have been cases in which such monsters (*Amyelencephalous*, Béclard), have had movements, either inside or outside of the uterus, and, without doubt, purely reflex, and which have been mistaken for voluntary movements, and admitted as a proof that sensibility existed. Among numerous cases collected by Isidore Geoffroy St. Hilaire[1] and by Ollivier d'Angers,[2] there are some which cannot be considered as entirely erroneous statements, and, to laugh at the believers in these facts, as Longet[3] does, cannot be an argument against their existence. What is to be done is, no more to deny, but to try to explain, and this I will do, after having related some extremely curious cases, recently published, and, perhaps, better authenticated than those of which Longet has spoken.

The first case I will relate is recorded in the very rich and interesting catalogue of the Boston Anatomical Museum, for which science is indebted to the zeal and activity of my learned friend Prof. J. B. S. Jackson.

Case 1.—A pregnant woman did not feel the movements of her child, until about the end of the fifth month, and they were always feeble and peculiar. In the last month, slight motions of the child were still occasionally felt, even after a profuse discharge of liquor amnii. Labor came on, and was accomplished with very little pain; the child was born *alive*, the mother having felt its motions for fifteen or twenty minutes after it was expelled. On the arrival of Dr. Hildreth, half an hour afterwards, the lower extremities of the child were still in the vagina.

Autopsy.—The spinal marrow was wanting, and the spinal column being open throughout, the nerves terminated in the membrane upon its posterior face. A very small bundle of nervous fibres was seen passing down over five or six of the processes upon the left side, and a few of the cranial nerves were found, among which, it was thought, was the par vagum. Nerves of the trunk and extremities well developed.

1 Hist. des Anomalies de l'Organisation, vol. ii. 1836, pp. 344–351, and 371–4.
2 Loco cit., vol. i. p. 146.
3 Anat. et Physiol. du Syst. Nerv., 1842, vol. i. p. 323.

The brain existed, weighing three ounces (the weight of the monster being three pounds and one ounce). It rested upon the expanded dorsal and lumbar vertebræ, and upon the integument which covered the depressed cranial bones. It was divided into two equal hemispheres, and, imperfectly, into convolutions, the arachnoid membrane being continuous about the base with the common integument. The whole mass was very soft, and of a dusky color, from congestion, and effused blood; there being in each hemisphere a cavity which was filled with coagula. No other parts of the brain were recognized, and no connection was traced between this mass and any of the nerves, either cerebral or spinal.[1]

It is to be regretted that some circumstances have not been pointed out in this case, and, for instance, the size of the ganglions of the sympathetic and of the spinal nerves.

The movements of the child, after birth, not having been ascertained by the physician himself, we cannot know whether they were respiratory, convulsive, or reflex. As to what took place before birth, if we can rely upon the assertion of the mother, there have been movements, but they began late, although much sooner than these uterine contractions, which are sometimes mistaken for movements of the child. The mother had had already two children, and therefore was able to distinguish the movements of a child.

I must say also that, in a physiological point of view, although the brain was existing in this monster, it is exactly as if it had been missing, because it was not connected with the nerves.

In the following case we will find that movements have existed, during pregnancy, in a case, the circumstances of which may lead us to explain how movements can exist.

Case 2.—A woman, pregnant for the sixth time, was not aware of the fact, although her abdomen had become large, and her menstruation had stopped, and she was much surprised when she felt the movements of her child, which were so strong, that even the hand of another person could perceive them. The 8th of May, she felt the movements for the last time; and after the expulsion of a very considerable quantity of water, she was delivered of a child,

[1] A Descriptive Catalogue of the Anatomical Museum of the Boston Society for Medical Improvement. By J. B. S. Jackson, 1847, p. 263. (Case by Dr. Charles T. Hildreth.)

who, out of the uterus, remained motionless. Its weight was from 3 to 3½ lbs. It had no neck, and the head—very small—appeared to be lodged in a cavity in the trunk. From the upper part of the orbitary arcade, the skin was missing all over the head. The spinal canal, open all along, from the cranium to the lumbar region, contained a spinal cord, being in shape like a band, flattened from behind forwards, and of about one line and a half in thickness; its beginning at the base of the cranium was somewhat bifurcated, and evenly cut. It was lying on a fatty and fibrous mass, which filled a deep excavation, found in the place where the neck should have been, had it existed. This medullary band was very loosely attached to the spinal canal, by some fibrous filaments. This band had no connection with the nerves, which terminated in the vertebral foramina by a swollen and ganglionary extremity. In the trunk and limbs, the nerves were well developed. There was no brain. The chest was large; no respiration had taken place, as the lungs showed. The upper part of the cranium was missing, and the basis was convex.

It is very much to be regretted that Dr. Olier,[1] to whom we owe the relation of this interesting case, has not given more details about the nervous system. He does not speak either of the cranial nerves or of the sympathetic.

I have now to examine the value of the two cases I have related, and of many other analogous to them, which are more or less authenticated.

The first question is, whether there has been any decided voluntary movement, and any perception of a sensitive impression in these monsters.

Nothing proves that sensibility exists, and the movements consecutive to an excitation, however regular or co-ordinate they may be, cannot give such a proof. Nothing in these circumstances proves that these movements are not reflex. It is now generally admitted, as Bischoff,[2] Prof. Simpson,[3] and others have established, that the movements of healthy children in the uterus, and even for some time after birth, are merely reflex. If it is so for them, *à fortiori*, is it so for the *pseudencephalic* monsters. These reasons against the existence of sensibility may be employed against that

[1] Observ. d'un fœtus Anencéphale, in Comptes Rendus de la Soc. de Biologie, 1850, vol. ii. p. 106.

[2] Traité du développement de l'homme.—Trad^{on}. françoise, 1843, p. 459.

[3] Edinb. Monthly Journal of Med. Science, July, 1849.

of a Will, in these monsters. Their movements are almost always consecutive to an external excitation. Nevertheless we admit that they have, sometimes, an *apparently* spontaneous movement; but, we well know that reflex movements may be excited by any irritation of the viscera, and that the respiratory movements of the chest may excite reflex movements in the limbs. Besides, the same excitation which produces respiratory movements, is able to produce movements in the limbs. I have tried to prove, in a work[1] which I published five years ago, that the nerves, muscles, and some other parts of the body, may be excited to act, by blood, containing a great quantity of carbonic acid. Very likely, respiratory movements, in monsters, as well as in healthy children and adults, take place in consequence of an excitation produced by carbonic acid, and an excitation, by this agent, may also be the cause of some of the falsely called voluntary movements in the pseudencephalic monsters.[2]

To conclude, we will say that, if there appears to be no doubt that movements may exist in these monsters, nothing proves that they are voluntary and that they result from true sensations. On the contrary they appear to be purely reflex or mere excited movements.

A second question now arises, much more difficult to be solved than the preceding. How to explain reflex movements, if there is no spinal cord, or if this organ, though existing, is not united with the nerves?

Let us examine alternately the different possible explanations.

1st. A man of genius, Etienne Geoffroy St. Hilaire,[3] has given credit to the idea that the liquid which is sometimes found in the pseudencephalic monsters, in the cranio-spinal cavity, and filling there a tube, formed by the meninges—may be considered as containing the elements of the brain and spinal cord, in their primitive state of development. In many cases this liquid is not found in the membranous tube formed by the meninges, but then it appears

[1] Experimental Researches applied to Physiol. and Pathol. New York, 1853, pp. 101–113.

[2] The pseudencephalic monsters compose the genus *Pseudencéphale* of the family of the *Pseudencéphaliens* of E. G. St. Hilaire. They correspond to the *Amyélencéphales* of Béclard. The characters of the genus are to have the spinal canal open and no spinal cord, and, besides (as family characters), no true encephalon, and, in its place, a vascular tumor, which may contain some nervous matter.

[3] Philosophie anatomique.—Des Monstruosités humaines, 1822, vol. i. pp. 125–153.

to have gone out, together with the liquor amnii, before parturition.

This theory is quite opposed to the well known doctrine of Morgagni,[1] who admitted that the production of the liquid, found in, or coming from the cranio-vertebral cavity, is the result of a morbid action, and that a true dropsy is the cause of the destruction of the nervous centres.

Of these two opinions, if we adopt the first, as regards the source and the nature of the liquid, we cannot, nevertheless, adopt entirely the view of E. G. St. Hilaire, that this liquid may act as the brain and spinal cord would. We know that as long as the nervous centres are in a liquid state, in the human embryo, there are no movements, and I have ascertained that this does not result from an insufficiency in the development of muscles. In embryos of rabbits, from eight to twelve days old, I have found the muscles irritable and producing movements when directly excited, and their nervous centres, then almost entirely liquid, appeared not to be endowed with any power of action. But it may be that the liquid we find in the vertebral canal of monsters, contains a sufficient number of soft nerve-fibres and cells, to produce some reflex movements. Micrographers, and they alone, may solve the question of the existence of these nervous elements in this liquid.

If we admit as true the doctrine of Morgagni, it belongs still more to micrographers to point out what nervous elements are left in the cases where the naked eye shows only a liquid.

2d. A second explanation might prove good for a number of cases, and especially those like the one of Dr. Olier, which I have related. A rudiment of the spinal cord exists, but is not found united with the nerves. For those who know how easily in fœtuses, healthy or not, the roots of the spinal nerves may become separated from the spinal cord and also from the ganglions, and, besides, may break in any part of their length, particularly when there is an unusual amount of water around them—it will be easy to understand that, in monsters, the roots of the nerves may not have been found, although they may have existed. It is known that a very able anatomist, Desmoulins, having vainly searched for the roots of the spinal nerves in fishes, concluded that they do not exist, and that the nerves, in these animals, are attached to the meninges. Desmoulins has been greatly mistaken, and if he has been so, in

[1] De sedibus et causis Morborum. Epist. 12.

such circumstances, it will easily be admitted that others, not so accustomed as he was to dissections, may commit the same error, in circumstances more favorable to a mistake.

In experiments, that I have performed on birds and other animals, I have found that reflex actions may exist after considerable alterations of the spinal cord. I will hereafter give the details of some of these facts and of some others proving that, not only then, reflex actions may exist, but also sensations and voluntary movements. We can, therefore, understand that a small stripe of the spinal cord, as in the case of Dr. Olier, if it is connected with the nerves, may be the cause of the reflex movements existing in the pseudencephalic monsters.

3d. We are led to propose a third explanation, based upon some anatomical facts, observed in amyelencephalians, and also upon the experiments we have just spoken of, and which prove that small parts or stripes of the spinal cord may be sufficient for reflex actions.

In some cases of anencephalia or of pseudencephalia, the roots of the nerves have been found hanging, apparently, as loose threads in the cranial and spinal cavity. In cases of this kind, reported by Dr. Lonsdale[1] and Prof. Paget,[2] it has been found that the nerve-fibres formed loops, imbedded in a filamentous tissue and surrounded by numerous granules. It is probable, and it is considered to be so by Prof. Paget, that this granular matter may be regarded as gray matter, in an early stage of development.

I am not prepared to say that these loops and this slightly developed gray matter are capable of producing reflex movements, strong enough to be observed, but I think that they may help other parts in the production of these movements.

An amount of gray matter, much greater than that found by Drs. Lonsdale and Paget, may certainly have existed, in cases of *amyelencephalia*, and no notice taken of it, by physicians who were not prepared to consider it as nervous matter. And this amount of gray matter, connected with the roots of the nerves, may have been able to produce reflex movements.[3]

[1] Edinb. Med. and Surg. Journal, January, '44.

[2] Brit. and For. Med. Rev., No. 48, p. 273.

[3] It is very much to be regretted that the recorders of the cases numbered 776, 778, 781, in the *Catalogue of the Boston Museum*, have not said if the mothers of the monsters they describe, had felt them move, during the last days of pregnancy. As regards the case No. 776, p. 254, the writer says: "A trace of brain only existed

The possibility of existence of reflex movements when the spinal cord is reduced to only a part of its substance, is well proved by the following experiments. Two pigeons had had their spinal cord divided transversely, at about the middle of its length. A metallic wire was passed in the spinal canal and pushed, from the place where the cord had been cut, until the level of the second or third caudal vertebra. In one of these animals there has been, a short time after the operation, weak but positive reflex movements, in the tail and the posterior limbs, whatever was the excited point. For many days and until the time when this animal was killed, reflex action lasted. The dissection of the animal was made at a meeting of the Society of Biology,[1] and all the posterior surface of the cord was found covered with coagulated blood; the cord was flattened from behind forwards, softened in all its thickness, and it had in many places a violet, reddish color, without doubt due to infiltrations of blood. This half liquid gray matter which, in birds, exists in the rhomboidal ventricle, was destroyed,[2] and the posterior columns of the cord were, almost everywhere, separated one from the other, so that the central gray matter was laid bare.

In the other pigeon there were evident, but weak, reflex movements, only in the left posterior limb and in the tail; excitations of the skin of the right posterior limb were absolutely without effect. Dissection being made, in presence of the Society of Biology, it was found that, in a great length, the right side of the spinal cord had been entirely destroyed, and that the other half, which existed, was red and softened, and in communication with the roots of the nerves and with the caudal part of the cord, which was but little altered.

I have performed other experiments of the same kind, on some mammals, and succeeded in obtaining like results, particularly on very young ones. Newly-born cats are the best animals for such experiments. Before my researches, experiments of this kind had

if any at all, but in the situation of the pituitary gland, there was found a soft, rounded, reddish mass; and there was some appearance, also, of a thin and superficial layer of medullary substance in place of the spinal marrow; and the same has been sometimes observed in other similar cases; spinal nerves and ganglia well developed, as they usually are in these cases."

[1] See Comptes Rendus, vol. ii. 1850, p. 47.

[2] I have already published, eight years ago, a very curious fact about this gray matter: it is that when it is taken away, a reproduction of a similar substance takes sometimes place in a very short time.

been made, but only on frogs and other cold-blooded animals, by Volkmann, Van Deen and Stilling.

The resemblance between what takes place in the animals I have experimented upon, and what exists in monsters, extends farther than the co-existence in both, of reflex movements and of a small amount of nervous matter, in the spinal canal. I have found[1] that, in animals, having had a part of their spinal cord crushed, there were, besides reflex movements, convulsions, and, in certain muscles, contractures producing deviations of different parts of the limbs. So that I had there, under my eyes, the phenomena which exist in the production of deviations, in the limbs of monsters, according to the theory of Dr. Jules Guérin.

4th. The last explanation I will propose, is founded on the fact that the ganglia of the spinal nerves and those of the sympathetic are generally much developed, in monsters deprived of a great part or of the whole of their cerebro-spinal axis, as Breschet, Lallemand[2] and others have pointed out.

In the case of Dr. Olier, above reported, we see that the spinal nerves had, in the vertebral foramina, a swollen and ganglionary extremity. In a very interesting case of acephalia, recorded by Prof. O. W. Holmes,[3] although the spinal marrow existed, the ganglia of the sympathetic nerve, and the filaments connecting them, were unusually developed in the thorax, abdomen and pelvis; in the thorax were two ganglia, which extended from the upper rib to about the eighth rib upon the right side and to the sixth on the left.[4] In this case the two upper limbs and the head were missing.

The increase in size of the ganglia in these monsters may easily be explained. The blood, containing the chemical elements, which are to be used in the formation of the nervous tissues, their deposition ought to take place, in the only parts of the nervous system which exist, and, the less there are of such parts, the greater, as a general rule, ought to be the accumulation of nervous matter in them.

It is to be regretted that in cases where the spinal cord was

[1] See Comptes Rendus de la Soc. de Biologie, vol. iii. 1851, p. 15.

[2] Observ. pathol. propres à éclairer plusieurs points de Physiol., 1818, p. 30.

[3] Catalogue Boston Museum, p. 245.

[4] It is interesting to compare this description with the statement of Antoine and Malacoune, who say that in acephalian lambs all the nerves originated from a ganglion in the abdomen. (See the already quoted work of I. Geoffroy St. Hilaire, vol. ii. p. 516.)

missing, and the ganglia of the sympathetic nerve were enlarged, it has not been examined if the branches of communication between the motor and sensitive spinal nerves were not larger than usual. The importance of such an examination becomes evident if we suppose a case of *amyelencephalia*, in which it would be positive: 1st, that there has been recently more or less reflex movements; 2d, that there is no trace whatever of the encephalon and of the spinal cord.

Then, we have either to give up all the teachings of daily experimentation and observation, about the necessity of nervous centres for the production of movements, after an excitation of the skin or of another surface—or to look upon the ganglia of the spinal nerves or of the sympathetic, or of both, as the nervous centres which, by their reaction, originate these movements. At first, we already know that these ganglia are larger than usual; but to admit the hypothesis to which we are forcibly led, some other things must exist. If the ganglia of the sympathetic alone are enlarged and are endowed with reflex power over the muscles of the limbs and trunk, of course, the nerves of these parts must be connected by many more nerve-tubes than usual, with these ganglia. In other words, the origin of the excito and reflecto-motor nerve-fibres of the limbs and trunk must be in these ganglia, instead of being, as normally, in the spinal cord. This implies, not only that the branches of communication, between the spinal nerves and the ganglia of the sympathetic, must be larger than usual, but, also, that the fibres come from the periphery of the spinal nerves into the branches of communication. If, instead of being in the ganglia of the sympathetic, the enlargement is in those of the spinal nerves, then the fibres of the motor roots, instead of merely passing along the ganglia, will penetrate them, and be connected there with the cells of the gray matter and with the excito-motor fibres, as, normally, in the spinal cord.

The four explanations, or rather the four hypotheses, which I have exposed, and by which I believe that we may understand how are produced the reflex movements in monsters, apparently deprived of the cerebro-spinal axis, may be solved by future examination. My object in relating these hypotheses was double; it was, 1st, to show, that there is possibility of explaining the movements of these monsters, so that we are not compelled to admit that our general ideas about the physiology of the nervous system are not grounded;

2d, to call the attention of future observers to what they will have to examine in *amyelencephalous* monsters, and to the causes of fallacies, in making such an examination. And, in view of this second object, I will sum up, here, what I think ought to be searched in such cases.

1st. The composition, chemical and microscopical, of the liquid, contained in or coming from the tube formed by the meninges, to ascertain the degree of analogy between this liquid and the nervous tissues, at an early period of development.

2d. The existence or absence of small masses of granular matter, connected one with another, and connected, also, with the spinal and cranial nerves. Of course, the nature of the granular matter must also be determined.

3d. The existence of communications between the nerves, and a more or less developed stripe of spinal cord; and, about this, it must be remembered that the nerves are so soft, so fragile, that they may be very easily separated from the spinal cord, as it may have been, in one of the two monsters, the case of which is above described.

4th. The enlargements of the ganglia of the spinal nerves and of those of the sympathetic and all what relates to the communication of these ganglia with the nerve-fibres coming from or going to the trunk and limbs, must be examined carefully.

There are some important facts relative to the pseudencephalic monsters, of which I must say here a few words.

As far as examination with the naked eye goes, it seems that the development of muscles and nerves in these monsters, born at full term, is, almost always, as perfect as in the most healthy newly-born children.[1] The fact that muscles are well developed, proves that they have been put in action, and as they can, hardly, have been acting, without having been excited by nerves, it follows that the nerves must have been able to act, at least, until a short time

[1] The theory of Tiedemann (Zeitschrift fuer Physiol., vol. i. p. 56, vol. iii. p. 1), that the nervous system is necessary to the development of the embryo is certainly not more exact than the analogous theory, according to which the nervous system is necessary to secretion and nutrition, in children and adults. As I have tried to show elsewhere (Exp. Researches applied to Physiol. and Pathol., New York, 1853, pp. 6-17), the numerous facts, which establish that the nervous system may have a great influence on nutrition and secretions, do not prove that this influence is necessary, and there are many other facts proving, on the contrary, that the functions may exist, without any intervention of the nervous system. Against the views of Tiedemann, see *Bischoff*, *loco cit.*, p. 468.

before the monster is expelled from the uterus. And as the nerves do not act spontaneously, but after an excitation, and, besides, as there is no known sufficient cause of direct excitation of the reflecto-motor nerves, it results that the action of these nerves is a secondary one, produced by a reflex action from a nervous centre, itself excited, in consequence of an irritation of some excito-motor nerves, in the skin or in the mucous membranes.

This series of deductions being right, it may fairly be concluded that even in cases where it is not known if a mother has felt the movements of her child, monstrous or not, it is probable that it has had reflex movements, if its muscles are well developed. In cases of monsters, in which the nerves have not been able to act on the muscles, either because there are no nervous centres at all, able to put them in action, by their reflex power, or because the nerves have not had their natural development, the muscles do not develop themselves, or if they have had a beginning of development, they become atrophied and changed into fibrous or fatty tissue, according to circumstances, which an eminent physician, Dr. Jules Guérin, has pointed out.

Alessandrini[1] has described two monsters, in which the inferior part of the spinal cord and its nerves were insufficiently developed, and the muscles of the posterior limbs were missing, although the bloodvessels, bones, and other parts, partly existed. In cases of absence, not only of the nervous centres, but also of the nerves, such as have been recorded by Clarke[2] and by Hempel,[3] the muscles had hardly any existence.

As a conclusion to all that we have exposed about the amyelencephalous or pseudencephalic monsters, we will say that their movements appear to be merely reflex, and that, although they are deprived of the greatest part of their nervous centres, there is, according to the greatest probability, enough of these parts remaining to produce reflex actions.[4]

Therefore, it cannot be concluded, from the facts observed in

[1] Novi Comment Scienc. Instit. Bonon, vol. iii., 1837.

[2] Philos. Trans., 1793.

[3] De monstris Acephalis, Hafniœ, 1850, p. 38, and Tabulœ 5 and 6.

[4] Another kind of movements may exist in monsters entirely independent from the nervous centres, and produced, as we have already said, by some local cause of excitation, just as those singular movements in the body of man after death by yellow fever or cholera, and described particularly by Dr. Bennet Dowler, of New Orleans, and by my pupil, Dr. Brandt, after his own observations and mine.

monsters, that the encephalon is not necessary for the perception of sensitive impressions and for the production of voluntary movements.

2. *Alleged existence of voluntary movements and sensibility, in parts of the body, considered as deprived of their natural connection with the encephalon.*

As I have already answered partly to objections of this kind in Lectures V. and VI., I will merely say here: 1st. That the cases of softening of the spinal cord, related by Velpeau,[1] Ollivier d'Angers and Abercrombie, in which no paralysis has existed, although there appeared to be an interruption of continuity, between the nerve-fibres of some parts of the body and the encephalon, are not fit to prove that this continuity is not necessary. Until it is demonstrated that the nerve-fibres and the cells of the cord lose completely their properties when they are softened, these facts will prove nothing against the necessity of the continuity of nerve-fibres, for sensation and for volition. But, it will be said that there are cases, where the softening was so considerable that the membranes of the cord contained only a liquid, which flowed out, when the membranes were opened. This also has no value: where is the proof that it was so during life? Is there any physician, knowing the facts, published by Calmeil,[2] and which demonstrate the extremely great rapidity of production of softening, which may take place in the spinal cord, a short time before or after death, and who will maintain that the liquefaction of the cord had existed previous to death, without causing paralysis?

2d. As to the cases of induration of the spinal cord, the same thing may be said as for cases of softening. Until it is shown that in cases of induration, in which voluntary movements and sensibility have continued to exist, there was a complete impossibility for the spinal cord to perform its functions, these cases will merely prove that the functions of this organ, may remain, although its organization appears to be much changed.

3d. We will show elsewhere that the same reasoning may be applied to the cases in which the transmission of nervous action from or towards the brain apparently continued to take place, in

[1] Archives Gén. de Médec., vol. vii.—1825.

[2] Journal des Progrès des Sciences Médic., 1828, vol. xii. p. 172.

the spinal cord, although it was much atrophied, in consequence of a compression or any other cause.

4th. There are cases in which it is said that the spinal cord had been, partly or entirely, cut across, and in which there was no paralysis of sensibility or voluntary movement. But in these cases, the section had taken place near the lower extremity of the spinal cord, as in the case so often spoken of, recorded by Desault,[1] so that almost all the nerves had their origin above the section. Besides, when a sword has been introduced into the spinal cord, as in a curious case related by Ollivier d'Angers,[2] we may understand that few of the fibres of the cord had been cut by the thin extremity of the sword.

We, therefore, will conclude that the facts of softening, induration, atrophy, or division of the spinal cord, cannot prove against the necessity of a communication of the encephalon with the different parts of the body, through the spinal cord, for the existence of voluntary movements and sensibility.

3. *Alleged persistence of sensibility and voluntary movements in men and animals, deprived of all the parts of the encephalon, except the medulla oblongata and the pons Varolii.*

The facts upon which physiologists and pathologists have grounded their opinion that the upper parts of the encephalon are not necessary for volition and for the perception of sensations are of two kinds: some are experimental, some clinical.

As to the experimental facts, they consist in showing that after the removal of the encephalon, except the pons Varolii and medulla oblongata, the animals manifest that they feel pain by their cries and agitation. "When," says Longet,[3] "rabbits and dogs have been submitted to this mutilation, upon their encephalon, although they seem to be in a deep coma, they are still able to agitate themselves and to cry plaintively, under the influence of the strong external irritations; but, if a sufficiently deep alteration is made, in the pons Varolii, there is an immediate cessation of the cries and of the agitation; it merely remains an animal, in whom circulation, respiration, and other nutritive functions are momentarily accomplished."

[1] Journal de Chirurgie, vol. iv. p. 137.

[2] Loco cit., vol. i. p. 354.

[3] Traité de Physiol., 1850, vol. ii., B. p. 38.

Longet concludes, from his experiments, that the pons Varolii is the *seat of general sensibility* (faculty of feeling pain, etc.), and *the centre for the perception of tactile impressions.*[1] Of these two deductions the second has no foundation whatever; there is not a single fact which may even appear to lead to it. As to the first deduction, if Lorry, Magendie, Desmoulins, Bouillaud, Gerdy, Serres, J. Mueller, have concluded, as Longet did, after them, that the existence of cries and of agitation, in animals, deprived of all their encephalon, except the pons Varolii and the medulla oblongata, proves that the general sensibility then exists—this merely shows that these eminent physiologists did not know how powerful may be the reflex power.[2] Of the two facts given as proofs of a perception of sensation, *i. e.*, agitation and cries, the first, certainly, cannot prove that there has been a perception of pain. It is exactly the same thing that we see in limbs, connected by their nerves, with a part of the spinal cord, separated from the encephalon. If, in this case, we call the agitation a reflex action, why shall we give to it another name, in the case where the spinal cord is connected with the medulla oblongata and the pons? The agitation, it will be said, is greater in this last case, but the extent of the nervous centre, able to produce reflex movements, is greater, so that these movements must be stronger and more extensive.

Now, as to the cries, we may also consider them as mere results of reflex contractions, taking place in certain muscles. The vocal cords, becoming fixedly stretched, and the expiratory muscles contracting strongly and suddenly, the column of air expelled from the chest passes along the stretched vocal cords, and vibrations take place, producing the sounds we call cries. I have seen two hysteric patients who cried suddenly (although they tried not to do it), after the slightest irritation of the skin, or after any kind of emotion.[3] It seems, then, that cries may be considered as mere

[1] These are his own words, loco cit., pp. 36 to 41.

[2] It may seem strange that I declare that Prof. J. Mueller, who has, in common with Marshall Hall, the glory of having called the attention of physiologists and physicians to the phenomena of reflex action, does not, nevertheless, know how great may be the power of the reflex faculty. But, to prove that I am right, I think it is sufficient to say that Prof. Mueller, at the time he published his view on the pons Varolii, admitted that reflex action is greater in cold blooded than in warm blooded animals, and also that he was not aware how much pure reflex movements may be harmonious and well co-ordinated.

[3] Dr. R. B. Todd has given some good reasons to show that the pons Varolii is the centre for emotional movements (Cyclop. of Anat. and Physiol., vol. iii. p.

results of reflex contractions. I must, nevertheless, say that I do not think that the question is positively decided. My only object now is to show that cries cannot prove that sensibility exists, because we may explain them, without admitting that pain has been truly felt.

All the writers on this subject, already named, had considered the pons Varolii as being the organ in which the perception of sensitive impressions take place, and they agree in saying that, after the removal of the pons, there are no more cries. They have been mistaken about this last fact, and I have obtained quite a different result, in performing this experiment on cats, rabbits, and guinea-pigs. After having removed, by slices, the whole encephalon, except only the medulla oblongata, I have observed that the animal, when pinched, is much agitated, and that it cries plaintively. Then, if the medulla oblongata is removed, there are no more cries, when the animal is pinched, but the agitation continues.[1] There is great appearance that, after this mutilation, cries would exist if the motor nerves of the larynx, instead of being connected with the medulla oblongata, were connected with the spinal cord. Of the two things necessary for cries, one exists: the animal, being pinched, not only has agitation of the limbs and trunk, but a contraction of the expiratory muscles. Flourens[2] had already seen that there may be a respiratory movement, in such cases, and he says that a true inspiration, producing a sound in the larynx, exists when the animal is pinched.

722, Q). I am ready to admit that the pons Varolii, particularly by its part connected with the roots of the auditive nerve, is a portion of the centre of emotional movements, but not the seat of the whole of this centre. The medulla oblongata, I think, is also a part of this centre. When a violent and sudden emotion causes death, it is in acting on the medulla oblongata, that it has such a powerful effect. An excitation is then produced on the roots of the *par vagum*, which appear to have their true origin in the neighborhood of the nib of the *calamus scriptorius*, and in consequence, the bloodvessels of the heart contract and expel the blood they contained, and with it, the natural excitant which causes the movements of the heart. So that a complete syncope and death take place. It is in acting on the branches of the par vagum, in the lungs, as I will prove elsewhere, or on the medulla oblongata, that chloroform sometimes kills suddenly. The stopping of the heart's action in the celebrated experiment of the brothers Weber, takes place in the same way, as I have tried to prove in my Exp. Researches, p. 77, and pp. 101 to 124.

[1] These experiments I had already published, in the Comptes Rendus de l'Acad. des Sciences, 1849, vol. xxix. p. 672.

[2] Rech. Expér. sur les Propr. et les Fonct. du Syst. Nerveux, 2d ed., 1842, p. 178.

Now we will conclude that, if cries prove that there is perception of pain, we must admit, it opposition to all the physiologists already named, that the medulla oblongata is a centre for that kind of perception. Besides, the view of these physiologists, as regards the pons Varolii, is erroneous. Still more, if agitation proves that sensibility exists, the spinal cord possesses this faculty, as well as the encephalon. But we repeat that the reflex theory explains the existence of agitation and of cries, and we are not, therefore, compelled to admit that the spinal cord and the medulla oblongata possess sensibility.

The *will*, or at least the faculty under the influence of the will, and by which the so-called voluntary movements are produced, is considered also by Gerdy, Mueller, Longet, and others, as having its organ in the pons Varolii and in the brain. The reasons given by these writers to prove their views are far from being satisfactory. They prove merely that there are energetic movements after an excitation of the animal, and these appear then to be mere reflex movements. Longet himself (*loc. cit.*, p. 39) says, that if the cerebral hemispheres have been removed, and also the corpora striata, in rabbits, they can stand up or move forwards, but that after the removal of the thalami optici, although the pons Varolii is left entire, there is no more possibility for the animal to walk or to stand up.

I have many times repeated these experiments upon rabbits and guinea-pigs, and uniformly obtained nearly the same results, which certainly are a deadly blow to the theory advocated by Longet. Not only standing and walking become impossible after the removal of the whole encephalon, except the pons and the medulla oblongata, but it seems also that the apparently spontaneous movements which sometimes exist there, are mere convulsive movements.

Besides, I have found that the reflex movements in this case are only a little stronger than in animals deprived of the pons Varolii. As to the regularity, the harmony, the direction of the reflex movements, they are alike in both cases.

The celebrated doctrine of Flourens, against which Bouillaud, Gerdy, Longet, and others had proposed the theory, which I have just proved to be erroneous, does not appear to be right. Flourens has gone too far, I believe, in thinking that the faculty of perception for all the sensitive and the sensorial impressions exists only in the cerebral lobes, and that the same parts are also the only seat of intelligence and volition. We will not discuss these questions here, but we will say, as regards the perception of sensitive impressions and volition, that experiments on animals, as well as pathological facts observed in man, and also microscopic anatomy, agree in showing that the thalami optici and the corpora striata, and also the crura cerebri, appear to be the centres for these actions. I am glad to agree almost entirely with Dr. Todd, as regards the corpora striata, which he considers as the principal centres for voluntary movements. But I do not agree with him as to the thalami optici, which, according to his views, are the centres for almost all the sensitive and sensorial nerves. Anatomy and pathology are opposed to this view, as I will try to show in a special paper.

There are on record many cases of acephalia or of anencephalia, which might be considered as proving that sensibility and voluntary movements may exist, when the whole encephalon is missing, except the medulla oblongata alone or with the pons Varolii. In all the cases of this kind which I have collected, I have found no evidence that the movements which existed were voluntary and not simply reflex or convulsive. I will give here a short analysis of two, among these cases, which appear to be the most favorable to the theory I reject.

CASE 1.—I have seen, says Lallemand,[1] an encephalous fœtus, born at full time, and which lived three days. During all this time it cried with a certain degree of strength, and tried to suck whenever anything was put between its lips. It made movements to some extent with its legs and arms. When anything was put in its hands, there was a flexion of its fingers, as though it would seize it, but generally all its movements were less energetic than those of a healthy fœtus of the same age.

The cerebrum and the cerebellum were entirely missing; there were only, on the basis of the cranium, the medulla oblongata and the pons Varolii, with the origin of the pneumogastric, trigeminal, and optic nerves.[2]

[1] Loco cit., p. 52.

[2] Lallemand, in this description, has not shown the accuracy which ordinarily characterizes his publications. He says that the optic nerves had their origin in the parts that remained of the encephalon; this implies, certainly, that some parts, at least, of the tubercula quadrigemina were also existing, although he does not mention it.

Although Lallemand concludes from this fact that sensibility and voluntary movements existed in this monster, no one acquainted with reflex action will accept these deductions.

CASE 2.—A fœtus nine months old was born perfectly well developed, except that it was anencephalous. Its eyes were constantly shut; it frequently uttered cries, that ceased when a finger was put in its mouth; it then sucked repeatedly.[1] Its limbs were agitated with some strength, and it pressed with its fingers the things that were placed in its hands. Three hours after birth, the number of respirations in a given time was diminished, and the cries were less frequent and less strong. Respiration diminished gradually and became convulsive. This state lasted for six or eight hours, during which the cries became weaker and weaker, and less frequent, as also the respiratory movements, which were accompanied with general convulsions, and at last it died in a true state of asphyxia. The cerebrum and the cerebellum were entirely missing, and of the basis of the encephalon nothing existed except a very irregular medulla oblongata, connected with a kind of pons Varolii, merely consisting in a square layer of gray matter only two lines and a half long and two lines broad. The membranes of the spinal cord were inflamed.

This case, recorded by Ollivier d'Angers,[2] and considered by him as proving that the spinal cord and the medulla oblongata possess the two faculties of perception of sensitive impressions and of volition, certainly cannot prove such things. Had Ollivier known reflex action, he would have considered this case quite in another light. But there is something important proved by this fact, and which is entirely opposed to the view of Gerdy, Mueller, Longet, and others; it is that the pons Varolii was so slightly developed, that we can consider it as missing, and, nevertheless, agitation and cries have existed as when the pons exist. If these phenomena prove that sensibility and volition exist, we must then admit that

[1] Suckling in anencephalic monsters may take place, as it takes place, also, in animals deprived of almost all their encephalon. This fact has been well proved by the experiments of Grainger (Observ. on the Struct. and Funct. of the Spinal Cord, 1837, p. 80), of J. Reid (Physiol. Anat. and Pathol. Researches, 1848, p. 183), and by my own (Exp. Res. applied to Physiol., etc., 1853, p. 5). Grainger has also well proved that sucking is a mere reflex action, by pointing out what takes place in the fœtus of the opossum, in which sensation and volition cannot exist, and the lips of which remain attached to the nipple by contraction and grasping.

[2] Loco cit., vol. i. p. 179.

the pons Varolii and the cerebrum are not the only centres for volition and for perception of sensitive impressions.

To conclude, we will say that both monsters and animals experimented upon, may cry and have movements, when they are deprived of almost all their encephalon (the medulla oblongata alone remaining), but that nothing proves that these movements and these cries are not mere reflex actions.

In other words, the facts, which have been considered by almost all the French physiologists of our day, as proving that the pons Varolii is a centre for volition and sensibility, cannot prove such a thing. Besides, it is clear, also, that these facts cannot prove anything against the theory that, in men and animals, having their nervous centres well developed, transmission, for both sensations and volitions, has to take place through the medulla oblongata and the pons Varolii.

4. *On cases proving that considerable alterations of the Pons Varolii and Medulla Oblongata may exist without producing paralysis either of sensibility or of voluntary movements.*

We have collected a large number of such cases, mostly relative to the medulla oblongata. It is strange that this nervous centre, which is considered so much more important than any other, is so frequently altered, and sometimes extremely, without producing either death or even a decided paralysis.

It is strange, also, that slow alterations of the pons Varolii, which is considered notably less useful than the preceding organ, produce more frequently a paralysis, and this even when these alterations are less considerable than alterations of the medulla oblongata, which do not produce paralysis. This seems still more strange when we remember that very rapid or sudden alterations kill more quickly when developed in the medulla oblongata than in the pons Varolii.

I will relate here as specimens, some few cases of alteration of both of these organs, to show how far such alterations may go without producing paralysis.

Case 1.—A patient had had—only during the last days of her life—all the symptoms of a cerebral compression, such as suspension of intelligence, stertorous respiration, sometimes deep groaning, slight spasms and involuntary movements.

Autopsy.—There was no alteration of the brain and cerebellum. The volume of the pons Varolii was almost doubled. It contained an encysted tubercle, with a smooth surface, not adhering to the nervous matter. The size of the cyst was that of a big walnut. A part of the tubercle was dense and lardaceous, the centre was softer.[1]

Case 2.—A man, aged 63, died of acute pnuemonia. He had been epileptic for twelve years; each fit began with very violent hiccups, lasting one or two minutes, and accompanied with a sensation of a ball going up from the stomach to the pharynx. All the liquids that were then given to him were violently expelled. To this state succeeded a loss of consciousness, which lasted two or three minutes, and then all the accidents passed away. This convulsive and momentary spasm used to come every fifteen days, and some physicians had considered it as very different from epilepsy. During the fits the loss of sensibility was complete.

Autopsy.—The brain and the cerebellum were normal; but, in the middle of the substance of the medulla oblongata, two tubercles were found: one as large as a small walnut, and the other the size of a filbert; they were adhering to each other, and each of them was in a very thin cyst. The medullary substance around them was not altered.[2]

These two cases show that, although there is a diminution in the number of fibres which establish a communication between the spinal cord and the parts of the encephalon anterior to the medulla oblongata and to the pons Varolii, sensibility and voluntary movements may continue to exist, at least until a short time before death. We are led by the fact that there is a number of fibres which are then destroyed in a part of their length, to admit one or the other of the two following opinions.

1st. The nerve-fibres of the pons and the medulla oblongata are not necessary channels of communication between the spinal cord and the parts of the encephalon anterior to the pons. I think no one will admit such an opinion, which is in complete opposition with almost all that is taught by physiology and pathology, as regards the nervous centres.

[1] Traité de la maladie scrofuleuse, par Lepelletier, p. 129.

[2] This case was recorded by Gendrin. See *Traité des Maladies de la Moelle épin.*, par Ollivier d'Angers. Vol. ii. p. 518.

2d. We can explain the facts by another hypothesis. Suppose that the divided extremities of the destroyed fibres become connected with either the tails or the envelop of some caudate or bipolar cells, and that by the means of the fibres originating from these cells, communication may continue from below upwards and from above downwards; if such a reunion takes place between the extremities of divided fibres, below and above the seat of the compression or of the alteration, although there is no decided paralysis, there must be much inaccuracy in the action of the will on the muscles, because certain muscles must be put in action at a time when the will does not wish for their contraction. As to sensations, if their intensity is not diminished, there must be a diminution in the faculty of determining from where an impression comes. These two kinds of changes, in voluntary movements and in sensibility, are very frequent in incipient paralysis, whatever may be the seat, in the encephalon, of the alteration which causes it. Very likely these changes are produced by the same anatomical causes, whatever is the seat of the disease.[1]

It may be said that when a tumor presses upon a nervous centre, it may not destroy the fibres and merely separate them one from the other and render them thinner. This certainly ought to take place; but besides this, a partial destruction must also exist in cases where a tumor becomes extremely large, and particularly if it exists in a relatively narrow place, as is the case in the vertebral canal, for the medulla oblongata and a part of the pons Varolii, compared to other parts of the encephalon. Another cause of the slight influence of tumors, in these nervous centres upon voluntary movements and sensibility, is that the conductors employed in the transmission of sensitive impressions and of the orders of the will to muscles are but a small part of these centres and that, therefore, a considerable alteration may exist in them, with but little injury to these conductors. (See Lecture XII.)

I wish I had room here to publish the very interesting and numerous cases I have collected,[2] and which show that the pons

[1] The cases of disordered movements, recently published by Landry and Duchenne, and which they explain in admitting that a pretended faculty of co-ordination has been lost, are most frequently due to the cause above mentioned.

[2] With the exception of two or three of these cases, I have borrowed them from modern writers. As a guarantee of the exactitude of observation, I give here a list of the most known among these writers: Bouillaud, Cruveilhier, Gendrin, J. Cloquet, Duverney, Gama, Esquirol, Stanley, Lieutaud, Lenhossek, Romberg, Aber-

Varolii and the medulla oblongata may be compressed, and sometimes as much as to be reduced to one-half or one-third of their size, if not more, although there is hardly any paralysis produced, except during the last days of life. These facts are extremely interesting in a pathological as well as in a physiological point of view.

There is one thing which appears to be well proved by these facts, and especially by those in which a layer only of white matter has been left either in the medulla oblongata or in the pons Varolii, it is that these organs are neither the centre nor an important part of the centre, for volition or for perception of the sensitive impressions; because if they were, these faculties should be lost. We may understand that the power of transmission of nervous actions (either for sensations or for volitions) may be kept in a part where there remains only some fibres, but the higher faculties of perception and volition would certainly be destroyed, had they their seat in organs so much altered as the pons and the medulla oblongata sometimes are.

As these pathological cases might be considered as proving that communications between the spinal cord and the parts of the encephalon anterior to the pons, are not necessary for the performance of voluntary movements and for the perception of sensitive impressions, and as such a conclusion might also be drawn from the result of certain experiments, recently published, I think I ought to examine here these experiments. It is certainly important to make this examination and to show that such a conclusion is not right, because, were it admitted to be correct, all the researches and conclusions exposed in our Lectures, concerning the region where the decussation of the voluntary motor and sensitive nerve-fibres takes place in the nervous centres, would almost become useless and without meaning.

Two French physiologists, Drs. Vulpian and Philipeaux,[1] relate some experiments, in one of which they had divided transversely a lateral half of the medulla oblongata, about one line in front of the nib of the *calamus scriptorius.* The result, as stated by the authors, was: conservation of the voluntary movements and of sensibility in the two sides of the body.

crombie, Velpeau, Guersant, Rilliet, Barthez, Bayle, Hutin, Pariset, Burnet, Ollivier d'Angers, Lebert, Bright, etc.

[1] Essai sur l'origine de plus. paires des nerfs craniens, 1853, p. 54.

As regards voluntary movements, the experimenters themselves say that the animals could not stand on their feet, but they consider as a voluntary action, a great agitation of the four limbs, consisting in alternative flexions and extensions. I will, first, remark that the experiment cannot prove much about voluntary movements, because the section has been made on the decussation of the pyramids, leaving there, undivided, a number of voluntary motor fibres belonging to the two sides of the body. We certainly might consider the agitation as voluntary and produced by the undivided fibres. But we have found that if the lateral hemisection of the medulla oblongata is made a little higher, *i. e.* above the decussation, so that only the voluntary motor fibres of the opposite side of the body have been divided, there is, also, agitation on both sides, though much more on the side of the section. But this agitation is not a *voluntary* action; it is *convulsive*, as will be shown hereafter.

Before any division of the medulla oblongata, and even before having laid it bare, the mere fact of having divided a number of the muscles of the posterior part of the neck, as Longet has found, is followed by a very great agitation in the whole body, at every time the animal attempts to move. This trouble comes from the fact that the head, being drawn, by the contraction of the anterior muscles of the neck, towards the sternum, the medulla oblongata is drawn upwards and excited, and so are the spinal cord and its nerves. Now, after the section of a lateral half of the medulla oblongata, this irritation of all the intra-spinal nervous system continues and only changes somewhat in nature, precisely because the will cannot act, as well as before, to diminish the agitation. This is one cause of agitation, but not the only one; there is another in the irritation existing in the wound. Besides, the animal, upon which a section of a lateral half of the medulla oblongata has been performed, is attacked with this peculiar and so curious convulsive affection, which manifests itself by a rotatory movement (see Lecture XII., and my *Exper. Researches*, p. 18 to 23), and we well know that, in man, this rotation is never voluntary, and that when it takes place in a man who has his consciousness entire, the rotation occurs, although the will tries to prevent it. Therefore the agitation of an animal, upon which a lateral half of the medulla oblongata has been cut, cannot be considered as a voluntary action. It may be partly voluntary, in one side of the body, when the section is made above the decussation of the pyramids, but then we have merely a confirmation of the facts and conclusions exposed in our Lectures.

As to sensibility, I need not say much. I had myself published, long ago, that a section of a lateral half of the medulla oblongata, above the roots of the pneumogastric nerves, does not appear to destroy sensibility, if we decide that the existence of this faculty is proved, there are cries and agitation, as have done Drs. Vulpian and Philipeaux. I had gone farther and shown that if, instead of merely cutting a lateral half of the medulla oblongata, we divide this organ entirely, where it unites with the pons Varolii (as we have already said in a preceding section of this paper), sensibility *appears* to exist everywhere, *i. e.* agitation and cries are observed after every excitation. But, as long as it will not be proved that cries and agitation are not mere reflex actions, we are entitled to consider them as such. Drs. V. and P. say that the animals, upon which they had cut a lateral half of the medulla oblongata, appeared to be more sensitive than normally. We agree partly with them: there is an apparent increase of sensibility, but much more marked in the side of the operation.

Nearly the same results are obtained, as regards sensibility, whether the hemisection is made on the medulla oblongata or on the pons Varolii.

It is known that there is a question, connected with our subject, which has been the cause of great discussion between Flourens, Calmeil, Ollivier d'Angers, Longet and others. This hitherto *quæstio vexata* is no more a question, after what we have said in our Lectures on the place of decussation of the nervous conductors for volition and sensation. The question was whether the medulla oblongata has a *crossed* action for sensibility and voluntary movement. The solution is, I believe, given in our Lectures III., VI. and XII., and as to the reasons for which there has been discrepancies of opinions, what we have just said of the experiments of Drs. Vulpian and Philipeaux, explains how the erroneous and contrary results of the various experimenters may have been obtained.

To conclude on this subject, I will say that the experiments of these two physiologists and the pathological cases, in which, although there was a considerable alteration of the pons or of the medulla oblongata, no decided paralysis existed—are certainly not able to prove against our admitting that a communication, by voluntary motor and by sensitive fibres, is necessary between the spinal cord and the parts of the encephalon anterior to the pons.

The number of fibres establishing the communication may diminish, without any notable diminution in the intensity of sensations and in the strength of voluntary movements. But, it seems that in such cases, there ought to be an alteration in the harmony and regularity of the voluntary movements, and in the power of judging from what place comes a sensitive impression.

5. *Cases in which an alteration in the two sides of the pons Varolii appeared to have produced a paralysis only in one side of the body.*

I know of no case where the pons, being much and equally altered, on both sides, there has been a mere hemiplegia; but there are some cases, in which an alteration, more considerable on one side than in the other, has produced paralysis in one side only of the body, which side has been that opposed to the most altered in the pons. Such facts cannot prove more than the facts above related, in which an alteration has existed on both sides of the pons without producing paralysis. There is a case, however, published by Mr. Huguier (*Bulletin de la Soc. Anat.*, 1829, p. 52) in which it is stated that a tubercle, the size of a walnut, was placed on the middle line against the anterior surface of the pons Varolii, separating the two crura-cerebri and producing paralysis only in the right side of the body. Had the autopsy been made with more care, it would have been observed that the alteration of the left crus was deeper than that of the right, or that there was some other cause to the hemiplegia.

6. *Cases in which an alteration existing in one side of the pons Varolii, or in the neighboring parts, appears to have produced paralysis in both sides of the body.*

There are some cases of this kind on record; but they cannot prove much, because an alteration in structure, sufficient to produce paralysis, may extend to a certain distance from the side of the pons, where is a tumor, to the other side. Now, many alterations may escape the search, made with the naked eye, and, as a tumor is found, observers have thought its existence was sufficient to explain the symptoms observed before death.

I will give here only a short analysis of two cases of this kind, which I find in the remarkable work of my friend, Prof. Lebert, on cancer.[1]

[1] Traité pratique des maladies cancéreuses, 1851, p. 806.

CASE 1.—Headache, blindness, pupils dilated, weakness and rigidity of the limbs, tetaniform contracture of the trunk, convulsions, respiration difficult and noisy, speech embarrassed, death.

Autopsy.—Tumor of the anterior part of the left lobe of the cerebellum, which had pushed the pons Varolii and made, in its anterior part, a cavity, in which it was lodged.

CASE 2.—Cephalalgia; not long before death, hemiplegia left side; incomplete paralysis of the right side; contracture, frequent shaking; lancinating and great pain in the left limbs; at last, involuntary expulsion of urine and fecal matters.

Autopsy.—A tumor, not larger than a pea, is found in the middle and inferior part of the right side of the pons.

No physician, acquainted with nervous diseases, will believe that in such a case there was no other alteration, besides the slight displacement or compression of nervous matter, in the immediate neighborhood of so small a tumor. The following fact will show that when an alteration appears to exist only in one side of the encephalon, when there has been paralysis, in the two sides of the body, the microscope is necessary to decide if there is no other alteration more able to give us the reason of the double paralysis.

This fact is so important, that I will give it with all the details, and in the very words of Prof. Hughes Bennett, who has related it. "Another well remarked case was that of a man who entered the Infirmary, under Dr. Paterson, in 1842. All the symptoms of acute softening were present; paralysis of the left side, including rigidity and contraction of the left arm, dulness of intellect, and tonic spasms of the muscles of the mouth and neck. The right side was also affected in a slighter degree. As the case excited considerable interest, great care was taken in examining the brain. When the lateral ventricles were opened, it became a question whether the right corpus striatum was softened. Several persons applied their fingers, and endeavored to ascertain the point. As the manual examination proceeded, the normal consistence of the part diminished, until at length it presented all the appearance of pultaceous softening. In this state it was shown to Dr. Paterson, who naturally enough considered it to be the result of disease. I differed from him in opinion: first, because I had carefully observed the gradual increase of the softening in the manner alluded to; and secondly, because disease of the corpus striatum, in one side of the brain, could not have explained the well-marked symptoms which existed on both sides of the body. When the pons Varolii was bisected, Dr. Peacock, who conducted the examination, conceived it to be softened; others who examined it, could perceive no difference in the texture; its color and consistence were unchanged. Reasoning from the symptoms, the lesion was very likely to exist. But how, it was argued, could a judgment be formed; we ought to reason from facts, not theories? Here, then, was an evident lesion of the corpus striatum, which explained nothing, and a problematical lesion of the pons Varolii, which, however, did it exist, would satisfactorily account for the symptoms. In this state of uncertainty the microscope was sent for, and I demonstrated, and made evident to Drs. Paterson, Peacock, and all the students present, that the corpus striatum contained no granular corpuscles, whilst in the pons Varolii they were very abundant. I have endeavored to describe what took place on this occasion, from which it must be evident that had not the microscope been appealed to, the right corpus striatum would have been pronounced softened; whilst the real lesion in the pons Varolii might have escaped observation. Under such circumstances, this case would have added another to the inexplicable observations with which the records of nervous diseases abound."[1]

After such a fact, we certainly are entitled to conclude that the cases, in which it is said that an alteration, only in one side of the pons, has produced paralysis, in both sides of the body, cannot prove anything, because the microscope has not shown that the other side of the pons was not altered.

7. *Cases in which an alteration, in one side of the pons Varolii or of the neighboring parts, has produced paralysis in the same side of the body.*

I regret not to have room enough to treat at length this subject, about which much has been said already in Lecture XII. I will merely give here, one only of the cases that are on record; then I will relate, shortly, the different modes of explanation of these facts, and, at last, I will show that these cases cannot be opposed to what I have said, as regards the place of decussation of the motor and sensitive nerve-fibres.

[1] Monthly Jour. of Med. Science. April, 1851, p. 365.

CASE.—Hemiplegia of the left side, without loss of sensation in the arm and leg, but in the left side of the face both sensation and motion were entirely lost. Loss of hearing in the left ear.

Autopsy.—A tumor was found in the left side of the pons Varolii, which compressed the origin of the 5th and 7th nerves against the base of the skull. The tumor was of the size of a walnut, of a firm consistence, and extended into the left crus cerebelli.[1]

This case is positive, and the co-existence of the paralysis in the face and the body, in the same side, points out, at once, a striking difference between the ordinary cases and this *extraordinary* one. In the ordinary cases, paralysis exists in the side of the alteration in the face, and in the opposite side of the trunk and limbs.

I will remark that in this case there was no paralysis of sensibility in the limbs, and I will add that it has been so, in all the cases, but one, that I know, in which paralysis has existed in the same side as the alteration.

Now, how to explain these facts?

1st. There is an explanation to which we are naturally led: it is, that in the men spoken of in these cases, there was no decussation at all of the sensitive and voluntary motor nerve-fibres. This would explain, not only the cases relative to the pons, but also the cases in which alterations have existed in one side of the cerebrum, of the cerebellum, of the corpora striata, or of the thalami optici, and in which hemiplegia has existed in the same side.

Longet[2] says that, sometimes, he has not found any appearance of decussation of the pyramids, in man, and I have also made the same observation on animals.

2d. It may be imagined that the decussation of voluntary motor and sensitive nerve-fibres, instead of taking place as usually, takes place, in some men, only in front of the pons, between the corpora quadrigemina and the crura cerebri.

3d. It may be, as it results from what we have related above, and what has been found by Prof. H. Bennett, that the true alteration which really produces the paralysis, and which can be detected only with the microscope, is in the side of the encephalon, opposite to the side where an alteration is seen, with the naked eye.

Now, I ought to say that, a few years ago (in 1855), by examining the circumstances of the cases in which there has been only a par-

[1] Stanley in Lond. Med. Gazette. Vol. i.

[2] Anat. et Physiol. du Syst. Nerv. Vol. i. p. 383.

alysis of movement, I was led to think that there was no decussation of the pyramids, and that the decussation of the voluntary motor fibres either did not exist at all, in these cases, or existed above the pons. As to the case in which there was together a paralysis of movement and of sensibility, I thought it might be explained by what results from Prof. Bennett's researches. But now, as it may be seen in Lecture XII., and with more details in the *Journal de la Physiologie*, Nos. 3 and 4, July and Oct., 1858, I have some other views concerning those cases. I shall not expose those views again here, as my object is now only to be able to state that those extraordinary cases may be explained.

Both the theories actually proposed about the place where exists the decussation of the voluntary motor and of the sensitive nerve-fibres, one which is the theory of Longet, Foville, Valentin and others, and the second which is mine—are, as much, in apparent opposition with these cases (of paralysis in the same side where is the alteration), one than the other. If it were true, as admitted by Foville, Valentin, Longet, etc., that the decussation of the voluntary motor and sensitive nerve-fibres, takes place partly in the pons and partly behind and before this organ, a considerable alteration of its sides, producing paralysis, should produce it, in both sides of the body; so that, if paralysis exists, only in one side, be it the side of the alteration or the other, the fact, in both cases, appears as much in opposition with the theory.

But we repeat that there is now an apparently well-grounded explanation of the cases of paralysis in the side altered in the encephalon, and we refer to the above quoted lecture and journal for the details on this subject.

8. *Cases and experiments which appear to prove that there are, in various parts of the encephalon and in the spinal cord, motor nerve-fibres, which are not voluntary motor.*

As to the spinal cord, the existence, in it, of fibres, which are motor but not voluntary motor, has already been pointed out by some physiologists. As it is not necessary for my object here to demonstrate the fact, I will merely state that I believe it is certainly true that there are such fibres. As to the encephalon, not only the doctrine of the existence of such fibres is a new one, but the proofs themselves, upon which it is grounded, are mostly new or presented here in a new light.

For a long while since Hippocrates, it was admitted that in wounds in the brain, the convulsions were always in the injured side, while paralysis was in the opposite side. Haller, though inclined to admit this doctrine, had remained in doubt about it.

Flourens[1] thought he had decided the question, and he gave the following conclusions:—

1st. The cerebral lobes and the cerebellum never give convulsions.

2d. The quadrigeminal tubercles give convulsions in the opposite side.

3d. The medulla oblongata and spinal cord give convulsions in the injured side.

Flourens has been led to erroneous conclusions, partly because he has not taken notice of what has been observed in man, partly because he has particularly experimented on birds.

Burdach, according to J. Mueller,[2] has given the following statistics: Out of 268 cases of alteration on one side of the encephalon, there have been 10 cases of paralysis in both sides of the body, and 258 of hemiplegia, of which 15 were in the side of the alteration. Convulsions took place in 25 cases in the side of the alteration, and in only 3 cases in the opposite side.

From many facts recorded by Andral, Rochoux, Rostan, Abercrombie, Serres, Bright, Bouillaud, Lallemand, and Romberg, it results that convulsions in the side of the alteration appear to be less frequent than convulsions in the opposite side. So that the results arrived at by Burdach are opposed to the results of these more recent writers. But whatever may be about this, it is sufficient, for my object now, that it is certain that convulsions may take place, either in the side where is the alteration or injury of the encephalon, or in the opposite side.

Now, there are other and very curious facts which also prove that contractions of certain muscles of the body may take place either in the side of the body corresponding to the injured side of the encephalon, or in the opposite side, exactly as in the cases of ordinary convulsions, as I have just said. And, in fact, this might have been foreseen, had it been known that a convulsive state of certain muscles is the cause of the phenomena of which I will now say a few words.

[1] Loco cit., p. 120.

[2] Manuel de Physiol. Ed. Littré, 1851, vol. i. p. 783.

If a puncture or rather a slight section is made, on mammals, in different parts of the encephalon, we see quite different effects, according to the part which has been injured. The animal *turns* round or *rolls* over itself (see my paper on *Turning* and *Rolling* in *Exp. Researches*, p. 18, and Lecture XI.), and this, as I will prove elsewhere, in consequence mostly of local convulsions. Turning or rolling takes place after an injury of the right side, sometimes on the right, sometimes on the left side of the body, as I have already shown.

In almost all these experiments, turning or rolling exists on the side where there are convulsions in certain muscles. The spasms exist in all cases, in the muscles of the neck, frequently in those of the trunk, and sometimes in those of the limbs. The convulsions of the muscles of the neck and trunk are sufficient, without the assistance of the limbs to produce rolling, as I have frequently seen, after the amputation of the four limbs.

It seems quite certain from these two series of facts (*i. e.*, pure convulsions in one side of the body and the local spasms coexisting with turning and rolling), that convulsions may be produced in muscles of one side of the body, by the same alteration which produces paralysis in the opposite side. From this it results that there are two different sets of motor nerve-fibres, which appear to originate from the same place, in many parts of the encephalon, one set being composed of voluntary motor-fibres, which then become paralyzed, and the other set composed of motor fibres, which are not voluntary motor, because, were they so, their alteration would produce paralysis, and we should, therefore, have then a paralysis in both sides of the body, although the alteration should exist only in one side of the brain. But what are these fibres, as they cannot be voluntary motor?[1] They certainly are able to produce muscular contractions, and, therefore, we are entitled to call them motor, but we do not know whether the irritation acts directly

[1] It is well known that no movement is produced in the limbs and trunk, when an excitation of any kind is brought upon the cerebral lobes or even the corpora striata. As the voluntary motor fibres extend into the encephalon, if not into the cerebral lobes, at least into the corpora striata, it is certain that there these fibres cannot be irritated by our means of excitation. It may be that these fibres remain so, *unirritable* all along, from these parts of the encephalon to their termination in muscles, and that the nerve-fibres which produce contractions when we irritate them, either in the encephalon, in the spinal cord, or in the nerves, belong to the other class of motor nerves, the existence of which I am now trying to establish.

upon them, or whether it is by a secondary, that is a reflex action that they become excited. It may be, and this seems very probable, that they are merely reflecto-motor.

But, whatever is the truth about their nature, they are motor, and they exist in great number, in all the isthmus of the encephalon, and particularly in the medulla oblongata. We can by this fact understand why there are so many motor fibres belonging to the anterior columns of the spinal cord which are not voluntary motor.

9. *Anatomico-pathological dissections which appear to prove that there are nerve-fibres, coming from the spinal cord, which decussate in parts above the medulla oblongata.*

The interesting facts discovered by Dr. Ludwig Türck, of Vienna,[1] showing that when there is an alteration of a part of the encephalon, the nerve-fibres which go from that part into and along the spinal cord, become very much altered in their structure, have proved that there is a decussation for these fibres in the Pons Varolii or in parts before it.[2] I do not think necessary to discuss at length the value of these researches, in relation to the subject of this paper. I believe it is sufficient to say that, as long as there are other fibres, besides the sensitive and the voluntary motor, which originate from the different parts of the encephalon, nothing in the curious facts described by Dr. Türck would prove against our admitting, that the decussation of the sensitive and voluntary motor fibres takes place where I have tried to show that it does.

This means of study of Dr. Türck will have the greatest value when (and only when) it shall be combined with all the other means that science already possesses to determine what are the kinds of

[1] See Braithwaite's Retrospect, Amer. edit., part xxvii. p. 344.

[2] Dr. Türck is disposed to consider the alteration produced, in these cases, in nerve-tubes, as a result of absence of action. I believe this view is partly right, but there is another cause of alteration, which is—according to what I have tried to show in a paper presented more than five years ago, to the *Société de Biologie*—that the nerve-tubes are endowed with capillarity, and that liquids, in which is placed a divided end of them, are absorbed, and conveyed very far in their canal, and there altering their contents. The spinal cord may become secondarily affected, in that way, by diseases of the different viscera, and this may prove to be a good means of finding the course of the roots of the nerves in the spinal cord. I had already made some researches about the disposition of these roots five years ago, and I intend to resume them as soon as possible.

nerve-fibres existing in the nervous centres, and what is their respective course.

General Conclusions.—In the first part of this appendix I have tried to prove successively:—

a. That reflex movements alone, and not sensations and volitions, exist in monsters, deprived of a great part of their cerebro-spinal axis.

b. That when the spinal cord, the medulla oblongata, or the Pons Varolii are altered, even considerably, sensibility and volition may continue to exist, because there are still communications by nerve-fibres through the altered part, between the nerves of the trunk and limbs, and the parts of the encephalon, in front of the Pons.

c. That if the reasons given by many physiologists to prove that the Pons Varolii is the seat of the centre for volition and for perception of sensitive impressions were true, we should have to admit that the medulla oblongata is the centre (or, at least, a part of the centre) for these faculties, because the same reasons appear to prove the same for this organ as for the Pons.

d. That very likely these faculties have not their centre (at least their principal centre) in the Pons Varolii, and, still less, in the medulla oblongata.

e. That there appears to be, in many places of the encephalon, nerve-fibres, which are not voluntary motor, and which, nevertheless, go to muscles, either in the same side of the body as the side of the encephalon, from which they originate, or in the opposite side, and that these muscular nerve-fibres are able to produce convulsions when they are irritated by an injury or an alteration in the encephalon, so that convulsions may take place either in the paralyzed side or in the other.

f. The results of the researches of Dr. Ludwig Türck cannot, in the actual state of science, prove against or in favor of any doctrine relative to the place of decussation of sensitive and voluntary motor nerve-fibres.

PART II. APPLICATION OF SOME OF THE FACTS AND VIEWS, EXPOSED IN THE PRECEDING LECTURES, TO THE TREATMENT OF DISEASE.

I will give here a short summary of several of the principal deductions for the practice of the various branches of medical science, that may be drawn from many of the facts and views presented in my lectures. I shall divide this second part of this appendix into several chapters, which will contain: 1st, application to surgery; 2d, application to medicine; 3d, application to obstetrics.

CHAP. I. *Application to Surgery.*—The first object to which I shall call the attention of my readers, concerns the *treatment of fractured spine*, and the first question I shall examine on this subject, is whether it may or not be useful to employ the trephine, with the view of removing a broken part of the bony ring of the vertebræ. I am convinced that the life of some patients might be saved by this means, and I hope the following discussion will give the same faith to others. I shall try to prove: 1st, that the laying bare of the spinal cord is not a dangerous operation; 2d, that death, after a fracture of the spine, is usually due to the effects of a pressure, or an excitation upon the spinal cord, and not the result of a partial or a complete section of this organ; 3d, that reunion may take place after a wound of the spinal cord, so that its lost functions may return; 4th, that the removal of some parts of the vertebræ may be followed by a production of new bone; 5th, that the cases of fracture of the spine in which the trephine has been applied show the usefulness of this operation.

1st. *The exposition of the spinal cord to the action of the atmosphere is not a dangerous operation.*—One of the principal objections raised against the use of the trephine, in cases of fractured spine, is that the laying bare of the spinal cord is a dangerous thing. This quite erroneous opinion has no other foundation, that I am aware of, than the well known fact that the laying bare of the brain or of its meninges is dangerous, and that in cases of tapping, for spina bifida, a meningitis is sometimes produced by the *supposed* irritation of atmospheric air upon the spinal meninges. But, as regards the first one of these grounds for an opinion that I consider entirely erroneous, it is sufficient to say, that it is only an inferential reason and not a direct proof, and as regards the second, I will say that certainly it is not the laying bare of the spinal cord, or its membranes, which causes a meningitis after tapping, in cases of spina bifida, as this inflammation occurs as frequently after the performance of the operation by the subcutaneous method, as after the use of the old method. We may add that the meninges of the spinal cord, in ordinary circumstances, do not become inflamed so easily as in cases of spina bifida, and that the meninges of the brain are much more liable to become inflamed than those of the spinal cord, as is proved by the relatively small number of cases of inflammation of the spinal meninges after they have been injured by a piece of bone, a sword, etc.

The opening of the spinal canal and the laying bare of the spinal meninges, or of the cord itself, are not dangerous operations in animals. I may safely say, that one dog, cat, or guinea-pig, out of ten, hardly dies from having the spinal cord laid bare, in the extent of an inch or even more. Of course, these facts cannot prove that in man the same innocuity would exist, as we know that certain membranes and organs are much more easily inflamed in man than in animals. But there are facts, of which I will speak hereafter (especially the similarity of results of fractures of the spine in men and in the animals already mentioned), which seem to show that there is no great difference between these animals and men, as regards the power of inflammation of the spinal cord, or its membranes; so that it is at least very probable, that what is found in the above experiments on dogs, cats, etc., would also be observed in man.

One of the most decisive reasons, however, for our admitting the truth of the proposition, that there is no danger in the laying bare the spinal cord in man, consists in the existence of several cases like the following in which there has been no ill effect at all, caused by the exposition of this organ to the contact of the atmosphere.

In a curious case of syphilitic caries of the spine, A. Mercogliana, an Italian surgeon, removed (through a deep ulcer of the throat) the body of the third cervical vertebra, leaving the spinal cord bare. The patient had no trouble whatever in the functions of this nervous centre, and recovered. (*Gazette Médicale de Paris*, 1832, pp. 589–90.)

In another case, analogous to the preceding, a part of a cervical vertebra was removed by another Italian surgeon, Marcacci. The patient was quickly cured. (*Gazette Médicale de Paris*, 1850, p. 268.)

In a case of acephalocystic cyst, in the spinal canal, the bones became altered, and the cyst having been opened, the spinal cord was laid bare. No ill effect is mentioned as the result of this operation. (*Traité des Maladies de la Moelle épin.*, par Ollivier d'Angers, 1837, vol. ii. p. 547.)

Three cases of exfoliation of the atlas, one observed by Mr. Robert Wade, the two others by Mr. Prescott Hewett, were communicated to the Royal Medico-Chirurgical Society of London in

February, 1849. The three patients got well. (*London Journal of Medicine*, April, 1849, p. 395.)

From these facts, and from several similar ones which have been published in various medical journals, it seems that we are entitled to draw the conclusion that the action of the air upon the spinal cord is not a dangerous one.

But it is still more important to state that there are no cases on record, so far as we know, of removal of broken parts of the spine, in which the operation has been followed by a meningitis. This assertion will be proved hereafter, when we give the principal details of all the cases we know of application of the trephine to the spine. In animals I never saw meningitis produced by injuries to the three membranes that surround the spinal cord.

It seems certain, from the facts above mentioned, that the laying bare of the spinal meninges, or even of the spinal cord after the section of the meninges, cannot be considered as dangerous operations either in man or in animals.

2d. *Death after a fracture of the spine is usually due to the effects of a pressure or some excitation upon the spinal cord, and not to the results of a partial or a complete section of this organ.*—It would be out of place here to enter fully into the demonstration of this proposition. We will only give a short account of the various causes of death after a fracture of the spine, which will sufficiently show what share a pressure or a mechanical excitation of the spinal cord has among these causes.

When the spine is fractured high up in the cervical region, if the spinal cord is crushed, death occurs instantaneously or after a very short time, on account, partly, of the cessation of respiration, and also, partly, of a peculiar influence on the heart similar to that influence exerted by the par vagum when it is galvanized by a powerful and interrupted galvanic current.[1] But when the fracture is in the lower part of the cervical region, or in the upper part of the dorsal region, the effects it produces are usually quite different. If the cord is partially crushed or incised, and if there is no pressure upon it, the patient's life may be saved. It is only when this nervous centre is completely or almost completely severed, that death seems to be unavoidable. But if there is pressure only, as

[1] For the influence of the medulla oblongata and spinal cord on the heart, see my paper in Journal de la Physiologie, vol. iii. 1860, p. 152.

is usually the case, life may be saved; and it is in such cases that the application of the trephine might be very useful.

When the fracture is in the middle of the dorsal region, there is a chance for the patient to have his life saved, even if the cord is completely severed; and, of course, the chance is still greater if only a part of the thickness of this organ is divided or crushed. If there be only pressure, we think there is a great probability of cure by the removal of this mechanical excitation.

The influence of a mechanical excitation of the spinal cord by a broken piece of bone deserves the full attention of both the physiologist and the practitioner. Among the alterations in the nutrition of the paralyzed parts in cases of that kind we will particularly notice the sloughs on the sacrum, and the various morbid changes that take place in the bladder and in the urinary secretion. These alterations in nutrition and secretion are certainly frequent causes of death after fractures of the spine. Therefore, it is of the greatest importance to find out the mode of production of these morbid changes, and to try to prevent or to cure them.

The production of sloughs on the sacrum cannot be considered as an effect of prolonged pressure of the trunk upon the parts of the skin where they appear, as they sometimes are produced in a few days and even in a few hours after the fracture. They result from a *morbid excitation* of the spinal cord, and not from the *loss of action* of that nervous centre owing to its partial or complete section, as proved by experiments showing that they never occur after section of the cord. The proof that pressure upon the sacrum has but a slight influence on their production is clearly given in the case of animals on which, after a fracture of the spine, I have seen sloughs occurring in parts that were not submitted to pressure. Besides, it is known that men who are confined to bed by other causes than a nervous complaint, may bear pressure upon some part of the body for a long while without the production of sloughs. Pressure on the sacrum is, therefore, only an additional cause of sloughs. For the mode of action of the nervous system in producing alterations of nutrition, I will refer to my lecture on the influence of the nervous system upon nutrition,[1] and I will only

[1] Lecture X. pp. 151–177. For more details on the capital point that it is chiefly owing to a morbid action of the nervous system that alterations of nutrition take place in diseases of that system, and not, as generally supposed, to a paralysis, *i. e.*, to the cessation of action of that system, see Journal de Physiologie, 1859, p. 112.

say here that an irritation and not a paralysis is the cause of these morbid changes.

It is an important fact that, after fractures of the spine in the dorsal or lumbar regions, it is very frequent that sloughs cause death by the propagation of the inflammation of the fibrous tissue lining the sacrum, to the membranes of the spinal cord, producing a very acute and quickly fatal meningitis. As a pressure upon the spinal cord by a fractured bone may produce sloughs and a fatal meningitis, it is important to try to remove such a mechanical excitation of the cord. We must say, however, that after the removal of the broken pieces of bone, the danger of the production of sloughs, though much diminished, would not be altogether removed, as a cause of them may remain, *i. e.*, a myelitis.

Another morbid change due to a mechanical excitation of the spinal cord may also cause death after a fracture of the spine; it is the alteration which takes place in the kidneys, an alteration sometimes amounting to a real inflammation. We hardly need to say that the changes in the urinary secretion, owing or not to an inflammation of the kidneys, and also the hematuria or the alterations in the mucous membrane of the bladder in cases of fracture of the spine, are morbid phenomena depending upon an irritation of the spinal cord, and not upon a paralysis due to a division of this organ. On the one hand, a section of the cord is never followed by these alterations in the kidney or the bladder; on the other hand, we often observe these alterations too quickly after the spine has been fractured, to admit that they are due to a paralysis.

Other causes of death besides the preceding exist in cases of fracture of the spine, depending also upon a mechanical excitation of the spinal cord. I will simply name the principal of these causes; they are, a myelitis, an increase in the amount of the cerebro-spinal fluid, and the influence upon the heart when the excitation exists in the cervical region. It is not a section of the spinal cord that usually produces these causes of death; it is the excitation of this nervous centre by broken pieces of bone. If we divide or crush the spinal cord in animals, we rarely find an inflammation occurring in this organ, and the beatings of the heart, instead of being diminished in frequency and force as when the spinal cord is irritated, increase in a more or less marked degree. It is, therefore, extremely important to remove, if possible, the pieces of bone that irritate the spinal cord, to avoid a myelitis, and the other causes of death above mentioned.

To complete the demonstration of the proposition that death after a fracture of the spine is usually due to the effects of the excitation of the spinal cord by broken pieces of bone, and not to the results of a partial or complete section of this nervous centre, we will only say that there are many cases on record showing that a section or even a crushing of the spinal cord has not proved fatal, and that in animals death is rarely caused by a partial or complete section of the cord in the dorsal region, while they die as quickly and as often as men after a fracture of the spine, if the broken pieces are not removed.

3d. *Reunion may take place after a wound of the spinal cord, so that its last functions may return.*—My experiments upon animals,[1] and also several pathological cases observed in man, prove the truth of this proposition. I must say, in addition, that I have sometimes seen a notable return of lost functions in animals the spine of which had been fractured and the spinal cord crushed.

4th. *The removal of some parts of the vertebræ may be followed by a production of new bone.*—This is a fact that I have observed a great many times in animals, even in cases when I had taken away the posterior half of the bony ring of five or six vertebræ. Generally the reproduction of bone is very slow except in young animals. The new bones are larger and thicker than those taken away. I never saw, but once, the reproduction of a spinous process. In man, after fractures of the spine, new pieces of bone have often been found round the callus, in cases when life has lasted more than one or two months.

5th. *The cases of fracture of the spine in which the trephine has been applied show the usefulness of this operation.*—Before mentioning these cases I must say a few words on the results of my experiments upon animals. I have found that if, after a fracture of the posterior arch of some vertebræ in the dorsal or lumbar region in dogs, cats, and guinea-pigs, I removed the broken pieces of bone, most of them were quickly restored to health. Some of them, in which the spinal cord had been either crushed or partially divided, remained more or less paralyzed either for a long while or permanently. A few died either of myelitis or some other cause. These experiments clearly prove the importance of the removal of fragments of bone in certain kinds of fracture of the spine in animals. No positive conclusion, however, could be drawn from

[1] Experimental Researches applied to Physiol. and Pathol., New York, 1853, p. 17.

these experiments alone as regards trephining in cases of fracture of the spine in man, as animals may be quite different from man. But, as I have ascertained that dogs, cats, and guinea-pigs almost always die after having presented the same symptoms that are observed in man, after a fracture of the spine, when the broken pieces of bone are not removed, it is fair to conclude, from the above experiments, that trephining might be a useful operation in man as it is in animals.

The first case of trephining of the spine in man, in which the operation was successful, is related by Louis, the most celebrated French surgeon of the eighteenth century. A man received a gunshot in the dorsal region of the spine, in consequence of which he became completely paralyzed in the lower limbs; the wound was enlarged at once, and the ball taken out. Louis saw the patient on the fourth day after the injury; he found that there were several fragments of bone pressing upon the spinal cord. He removed these fragments, and, although there was a considerable suppuration after this operation, the paraplegia slowly but gradually disappeared, and the patient was completely cured, excepting, however, a slight weakness which remained in his lower limbs.[1]

In the above case we have a proof that the removal of broken pieces of bone may be quite successful, at least when the fracture of the spine is due to gunshot, and limited to the posterior arch of a vertebra.

Another important case of cure of fracture of the spine, obtained by surgical interference, is mentioned in the following terms in the *British and Foreign Medical Review*, for 1838, p. 162: "We know only four cases, and of these one was performed successfully, as we are informed, only a few months ago, by a surgeon of the name of Edwards, living at Caerphilly, in South Wales. There were present the usual symptoms of compression, paralysis of the organs of locomotion, the rectum, and the bladder. The situation (of the fracture), as far as the operation was concerned, was unfavorable—the lumbar region. The posterior arch of the bone was raised, the symptoms of compression relieved, and the patient did well." It is a pity that the details of this fact have not been published. However, we have there a clear proof that the most happy result may be obtained by the elevation of a depressed bone in a case of fracture of the spine.

[1] Mémoire posthume, in Archives Gén. de Médecine, etc., Août, 1836, p. 397.

A third successful case of surgical operation on the spine after a fracture, has been published by Dr. Alban W. Smith, of Kentucky. (*North Amer. Med. and Surg. Journal*, July, 1829, p. 94.) Two years after a fall that was followed by complete paralysis of the four limbs, except the muscles above the elbow on each side, it was supposed that there was a fracture of the base of the spinous process, and that there was compression of the spinal cord by the broken piece of bone. "The diagnosis," says Dr. Smith, "was confirmed by the operation." The fragments were found displaced laterally, but so completely fused and offering so smooth a surface that the line of separation was not well marked. With a Hey's saw the operator divided first each side of the second dorsal vertebra, as near as possible to the bases of the transverse processes; and resected and raised up a portion of the spinous processes of two vertebræ, half that of the third and all that of the fourth, which seemed most deeply driven in. *No bad symptoms ensued; sensibility was regained in the thighs and in the hands*, auguring well for the re-establishment of motion.

It is much to be regretted that the further history of this case has not been published; but, so far as it goes, it proves, like the two preceding cases, that in man as in animals, the exposition of the spinal meninges to the atmospheric air is not a dangerous operation; it shows also that good results may be quickly obtained by the removal of a bone compressing the spinal cord. The account published by Dr. Alban W. Smith has been severely criticized by several writers. We agree with Malgaigne[1] when he says that the diagnosis was made out carelessly, and the operation rashly undertaken; but he certainly is unjust when he says that "all the dates are omitted, and the seat of the lesion not stated." True, the dates are omitted, but it is said that it was two years after the fracture that the operation was made; and, as regards the seat of the lesion, the second, third, and fourth dorsal are clearly designated.

If we now study those cases of trephining applied to the spine, in which the operation has not saved the life of the patients, we find, in the first place, that the operation has not proved injurious, and, in the second place, that it has been often followed by an amelioration in the condition of the patient. We also find that those cases were all very bad ones, and that death was to be expected in

[1] See the excellent translation published by Dr. J. H. Packard, of Philadelphia, of Malgaigne's Treatise on Fractures, Philad., 1859, p. 336.

all. Still more, in some cases besides the fracture of the spine, there were other injuries sufficient to cause death. We will mention some of the most interesting of those cases, and also those the authenticity of which is most certain.

In 1822, a patient with a fracture of the ninth and tenth dorsal vertebræ was admitted at St. Thomas's Hospital. There was a complete paraplegia of the lower limbs, the bladder, and the rectum. The posterior arch of the two broken vertebræ was removed, so that three inches of the spinal meninges were laid bare. A few hours after the operation, the patient felt when he was pinched, which had not been the case previously; he recovered at least partly the voluntary power over the lower limbs, the bladder, and the rectum. However, the patient died a fortnight after the operation, but from a peritonitis and an enteritis, which seem to have been produced by the cause of the fracture.[1]

Mr. J. F. South, in one of the important notes he has added to his excellent translation of Chelius,[2] says of the above case: "The result of Tyrrell's case, which was certainly most favorable for operation, the cord not having been subjected to other injury than pressure, was most highly encouraging, and I cannot but think that if the after-treatment had been different he would probably have recovered."

Dr. J. Rhea Barton performed the operation with as good results as those obtained by Tyrrell, as shown by the following account: "J. P. was received in the Pennsylvania Hospital, August 18, 1824, with a fracture of the spine, caused by a fall from the mast-head of a brig. The lower part of the trunk and the inferior extremities were totally paralyzed. He continued in this state, discharging his feces and urine involuntarily, until the 30th of August, when Dr. Barton performed the following operation: An incision was made, about eight inches in length, immediately over the injured vertebræ. He found the spinous process and arched portion of the seventh dorsal vertebra broken off and depressed on the spinal marrow. When this was done, it was ascertained that the bodies of the seventh and eighth dorsal vertebræ were dislocated from each other, without any fracture but that above mentioned. Lint

[1] See the account given of this case by Georgii, who witnessed the operation, in the work of Ollivier d'Angers, Traité des Maladies de la Moelle épin., 3d ed., 1837, vol. i. p. 381.

[2] A System of Surgery, by J. M. Chelius, translated by J. F. South, London, 1845, vol. i. p. 540.

was laid over the wound. The paralysis not being immediately relieved, it was inferred that compression was kept up by blood effused within the spinal canal, which would possibly escape with the suppuration from the wound. About forty-eight hours from the time of the operation, sensibility began to return below the injured vertebræ, and gradually extended toward the toes until the third day, when he was attacked with a violent chill, which continued, notwithstanding all the stimulant medicines given, until his death, which occurred in twelve hours from its commencement. On opening the thorax, the posterior mediastinum was found filled by about half a gallon of coagulated blood, which accounts for the difficulty of respiration, especially when he lay on his back. This being cleared away, the condition of the vertebral column was seen. The seventh and eighth dorsal were injured as before stated, the body of the ninth was fractured, and blood was effused throughout the spinal canal."[1]

In this case death was most likely due to the loss of blood combined with the difficulty of breathing. In the following case we will find also that the operation was followed by good results as regards the functions of the spinal cord.

In the next case the result of surgical interference was extremely marked. A strongly-built young man, having been struck on the neck, was brought to a hospital. Symptoms of fracture of the spine were observed. Three months and a half after the accident, Dr. A. Potter, of New York, saw the patient and found him paralyzed both as to sensibility and motion in all the parts below the seat of the fracture. Dr. Potter thought that there was compression of the spinal cord by the broken pieces of bone, and proposed to raise or extract these pieces. The next day he performed the operation, and took away several pieces belonging to the last four cervical and the first two dorsal vertebræ. *The patient recovered sensibility almost immediately, and a few hours after he could easily say what foot and what toe were touched.* The wound was in the way of healing, when a thoracic inflammation, which existed before the operation, increased rapidly, and caused the death of the patient, eighteen days after the operation.[2]

This case is a most important one, as it clearly shows, 1st. That

[1] J. D. Godman's edition of Sir A. Cooper's Treatise on Dislocations and Fractures, p. 421; see also Packard's translation of Malgaigne, p. 343.

[2] See Gaz. Méd. de Paris, 1845, p. 748, or New York Journal of Medicine, March, 1845.

the extraction of broken pieces of vertebræ has been followed by a complete return of sensibility; 2d. That cicatrization of the wound due to this operation may proceed rapidly; 3d. That the operation had proved in a great measure successful, and that the cause of death was altogether independent from it. The following case, though less important than the preceding, is a very interesting one.

A man fractured his spine in the cervical region. His breathing was performed by the diaphragm alone; sensibility and motion were lost everywhere in the trunk and lower limbs; the bladder was paralyzed; pulse very low. He became gradually worse, and, five days after the accident, Mr. G. M. Jones, of Guernsey,[1] took away the posterior arches of the fifth and sixth cervical vertebræ. "The pulse after the operation rose to 80, and no longer intermitted. At 8 P.M. the patient had entirely recovered from the effects of chloroform; merely complained of smarting pain in the neck and back; *was perfectly cheerful, and had entirely recovered sensation as low down as the umbilicus.*" He recovered also the power of raising his arms, and he could, without inconvenience, throw them across the chest. During the first succeeding days the improvement continued, and Mr. Jones had some reason to hope that recovery might take place, when suddenly, after the nurses had changed the linen of the patient, he was attacked with "coma," and died shortly after. The autopsy showed that there was considerable effusion at the base of the skull.

Whatever may have been the real cause of death in the above case, it is certain that it is not to be found in the operation or any of its effects. We find, in this last case as in all the preceding, that the laying bare of the spinal cord, instead of being followed by any grave symptom, was followed by a return of some of the functions of this nervous centre, especially as a conductor of sensitive impressions.

Two cases of operation upon the spine after a fracture have been published in Germany; they both show the importance of this operation. In one of them, the patient was operated upon by Dr. A. Mayer, of Wurzburg.[2] There was a notable amelioration in the symptoms, but the patient, after a fortnight, died from disease of the lungs. In the other case the patient, after a fracture of the

[1] See Medical Times and Gazette, July, 1856, p. 86.

[2] Journal der Chirurgie, von Walther und Ammon, vol. xxxviii. 1848, p. 178.

eleventh and twelfth dorsal vertebræ, had a complete paraplegia, with retention of urine, vomiting and vertigo. He was seen first on the thirteenth day by Dr. Holscher. He found a slough beginning on the sacrum, and a notable depression at the level of the fracture. After having made a crucial incision, and exposed the bones to view, he took away the posterior arch of the eleventh and twelfth vertebræ, and removed a little coagulated blood. The sloughing healed after considerable exfoliation. In six weeks the wound of the operation had healed well. Eight weeks after the injury, sensibility reappeared in the dorsum of the foot, and afterwards higher up. A few weeks later, the patient moved the legs a little. After twelve weeks, he was capable of raising himself up in his bed, and of moving slightly the lower limbs; but after that time his strength diminished. He had œdema in his feet, ascites, and hydrothorax. He died fifteen weeks after the fracture, and besides the anasarca, there was found pericardial dropsy. The spinal membranes were denser and more vascular at the place of the operation, and there were ligaments uniting the bony parts; the spinal cord seemed healthy.[1]

We will mention but one more case, that of a man who had a fracture of the ninth dorsal vertebra, and on whom Professor Laugier[2] practised trepanation. In this case the spinal cord had been ruptured, and therefore there was no chance of a return of sensation and motion in the lower limbs, but *respiration became easier, he felt desire of voiding the bladder, and had abundant stools.* Four days after the operation the patient died, chiefly from a pleuro-pneumonia caused by a fractured rib.

We cannot but agree with Jæger,[3] who, concluding from some of the above facts, and also from some others recorded by Attenburrow, Holscher, Wickham, and Rogers, declares that after the operation of trephining or removing broken pieces of bone, there is not any aggravation, but rather, in most cases, a notable improvement, with restoration of motion or sensibility.

To the above cases I might add an interesting one, not of fracture, but of dislocation of the fourth cervical vertebra. An incision was made, and it was found that there was no fracture. The reduction of the luxation was performed, and the patient improved

[1] Hannoverschen Annalen, vol. iv. p. 330, 1839.

[2] Bulletin Chirurgical. 1839, vol. i. p. 401.

[3] Cited by Chelius (A System of Surgery, translated by J. F. South, 1845, vol. i. p. 538).

after it. He died, however, on the sixth day, from a hemorrhage in the spinal cord.[1]

The objections brought forward against trephining in cases of fractured spine by Sir Charles Bell, Sir Benjamin Brodie, and others, have probably prevented many surgeons performing this operation. Already Mr. J. S. South[2] has convincingly refuted some of these objections; consequently, we will say but little of them, inasmuch, also, that any reader who will weigh carefully the arguments we have advanced in favor of the operation, will find in them a sufficient reply to most of the objections of Bell, Brodie, and others. The following objections are those which alone deserve to be noticed :—

1st. It has been said that it is dangerous to expose the spinal cord or its membranes to the action of the air. We have at length shown how erroneous is this opinion.

2d. It has been objected that the parts divided to lay bare the spinal cord will necessarily become inflamed, and that the inflammation may be propagated to the membranes of the cord. Experiments on animals and the cases of trephining in man, do not show any case of meningitis due to such a cause. Besides, there is much more danger of inflammation from the laceration existing in a fracture than from a clean cut.

3d. It has been objected that we often do not know whether there is a fracture of the posterior arch of the vertebræ or only of their body. Surely a mistake may be made in that respect, but the laying bare of the spinal cord may be useful in allowing the escape of the bloody fluid effused in the vertebral canal. At any rate, the worst would only be that an operation, which is not dangerous, has been performed without profit.

4th. It has been said that the pressure upon the spinal cord, after a fracture of the spine, being due, in a great many cases, to the body of the vertebræ, sometimes even when some other part of these bones are fractured, the removal of a portion of the posterior arch or its raising up would not change the situation of the body of the vertebræ. It is true that there would be no change, but certainly we need not insist upon the fact that if there is no resistance on the back part of the cord, there will be no compression by a displaced bone forward, as the cord, being movable, will simply be pushed backward.

[1] Catalogue of Boston Museum, 1847; case of Dr. William J. Walker, p. 25.

[2] Ibid.

5th. It has been objected that, in many cases of fractured spine, we do not know whether the spinal cord is considerably injured or not. It is true that if the paralysis of movement and sensibility is complete, it will be very difficult and sometimes impossible to say what is the extent of the injury to the spinal cord. But there is no reason not to perform the operation on account of our ignorance of the condition of the spinal cord, as the object of the operation is to give a chance of saving a life which otherwise would be lost.

6th. It has been said that, after having taken away the posterior arch of one or two vertebræ, the spine would not be sufficiently strong to support the body. The three cases of cure we have reported show that this objection should not be minded.

7th. Mr. Malgaigne calls this operation "a desperate and blind one,"[1] and he adds that he would not advise any one to perform it. He does not give the reasons of his opinion against it, and contents himself with simply asserting that "it has *always* been undertaken *at great risk, and has never been justified by the results.*" As clearly shown by the facts we have related, the truth is that *this operation has always been undertaken without any great risk, and that it has frequently been quite justified by the results.* Mr. Malgaigne says, in answer to Sir Astley Cooper, who has written in favor of trepanation of the spine, that "it is not accurate to call it our only scientific resource. In every fracture with displacement, the most scientific and rational plan is first to attempt reduction by the ordinary methods; and to this rule fractures of the vertebræ do not constitute an exception." We know full well that several surgeons (Ehrlich, Schub, Wittfeld, Tuson, Stafford, and others[2]) have related cases of fracture and luxation of the spine successfully treated by extension and reduction; but we know also that there is on record at least one case of sudden death caused by the efforts at reduction,[3] and we feel very much inclined to repeat with Mr. South,[4] "that the attempt to set a fracture through the body of a vertebra, accompanied, as it almost invariably is, with displacement, and most commonly with fracture of the vertebral arch, or articular processes, is, as Chelius says, most highly dangerous and ought never to be attempted." No doubt that the reduction may some-

[1] Packard's above quoted translation, p. 345.

[2] See the good dissertation of Richet: Des Luxations Traumatiques du Rachis, 1851, p. 85.

[3] See Traité des Maladies Chirurgicales, par Boyer, 5th ed., vol. iii. p. 650.

Loc. cit., p. 538.

times succeed admirably, but in some cases this operation might be the cause of a more or less extensive crushing or laceration of the spinal cord.

Conclusions from the above Clinical Facts and Experiments.—It is quite evident that the laying bare of the spinal cord is not a dangerous operation. Experiments upon animals, and clinical facts observed in man, agree completely in giving a demonstration of the exactitude of this assertion. It is evident, also, from the results of experiments and from clinical facts, that the operation of trephining gives a chance of saving the life of patients in whom one or several vertebræ are broken, so that if we take notice of the fact that most patients are sure to die after a fracture of the spine, especially in the neck or in the upper part of the dorsal region, we cannot understand why this operation has been so rarely performed. Indeed, it is surprising that a man is allowed to die without any attempt to save his life, by an operation which is neither dangerous nor very difficult.

It is evident, also, that operations which are not dangerous, and which *may save the life of three or four*[1] *patients out of a number of sixteen or seventeen, i. e., nearly* 20 *per* 100, should not be neglected. The percentage of cure after these operations, compared to the percentage of cure (perhaps less than 1 per 100) when neither of them is performed, shows clearly the importance of such kinds of surgical interference after fracture of the spine.

Three distinct operations may be performed on the spine in cases of fracture: 1st. The extirpation of broken pieces of bone; 2d. The raising up or lifting out of the posterior arch of one or several vertebræ, when they press upon the spinal cord; 3d. The

[1] To the cases of cure above recorded, I would have added the interesting case published by Dr. J. B. Walker, of Boston, had the seat of the fracture been indicated with more precision. A man was struck upon the back of the neck, and immediately lost all power of motion and sensation below the middle of the chest. The next day an incision was made over the back of the neck, and, the muscles having been dissected away, it was found that the spinous process of the sixth cervical vertebra was fractured and quite loose, though not driven in; the bone was seized and twisted away. The wound was closed by four sutures, and healed without any trouble. On the third day from the operation, there was some return of sensibility, and twelve days later it was reported as quite natural. The power of the bladder partly returned, and, although symptoms of myelitis appeared, he recovered some power upon the lower limbs. Two years afterwards, his condition was stationary. His general health was very good. (*Catalogue of the Museum of the Boston Society for Medical Improvement*, by J. B. S. Jackson, 1847, p. 31.)

application of the trephine. Examples of each of these three operations have been reported above. These various operations, or one or two of them, ought to be employed in almost all cases of fracture of the spine, especially in the cervical region, and in the upper parts of the dorsal region, where pressure upon the spinal cord is attended with so much danger. The operation should be performed as quickly as possible after the fracture, and before inflammation has set in. If, after having laid bare the spinal cord, it is found necessary to reduce a fracture of the body of one or several vertebræ, the reduction will then be much easier, and attended with much less danger than if the vertebral canal had not been opened in its back part.

In concluding these remarks upon trephining in cases of fractured spine, we cannot do better than to repeat these sentences of Sir Astley Cooper: "The proposal is laudable, and the *operation is not severe*, nor does it increase the danger of the patient; time and experiment can only determine its value. If we could save one life in a hundred by it, we should deserve well of mankind; and if any good does ultimately result from it, Henry Cline has the merit of proposing it."[1] To this we will only add that three or four lives have been saved already by that or by kindred means, and it is high time that surgeons should put aside their fear of compromising themselves, and rather expose their reputation than allow a man to die whom they have a chance to cure.

II. *Prevention and Treatment of Sloughs on the Sacrum, Nates, etc., in Cases of Fracture of the Spine, Myelitis, Meningitis, etc.*—I will not insist upon this point: I only wish to say that, led by the knowledge of facts showing the influence of nerves upon nutrition through their action upon bloodvessels, I have tried to prevent or to cure those sloughs which are an evident result of disturbance of nutrition due to an irritation of nerves of bloodvessels, by acting upon the bloodvessels of the part where sloughs exist. I have made many experiments upon animals, showing that by applying alternately two poultices, one of pounded ice, the other a very warm bread or linseed poultice, there is a rapid cure of sloughs due to a nervous irritation. Several medical men have already obtained the same result in man that I have obtained in

[1] Lectures on Surgery, p. 16. Sir Astley is mistaken in saying that Cline has the merit of having proposed this operation. Many surgeons had made the proposition long before Cline.

animals, in following the plan of treatment that I have proposed. The pounded ice, kept in a bladder, is applied for eight or ten minutes, and the warm poultice for an hour or two, or even a longer period. It is especially in cases of fracture of the spine, or of myelitis, that this mode of treatment would be employed with great success. As it is certain that when they are not quickly the cause of death, fractures of the lower part of the spine destroy life chiefly through the production of sloughs, and the propagation of the inflammation to the fibrous structures of the sacrum, and thence to the spinal meninges, it will easily be understood how important it would be to make use of the means I have just spoken of, against sloughs. I think I can safely say that, in cases when a slough is beginning, its progress will always be stopped by the means I propose.

III. *Rational Treatment of Burns.*—I have shown, in one of the preceding lectures, that burns are very often fatal, on account of the reflex disturbance of nutrition that they produce, by a reflex action in one or several of the thoracic, abdominal, or cranial viscera. (See LECTURE X., pp. 161, 171, and 175.) I will only say now, that of the various modes of treatment of burns there is one which has given admirable results at the great military hospital of Paris, the *Val de Grâce*, and theoretically there is no better means. As the principal object of the treatment is to prevent reflex influences and pain, the best therapeutical means consists in applications of ice upon the burnt part. But, as it has been found long ago, applications of cold, if once made, must be continued without interruption.[1] Cold, by diminishing considerably the vital properties of the nerves, will prevent pain, and, what is more important, those reflex influences which are so often the causes of death after burns. I need not repeat here what I said (pp. 175, 176), that belladonna is the best narcotic to be employed in cases of burns, as it is the most powerful agent to diminish the reflex power of the spinal cord. Opium must be avoided, not only because it produces congestion of the brain, but also because it increases the reflex power of the spinal cord.

IV. *Rational Treatment of Hydrophobia.*—We only wish to say a few words on this most important subject. The facts and views exposed, in several of our lectures, on the production of nervous

[1] See the Notes of Mr. South, in his translation of Chelius' Surgery, vol. i. pp. 112, 113.

diseases by an irritation starting from the periphery of the body, tend to show that tetanus, epilepsy, hysteria, catalepsy, chorea, etc., may have their origin in an irritation on some peripheric part of a nerve. We think it is so, also, as regards hydrophobia, and if really such is the origin of symptoms, it seems rational to employ in this affection, as well as in certain cases of tetanus and other convulsive diseases, the section of the nerve through which the excitation is transmitted to the nervous centres.

This view will certainly seem very strange to those persons who look upon hydrophobia as the result of the absorption of a poison, which acts upon the nervous centres, through which it circulates with the blood. But if we observe: 1st, that an alteration takes place in the part of the body that has been bitten by a rabid dog, before the convulsive and other phenomena of hydrophobia appear; 2d, that the convulsions of hydrophobia occur by fits following a kind of *aura* (pain or other sensations) starting from the wound of the bite or its cicatrix (which very often then gives way and is replaced by a bleeding or suppurating wound)—we are forcibly led to think that the cause of hydrophobia is in the irritation of the wounded nerves, and cannot be an action of a poison on the nervous centres.

Many other facts lead to the same conclusion. The following is the most important. An eminent physician, Dr. W. Stokes, of Dublin, after having heard a lecture I delivered last year on this subject, told me that his father was led by the following fact to admit the view I hold. A tourniquet having been applied on a limb of a patient attacked with hydrophobia, the symptoms were quickly improved, and even seemed to cease altogether. The surgeon then proposed to his colleagues to amputate the limb, but they declined giving their assent to this operation. It was ascertained several times that so long as the tourniquet was applied there were no convulsions, and that they occurred at every time it was taken away. As the danger of producing gangrene prevented a constant application of the tourniquet, the patient ultimately died.

We admit as everybody that there is a poisonous principle in the saliva of rabid animals, but we think that it is in consequence of changes produced locally in the nerves wounded by the bite, that the phenomena of hydrophobia occur. We are told that this hypothesis has been already put forward by a London surgeon in an article published many years ago in the *Lancet*, and that the author of this article has proposed the division of the wounded nerve as a means of treatment.

I think that the first thing to be done in a case of hydrophobia, owing to a bite in a limb, would be to apply the tourniquet upon the principal artery of the limb, above the wounded part, and if there is no tourniquet at hand, to apply a very tight ligature round the upper part of the limb. If the symptoms cease in consequence of either of these means, then I would advise the resection of two inches of the trunk of the nerve that gives fibres to the wounded part. But if the patient is seen a short time after the bite, I would advise, besides the application of the heated iron to the wound, the resection of a part of the nerve at a small distance above the wound. If the bite has been made on some part of the head or trunk, I would advise also the resection of the nerve that gives fibres to the wounded skin or flesh.

It may be that patients will only be temporarily cured by this mode of treatment, and that the parts of the poison that are absorbed and circulate in the blood, will, after a time, act upon other nerves than the one that has been wounded and resected; but as there is no certainty, and, I might say, no probability of such a recurrence of hydrophobia, and I do not hesitate in urging the trial of this mode of treatment. In a fatal affection like hydrophobia, anything that gives even the slightest chance of a cure should be eagerly tried.

PART III.—ADDITIONAL FACTS IN PROOF OF SOME OF THE VIEWS OF THE AUTHOR.

We have stated in Lecture XII. (see p. 201), that there is a peculiar kind of paralysis quite distinct from the ordinary cases of paralysis, produced by lesions of the encephalon, and characterized essentially by its being *on the side of the seat of the lesion,* instead of being on the opposite side, and we have tried to prove that this special kind of paralysis is due not to any immediate alteration of voluntary motor conductors, but to an irritation of some parts of a crus cerebelli (Fig. 25, *h*, *p*), producing a paralysis by a reflex action upon some other part of the nervous centres. It is probable that the mechanism of production of this paralysis is just the same as that which we have described in our "*Lectures on Paralysis of the Lower Extremities*, Philadelphia, 1860, Lectures I. and II." We will not enter into any discussion on this subject here. We only intend to refer the reader to several articles in which we have related facts in favor of our view (see *Journal de la Physiol.*, 1858, vol. i. p. 531 et seq., and 1859, vol. ii. p. 121), and to give a short account of a case recently published by Dr. J. W. Ogle.

CASE.—Mrs. S., æt. 46, had enjoyed good health until 1848, when she occasionally lost her sight for a few seconds at a time, and had pain at the front and vertex of the head; afterwards she had epileptic seizures and became totally blind. Dr. Ogle saw her in December, 1851. She was pale; had her mouth drawn to the right side; pupils dilated; no ptosis; left ear deaf; very intelligent; incomplete loss of power on the whole of the *left* side of the body, with hyperæsthesia of the face on that side. At times twitching of the left arm (in March, 1852); the paralysis was then less than it had been. In April, pain, with a feeling of numbness and stiffness in all the limbs, but no anæsthesia anywhere; sense of smell lost in the left nostril. In September, loss of taste in the left side of the tongue. She remained in pretty much the same condition until September, 1856, when she died, after a violent fit of convulsions, which were almost entirely limited to the *left* side of the body.

Autopsy.—Connected with the anterior cerebellar artery on the *left* side of the brain, there was an aneurism (see Fig. 26, *a*,) of about the size of a small nutmeg, *resting immediately upon the inferior surface of the left middle crus cerebelli*, and indenting, although very slightly indeed, the contiguous structures of the pons Varolii and left lobe of the cerebellum, which parts, at the point of contact, were very superficially softened. The root of the fifth nerve was pressed upon by the aneurism, and the facial nerve was stretched by it.[1]

We give this summary of this case, both because it has been recorded by a most accurate observer, and because it may serve as a type of analogous cases. This case offers all the principal features that may exist in consequence of *irritations* of the cerebellum, of the trigeminal nerve, and of the middle crus cerebelli; *i. e.*, loss of sight in both eyes; loss of the senses of smell, taste, and hearing in the corresponding side; incomplete paralysis and spasm in the limbs of the corresponding side; and, also, epileptic seizures. We have tried to show elsewhere that all these symptoms are simply the results of a reflex action of these irritations.

[1] See the interesting paper of Dr. Ogle, in vol. xlii. of the "Medico-Chirurgical Transactions of the Royal Med. and Chirurg. Soc. of London," 1859.

We will call the reader's attention to the figures in Plate III. (Figs. 25 and 26), representing the part of the base of the brain which, being irritated, may produce the phenomena just mentioned. The part marked *h*, in Fig. 25, is the centre of the zone, the irritation of which produces a reflex paralysis on the corresponding side.

My friend, Dr. Ogle, has also published two other papers, which contain many facts proving the correctness of several of the views held in my Lectures. In one of these papers he gives a number of clinical cases, showing the effects of the paralysis and of the irritation of the cervical sympathetic nerve in man.[1] In the other paper, he gives many facts showing that the posterior columns of the spinal cord are not the conductors of sensitive impressions to the brain, and also that the gray matter is endowed with that function. He relates, also, a most important case, similar to those I gave in Lecture VII. p. 93, showing the conductors of sensitive impressions decussate in the spinal cord. The number of cases of that kind (loss of sensibility in one side, and loss of movement in the other side) will soon be considerable. Besides the case of Dr. Ogle, I could add three others to those I have published: one lately observed by myself,[2] one by Dr. Lente,[3] and a third by Dr. T. Chew, of Baltimore.[4]

[1] The Medico-Chirurg. Transactions, 1858, vol. xli.
[2] The Brit. and For. Medico-Chirurg. Rev., 1859.
[3] The American Journal of the Medical Sciences, Oct. 1857, p. 742.
[4] North American Medico-Chirurg. Rev., July, 1860, p. 711.

LIST OF AUTHORS REFERRED TO.

EXPLANATION OF THE PLATES.

PLATE I.

FIG. 1.—*A*, anterior roots; *P*, posterior roots; *g*, ganglion on the posterior roots; *c*, central parts of the divided roots; *d*, distal parts of the roots. The arrows show the direction of nervous action in the anterior and posterior roots. (Lecture I., pp. 4 and 5.)

FIG. 2.—*W*, a weight attached to *l*, the tendon of *m*, a muscle attached to a ring by its other extremity; *n*, the nerve of m^2, another muscle which contracts, when the muscle *m tends* to contract. (Lecture I., pp. 6 and 7.)

FIG. 3.—Spinal cord of a frog.—*A*, anterior roots; *P*, posterior roots; *l*, left, *r*, right side; *s*, transversal section of the spinal cord; *c*, central, and *d*, distal parts of the divided anterior root on the left side. An irritation upon *d*, the distal part of anterior root, produces in some muscles a spasmodic contraction, which excites the sensitive or excito-motory nerves of these muscles; the spinal cord receives the excitation of these nerves, and, through other anterior roots, reflects it to some muscles of the right side, which then contract. The arrows show the direction of nervous action. (Lecture I., p. 6, and Lecture III., p. 35.)

FIG. 4.—Spinal cord of a mammal.—*s*, a transversal section of a lateral half of the cord; *P*, sensitive roots decussating in the spinal cord; *A*, anterior roots on the right side; *l*, left, and *r*, right sides. The arrows indicate the direction of nervous action. It sometimes occurs that, in irritating the sensitive nerves on the *left* side, which has lost its sensibility, there is a spasm on the *right* side, due to a reflex action, and as the spasmodic contraction excites the sensitive nerves of the muscles in which it takes place, and as, besides, these nerves are in a state of hyperæsthesia, there is a sensation of pain. When the posterior roots are divided on the *right* side, there is no sign of pain when the left side is irritated. (Lecture I., p. 6, Lecture III., p. 35.)

FIG. 5.—*c*, cerebellum; *p*, a pin, part of which has passed through the left restiform body, the descending fibres of the large or sensitive root of the trige minal nerve, and the left anterior pyramid; *v*, the *V* of gray matter, the pretended vital knot; *f*, the floor of the fourth ventricle. (Lecture II., p. 18.)

FIG. 6.—Sections of the posterior columns of the spinal cord, and formation of upper and lower segments of these columns.—In the four figures, *a* is the upper or cephalic segment, and *b* the lower or caudal. In the 2d, 3d, and 4th figures, *s* is a section of the posterior columns. In the 4th figure, *s* is a section of the anterior columns. In the four figures, *a′* represents the anterior columns, *p*, the posterior, and *g*, the gray matter. (Lecture II., pp. 24–26.)

FIG. 7.—Two figures, 1 and 2, showing a double section of the posterior columns, *p*. In the figure on the left side, the two sections *s*, *s*, are far one from the other; in the figure on the right side, they are very near, and the roots of only one pair of nerves are between them. (Lecture II., p. 26.)

FIG. 8.—*p*, *p*, posterior columns of the spinal cord; *s*, transversal section of these columns; *d*, a transversal section of the whole cord, except the posterior columns; *r*, *r′*, *r″*, the posterior roots of the three pairs of nerves below the last section. (Lecture II., pp. 21, 28.)

PLATE II.

FIG. 9.—*s*, *s′*, transversal sections of the right and left lateral halves of the spinal cord; *f*, *f′*, conductors of sensitive impressions decussating along the median line; *l*, left, *r*, right sides. (Lecture III., p. 31.)

FIG. 10.—*p*, posterior columns; *r*, right side, *l*, left side; *s*, section of the whole right lateral half of the cord; *s′*, section of the left posterior column at the level of the preceding section; 1, 2, 3, pairs of nerves below the sections. (Lecture III., p. 32.)

FIG. 11.—Spinal cord of a rabbit.—*l*, left side; *ri*, right side; *f*, longitudinal section of the brachio-cervical enlargement of the cord; *s*, transversal section of the right lateral half of this enlargement; *r*, *r′*, *r″*, posterior roots of nerves decussating along the median line. (Lecture III., p. 34, and Lecture VI., p. 90.)

FIG. 12.—*l*, left side, *r*, right side; *l′*, longitudinal section of the spinal cord; *s*, transversal section; 1, 2, 3, 4, the posterior roots of the spinal nerves behind the transversal section. (Lecture III., p. 36.)

FIG. 13.—Transversal sections of the spinal cord of the guinea-pig, magnified four diameters.—*P*, posterior columns; *A*, anterior columns; *p r*, posterior roots; *a r*, anterior roots. In Nos. 2, 3, 4, 5, the black surfaces represent the divided parts of the spinal cord. (Lecture IV., pp. 46, 48.)

FIG. 14.—Transversal section of the spinal cord.—*P*, posterior, and *A*, anterior columns; *L*, lateral column; *p r*, posterior, and *a r*, anterior roots of a pair of nerves; *g*, ganglion. The dark lines show the passage of the posterior roots into the posterior and lateral columns, and of the anterior roots into the anterior and lateral columns, through the gray matter. Some of the anterior and of the posterior roots decussate in the gray matter. (Lecture V., p. 54.)

FIG. 16.—Transversal section of the spinal cord of man.—*f*, posterior roots; *a*, anterior roots; *a l*, altered part of one of the posterior and lateral columns. (Lecture V., p. 73.)

FIG. 17.—Transversal section of the spinal cord of man.—*p*, posterior, and *a*, anterior root; *a l*, altered parts of the two posterior columns. (Lecture V., p. 73.)

FIG. 18.—*c*, the right lateral half of the cerebellum. The floor of the fourth ventricle is seen. The dotted lines, *f, f*, represent the conductors of sensitive impressions, according to the hypothesis of Longet; *f'*, fibres which do not pass through the cerebellum; *n, t*, tubercula quadrigemina; *r*, left and *r'*, right restiform body. (Lecture VI., p. 77, and Lecture XII., pp. 198 and 200.)

PLATE III.

FIG. 19.—Represents a tumor on the spinal cord.—*t, t*, tumor in one part entire upon *p*, the posterior surface of the cord, and in the other part divided longitudinally; *a*, the atrophied part of the spinal cord; *m*, the meninges. (Lecture VI., p. 86.)

FIG. 20.—In these three figures, the black part represents the blood effused in the gray matter. At 1, the section has been made immediately below the cervico-brachial enlargement, at the upper limit of the effusion; at 2, the middle part of the effusion; at 3, its lower extremity, above the dorso-lumbar enlargement. (These figures are taken from Ollivier's work; by a mistake, the effusion is represented in the *left* side of the cord, instead of the *right*.) (Lecture VII., p. 96.)

FIG. 21.—Represents the decussation of the conductors for voluntary movements and of those for sensations. *a r*, anterior roots continued by dotted lines in the spinal cord, where they decussate; *p r*, the posterior roots and their decussation; *g*, the ganglion; *m o*, the medulla oblongata; *r*, the right, and *l*, the left side; 1, 2, 3, transversal zones of alteration in one lateral half of the medulla oblongata and spinal cord; 1, above, 2, at the level, and 3, below the decussation of the voluntary motor conductors. The arrows show the direction of nervous action in the motor and sensitive conductors. (Lecture VII., p. 111, and Lecture XII., pp. 199 and 200.)

FIG. 22.—Represents the decussation of the anterior pyramids.—*P, D*, decussation; *A, A*, the *right anterior* column of the spinal cord passing into the *right* (the same) side of the medulla oblongata; *L, L*, the *right lateral* column of the spinal cord forming the *left anterior* pyramid of the medulla oblongata. (Lecture VIII., p. 122.)

FIG. 23.—Represents the three kinds of reflex actions; *p r*, posterior root of a spinal nerve entering into the spinal cord, and connected by a dotted line with three nerves; one going to a gland, *gl*, another to a muscle, *m*, and the third to a bloodvessel, *v*. The arrows indicate the direction of nervous action, which, on reaching the gland, produces a secretion; the muscle a contraction, and the bloodvessel and surrounding tissues a modification of nutrition. (Lecture X., p. 152.)

FIG. 24.—Posterior surface of the pons Varolii and medulla oblongata, partly divided all along the median line, to show the decussation described by Valentin and Foville. *C, C* (instead of *B, B*, as stated in the text, p. 198), the pretended decussation of the olivary columns in the pons Varolii, and between the crura cerebri; *D, D* (instead of *M, N*, as in the text, p. 198), the posterior tubercula quadrigemina; *S*, pineal gland; *T*, optic thalami; *F*, the nib of the calamus scriptorius; *j*, valve of Vieussens; *U*, processus cerebelli ad testes; *U'*, processus cerebelli ad medullam oblongatam; *U''*, crus cerebelli (processus cerebelli ad pontem); *Y*. restiform body; *R*, *R*, corpora geniculata. (Lecture XII., pp. 198–200.)

FIG. 25.—A part of the inferior surface of the encephalon.—*V*, pons Varolii: *h*, the part of the anterior surface of the crus cerebelli (*processus cerebelli ad pontem*), which causes a paralysis on the corresponding side, when irritated (marked *c*, *c*, in the text, p. 201); *a*, anterior pyramid: *o*, olivary body; *p*, a section of the crus cerebelli of the left side; *c*, cerebellum dissected, so as to show the passage through it of the fibres of its peduncle, the crus cerebelli; *t*, the trigeminal nerve; *n*, the chiasma of the optic nerve. (Lecture XII., pp. 198–201, and Appendix, pp. 263, 265.)

FIG. 26.—*V*, the pons Varolii; *c*, the cerebellum; *a*, a tumor upon the crus cerebelli; *p*, the anterior pyramid; *m*, a transversal section of the medulla oblongata. (Appendix, pp. 264–5.)

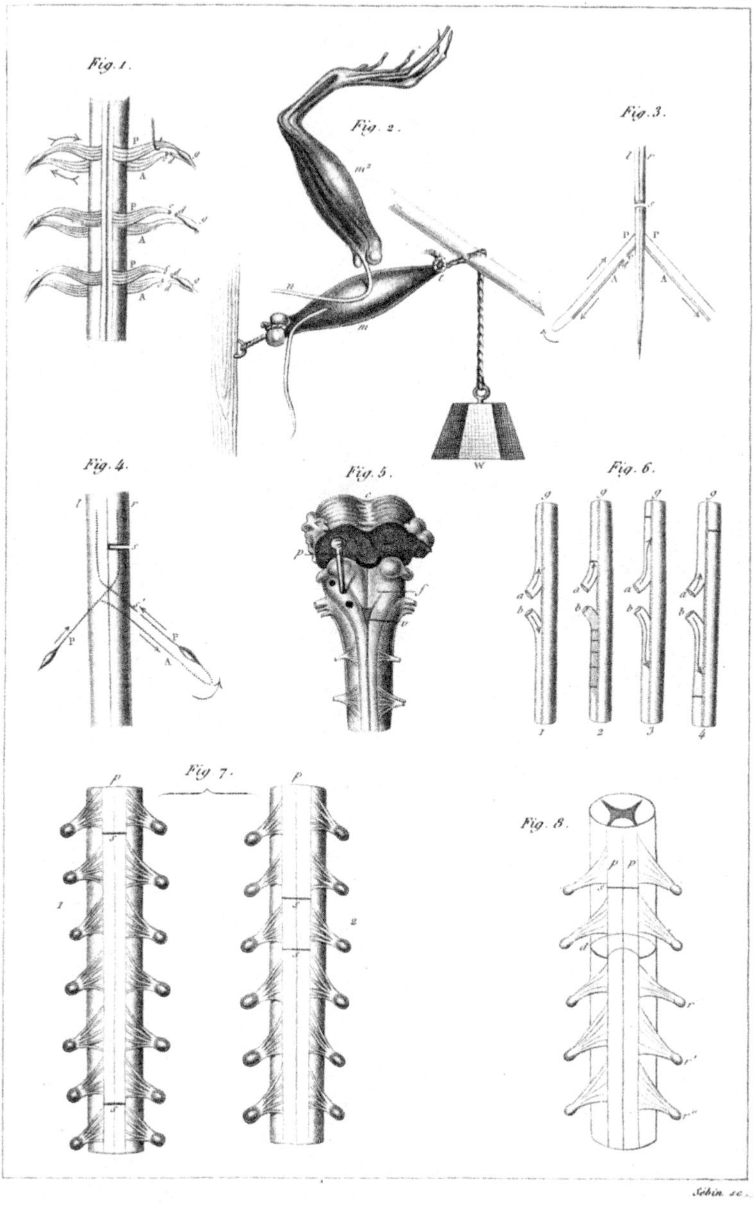

Sébin sc.

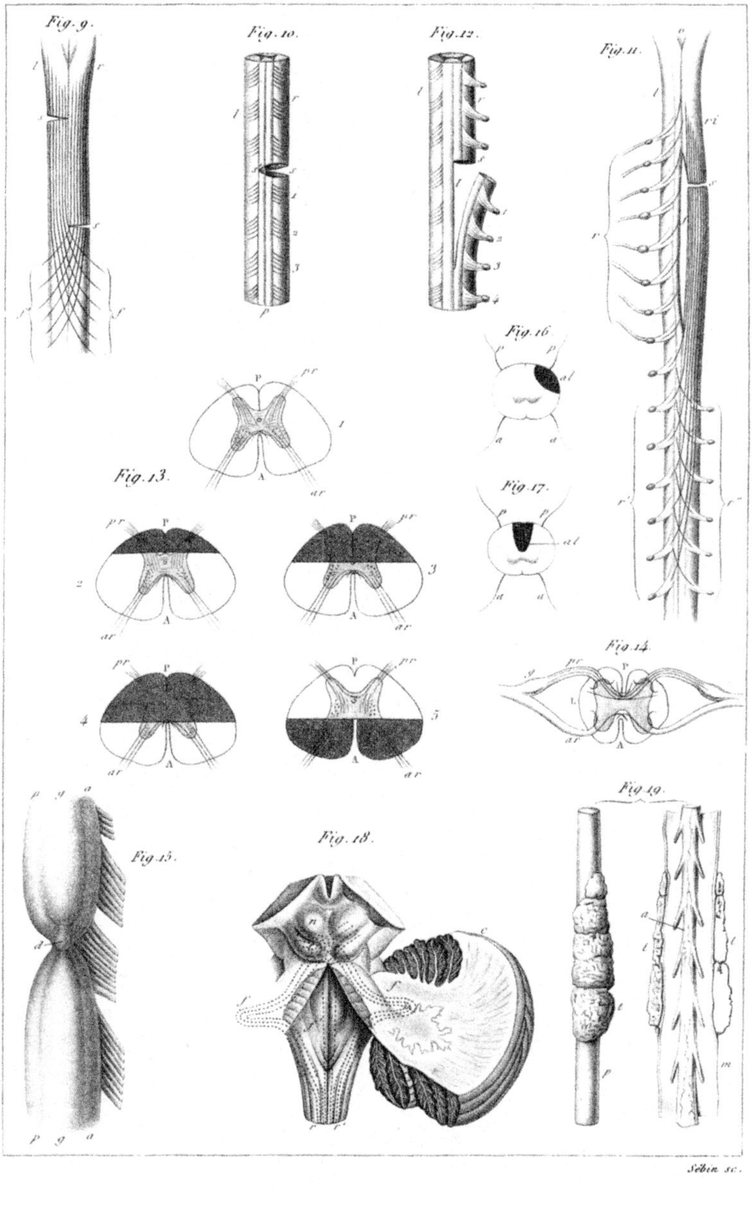
Fig. 9.
Fig. 10.
Fig. 12.
Fig. 11.
Fig. 16.
Fig. 13.
Fig. 17.
Fig. 14.
Fig. 19.
Fig. 18.
Fig. 15.

Sébin sc.

Fig. 20.

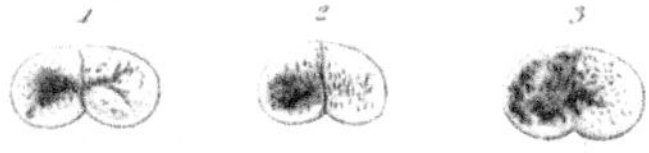

Fig. 21.

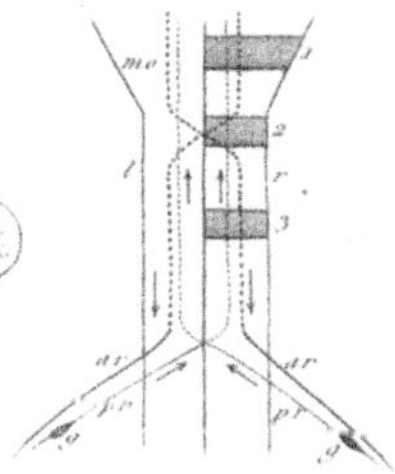

Fig. 22.

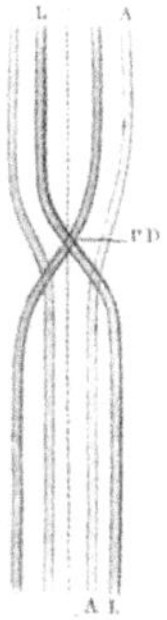

Fig. 23.

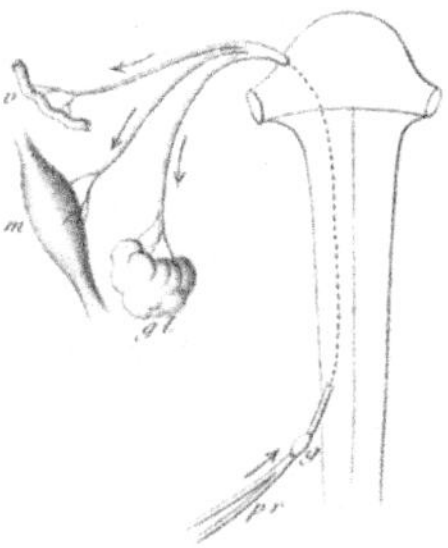

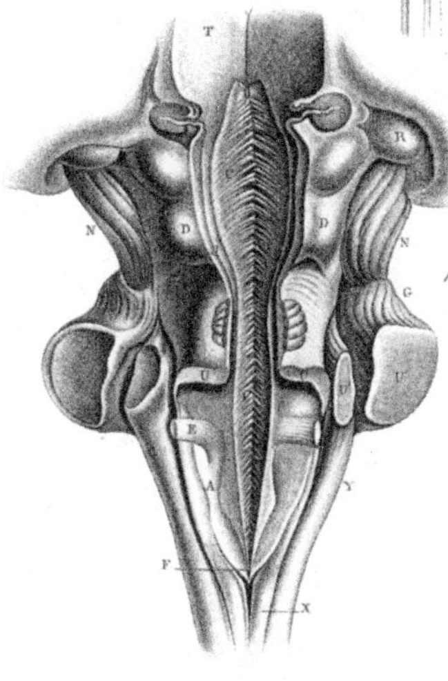

Fig. 24.

Fig. 25.

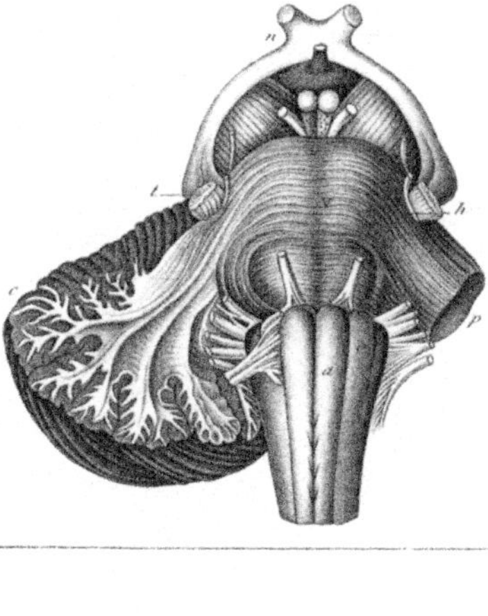

Fig. 26.

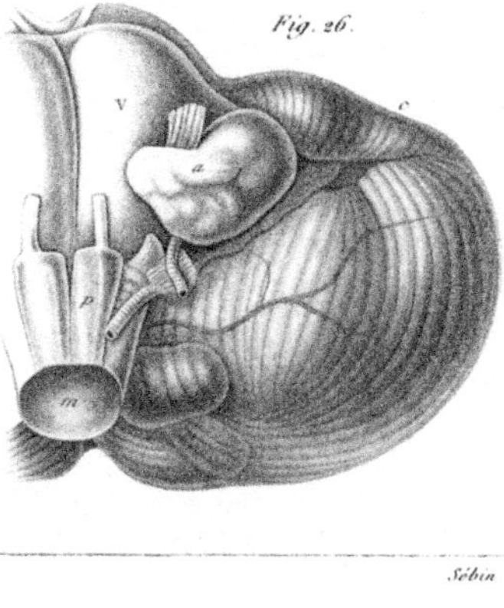

Sébin sc.

Printed in Dunstable, United Kingdom

91220014R00167